Progress in
Clinical Psychiatry
Number 1

Progress in Clinical Psychiatry Number 1

Edited by

Malcolm P.I. Weller MA (Cantab), MB, BS,
FRCPsych, FBPsS
Consultant Psychiatrist,
St Anne's Hospital, and
Honorary Research Professor,
Middlesex University,
London, UK

and

Daniel P. van Kammen MD, PhD
Chief of Staff,
Department of Veterans Affairs,
Medical Center Pittsburgh (Highland Drive Division),
and Professor of Psychiatry,
University of Pittsburgh School of Medicine,
Pittsburgh, USA

W.B. SAUNDERS COMPANY LTD
London · Philadelphia · Toronto
Sydney · Tokyo

W.B. Saunders Company Ltd   24–28 Oval Road
London NW1 7DX, England

The Curtis Center
Independence Square West
Philadelphia, PA 19106–3399, USA

55 Horner Avenue
Toronto, Ontario M8Z 4X6, Canada

Harcourt Brace
(Australia) Pty Ltd
30–52 Smidmore Street
Marrickville, NSW 2204, Australia

Harcourt Brace Japan Inc.
Ichibancho Central Building
22-1 Ichibancho
Chiyoda-ku, Tokyo 102, Japan

British Library Cataloguing in Publication Data is available

ISBN 0–7020–2270–5

This book is printed on acid-free paper

Typeset by Florencetype Ltd, Stoodleigh, Devon
Printed and bound in Great Britain by Hartnolls Ltd, Bodmin, Cornwall

Contents

Contributors

Anthony W. Bateman Consultant Psychotherapist, Clinical Director, St Ann's Hospital, St Ann's Road, London N15 3TH, and Honorary Senior Lecturer, University College, London, UK.

Timothy G. Dinan Head of Academic Department, St Bartholomew's Hospital, London, UK.

Earl L. Giller Jr Senior Associate Director, CNS Clinical Research, Pfizer Inc., Groton CT 06340, and Associate Professor of Psychiatry (Adjunct), Yale University School of Medicine, New Haven, CT, USA.

Angelos Halaris Professor of Psychiatry and Pharmacology, Department of Psychiatry and Human Behavior, University of Mississippi, Medical Center, Jackson MS 39216, USA.

Uriel Halbreich Professor of Psychiatry, Research Professor of Gynaecology/Obstetrics, Director of Biobehavioural Research, State University of New York, SUNY Clinical Center, BB170, 462 Grider Street, Buffalo NY 14215, USA.

Eric Johnson-Sabine Medical Director, St Ann's Hospital, St Ann's Road, London N15 3TH, Honorary Senior Lecturer, Royal Free Hospital School of Medicine, University of London, London, UK.

James V. Lucey Senior Lecturer, Joint Academic Department of Psychological Medicine, St Bartholomew's Hospital, London EC1, UK.

Sahebarao P. Mahadik Professor of Psychiatry, Department of Psychiatry and Health Behavior, Medical College of Georgia, 1515 Pope Avenue, Augusta GA 30912-3800, USA.

Stephen R. Marder Director of Mental Health Services, West Los Angeles Veterans Affairs Medical Center, 11301 Wilshire Boulevard, Los Angeles, CA 90073, and Professor and Vice Chair, Department of Psychiatry and Behavior Sciences, UCLA School of Medicine, USA.

Sukdeb Mukherjee (deceased) Department of Psychiatry and Health Behavior, Medical College of Georgia, 1515 Pope Avenue, Augusta GA 30912-3800, USA.

Robin Murray Professor of Psychological Medicine, Department of Psychological Medicine and Social, Genetic and Developmental Research Centre, Institute of Psychiatry, De Crespigny Park, London SE5 8AF, UK.

Hans Rommelspacher Professor of Pharmacology, Department of Neuropsychopharmacology, Free University, Ulmenallee 30, D-14050, Berlin, Germany.

Janice R. Stevens Professor of Neurology and Psychiatry, Oregon Health Sciences University, 3181 S.W. Sam Jackson Park Road, Portland OR 97201-3098, USA.

Jogin H. Thakore Lecturer, St Bartholomew's Hospital, London, UK.

Daniel P. van Kammen Chief of Staff, Department of Veterans Affairs, Medical Center, 7180 Highland Drive, Pittsburgh PA 15206-1297, and University of Pittsburgh School of Medicine, Pittsburgh, Pittsburgh PA, USA.

Jim van Os Associate Professor, Department of Psychiatry and Neuropsychology, University of Maastricht, PO Box 616, 6200 MD Maastricht, The Netherlands and Honorary Senior Lecturer, Department of Psychological Medicine and Social, Genetic and Developmental Research Centre, Institute of Psychiatry, De Crespigny Park, London SE5 8AF, UK.

Malcolm P.I. Weller Consultant Psychiatrist, St Ann's Hospital, St Ann's Road, and Honorary Research Professor, Middlesex University, London, UK.

Simon Wessely Reader in Psychological Medicine, Honorary Consultant Psychiatrist, King's College and Maudsley Hospitals, London SE5 9RS, UK.

Padraig Wright Honorary Lecturer, Department of Psychological Medicine and Social, Genetic and Developmental Research Centre, Institute of Psychiatry, De Crespigny Park, London SE5 8AF, UK.

Preface

This is the first of what we hope will be bi-annual reviews of advancing areas of psychiatric research that impinge on clinical practice. We have tried to strike a balance between depth and scope, an interesting level of discussion and a reasonably succinct and clinically relevant overview.

The present health care revolution requires that we practise a different kind of psychiatry, more focused on outpatient care, more consultative and more in an educative role. Soon we will be using practice guidelines. Just when psychiatric knowledge and insights are at an all-time high, psychiatric beds are closing. Although patient advocates and consumer representatives have become more sophisticated, managed care may prevent psychiatric patients from getting the timely care that they need. We can read in the lay press every day about new information on how the brain functions. Psychiatric clinicians need to absorb more information than ever. We choose our topics because we believe that they are neglected or that recent developments require a closer look. In many ways, this is a most exciting and challenging time for both our patients and us, their care providers.

Schizophrenia remains our most baffling disorder. However, neuro-developmental risk factors (Dr van Os, Chapter 6), new neuropathological findings (Prof. Stevens, Chapter 7) and new and more effective pharmacological treatments with fewer side-effects (Prof. Marder and Prof. van Kammen, Chapter 8) provide new answers and raise new questions about the pathophysiology of schizophrenia. Psychiatry tended to neglect women's issues for a long time. These issues get some special attention in this book, either in a specific chapter dealing with specific psychiatric conditions concerning women (Prof. Halbreich, Chapter 4), or as part of different chapters (borderline personality disorder (Dr Bateman, Chapter 5) and post-traumatic stress disorder (PTSD) (Prof. Giller, Chapter 1)). Sexual dysfunction, whatever the cause, is present in many of our male and female patients, but as a topic is often avoided. Dr Halaris (Chapter 10) writes about what is presently known about its treatment.

Post-traumatic stress disorder has finally gained its status among established psychiatric diagnoses. Although biological measures have not yet led to diagnostic indicators, the findings show that biological changes are present in well-established cases. The horror of having been a death camp survivor or a prisoner-of-war and the enduring problems of the Vietnam veterans brought the concept into sharp relief, with a halo effect on the recognition of the impact of catastrophic events in civilian life. We also expect that current terrorist activities, ethnic wars, aeroplane, fire or natural disasters will leave another generation to deal with the aftermath of such events. Although sporadically presented in the psychiatric literature, the topic has achieved a much more central place in current psychiatric thinking which the editors thought merited exploration (Prof. Giller, Chapter 1).

Alcoholism remains a major scourge for many of our patients, particularly if the diagnostic picture is confounded with other psychiatric diagnoses. Prof. Rommelspacher (Chapter 9) discusses the pharmacology of this agent.

Obsessive–compulsive disorder has now been shown to have biological changes in the brain that we can treat with serotonin enhancing drugs and also with behaviour therapy (Dr Lucey, Chapter 3).

The public has rediscovered neurasthenia. Malaise, weakness, fatigue, headaches, intolerance to noise, and lack of concentration, commonly follow influenza, typhoid, dysentery and hepatitis. Recent studies suggest that chronic fatigue syndrome has biological findings that require follow-up. We felt that this area needed more attention (Dr Wessely, Chapter 2).

Recently, vitamin E and other antioxidants are among over-the-counter compounds that are widely taken as alleged anti-ageing agents. A growing literature suggests that antioxidants may have a place in psychiatric treatment. Dr Mukherjee (Chapter 11) reviews this area. He died unexpectedly while writing the chapter. Dr Mahadik finished it.

With increasing diversity of our societies, transcultural psychiatry has something new to tell us (Dr Sabine, Chapter 12).

We enjoyed putting this book together, knowing quite well that many other topics are waiting to get a similar treatment. Our authors are from both sides of the Atlantic Ocean, as we expect our readers to be. We hope that our readers, whether they are psychiatrists, internists, family or other general practitioners, neurologists, clinical psychologists, managed care providers, residents or medical students who are intrigued by the same topics, will find the same enjoyment. We welcome feedback and suggestions for a second volume.

Malcolm P.I. Weller
Daniel P. van Kammen

1

Post-Traumatic Stress Disorder

Earl L. Giller Jr

INTRODUCTION

The evaluation of patients for traumatic stress response disorders involves establishing the nature of the traumatic event(s) and the ascertainment of the presence of specific symptoms to determine whether or not criteria are met for the currently recognized diagnoses of acute stress response or post-traumatic stress disorder (PTSD). Even if patients do not meet the criteria for either of these two diagnoses they may still have a disorder related to their response to traumatic stress, i.e. a traumatic stress response disorder. A historical perspective is helpful for understanding the current concept on when stress becomes classified as traumatic, which symptoms contribute to the diagnosis, the nature of the spectrum of traumatic stress response disorders and where our knowledge is incomplete and controversy exists. PTSD is the current label of a concept emergent in classical times. Based on an analysis of *The Iliad*, Jonathan Shay (1994) has eloquently and convincingly demonstrated not only the symptom profile of what we today call PTSD, but also the profound personal and social impact of combat PTSD in the Trojan War. Other portrayals of the effect of combat PTSD on the individual and society can be found in *All Quiet on the Western Front* (Remarque, 1929) and Mark Helprin's *A Soldier of the Great War* (1987).

Because this syndrome has such an impact on our very concept of self and society, it has been subject to a cycle of retrieval and denial, a veritable Phoenix of a disorder. For example, many of these patients carried the diagnosis of neurasthenia, hysteria, and, most recently, borderline personality disorder. Now many (but not all) of these patients are understood as having complex PTSD (Herman, 1992). Freud struggled with the controversy of reality versus fantasy of childhood sexual abuse. Today we have the battle between the believers of all childhood trauma and the false memory camp. Both perspectives have some truth, so the charge to today's clinicians is to nurture the dialectic and to sustain the debate, rather than allow the zealous, dogmatic defence of one or the other points of view to again bury the concept.

Knowing the history of a disorder is important and helpful not only in understanding the current conceptualization of the problem, but also having a sense of the historical trajectory of the disorder gives an idea of how future concepts are likely to develop. Understanding the history of PTSD in particular is even more important to avoid the pitfalls and landmines that overwhelmed those in the past who were not armed with such knowledge.

HISTORY: THE CYCLE

As mentioned above, indications of combat PTSD can be found as far back as the Trojan War. As a discrete clinical entity in veterans, irritable heart was described in Civil War soldiers, and the World Wars had combat fatigue and shell shock, best articulated by Kardiner and Spiegel (1947). Freud recognized stress disorders as being different from neurotic disorders, but his initial focus on the effects of actual childhood trauma moved to psychological rather than historical reality. What remained, however, is the formulation that traumatic stress disorders could be treated like neurosis with psychoanalysis. This perspective is correct (Marmar et al., 1993) for the unreasonable, nonadaptive, overgeneralization of the traumatic experience, but not necessarily for the core intrusive, avoidant and hyperarousal symptoms themselves that may be direct biological changes in an organism tuned to record and then interpret the world through that lens; i.e., it is adaptive to be vigilant. The assumption of invulnerability is likely more unrealistic than the assumption that the world is a dangerous place.

Another imprecision that discouraged a focus on traumatic stress is the attempt in the 1950s to formulate a connection between psychological aspects of stress and particular medical disorders like ulcer and myocardial infarction. The idea of traumatic, catastrophic stress was not distinguished from day-to-day stress or problems of living. Also, the neurotic amplifications of stress seen in adjustment disorders was not differentiated from the subjective response to traumatic stress and the impact of that mediating variable on the association between the traumatic stress and the development of the traumatic stress response disorder. This direction foundered on the lack of an operational formulation of the spectrum of stress, relying too much on the subjective response to any environmental perturbation. Our current formulation has developed from the writings of engaged clinicians like H. Krystal, Y. Danieli, J. Herman and D. Laub. The challenge to us today is to keep this exploration alive through our clinical, research and theoretical work.

CURRENT DEFINITION OF PTSD: STRENGTHS AND WEAKNESSES, AND IMPACT ON TREATMENT

Pure PTSD

While controversy existed about the very diagnosis of PTSD in the late 1970s and early 1980s, we now see acute stress response and PTSD itself in adults in 'pure culture' as being relatively straightforward disorders that occur after a catastrophic stress in individuals without previous trauma and without other psychiatric disorders. These individuals, while possibly the minority of subjects with traumatic stress response disorders, do exist and help to define the diagnosis. While our knowledge of traumatic stress disorders has increased, differences about necessary and sufficient diagnostic criteria remain.

The DSM-III-R, and now DSM-IV, provides the most specific and extensive list of criteria, which is helpful for identifying target symptoms and for research. PTSD and acute stress disorder are still classified as anxiety disorders, although they have many elements of a dissociative disorder, which is where some experts feel they should be classified.

The Traumatic Event

The first criterion is 'exposure to a traumatic event' involving actual or threatened physical harm. DSM-IV has now added the necessity of a subjective response to such an event involving 'intense fear, help-lessness or horror', and removed the statement that the event had to be 'outside the range of usual human experience'. Clinically, some-times patients may present with the remaining criteria for PTSD in response to what might be considered a less than traumatic event. In such cases, a lifetime trauma history often uncovers a previous, more clearly traumatic event, for which the current event is a reminder. For treatment purposes, however, intrusive, avoidant and hyperarousal symptoms need treatment even if the event is not considered traumatic. For legal purposes like liability, on the other hand, whether or not the event was 'traumatic' is of much more importance.

Intrusive symptoms

These are the most traumatic response disorder specific. Psycho-logical and physiological reactions to reminders of the trauma may have the most impact on function. The patient may not recognize the relationship of the reactivity to the traumatic event, so this connection can be one of the major foci of the psychological treat-ment. An important balance in the psychological treatment is to help the patient come to grips with the emotional and cognitive sequelae of the trauma without simply re-traumatizing the patient. The feeling of actually re-experiencing the traumatic event ('flashbacks') seems to be rarer than the other intrusive symptoms.

Avoidant symptoms

Whether symptoms in this cluster are a primary response to the trauma or secondary responses to the intrusive symptoms is not clear. Some think that numbing of general responsiveness and detachment may be primary, and active avoidance of reminders secondary. The sense of a foreshortened future may be less common than other avoidant symptoms.

Hyperarousal symptoms

The exaggerated startle and hypervigilance may be more specific to PTSD than the other symptoms in this cluster, which can also be seen in anxiety and mood disorders.

Impairment

DSM-IV has added as a severity criterion that the disorder must have a clinically significant effect on function, which should be documented in the history and formulation.

Course of illness

DSM-III-R required the presence of symptoms for one month before the diagnosis could be made, did not differentiate between acute and chronic PTSD and did not recognize an acute stress disorder. These deficits have been corrected in DSM-IV. An acute stress disorder has many of the features of PTSD plus some acute dissociative symptoms. Not all people with acute stress disorder develop PTSD, and PTSD can develop without an initial acute stress disorder. Since PTSD can be a lifetime diagnosis for some people, when symptoms abate it is not clear whether the individual is cured or simply in remission; the same problem is found in mood and some other psychiatric disorders. Thus, a return of symptoms could be a relapse (of the same episode), which is at times seen in individuals in stressful, but not traumatic stress, situations, or, especially after another traumatic event, a recurrence (new episode) of PTSD.

For treatment, the goal is to record all symptoms in terms of frequency and intensity, which together give an estimate of severity. DSM-IV is insufficient for this because it only records presence or absence of symptoms for a threshold duration of time. Instruments such as the Clinical Assessment of PTSD Scale (CAPS; Blake et al., 1990) and self-rating scales like Davidson's are better for initial and follow-up measures. Other scales like the Mississippi for combat veterans (Keane et al., 1988) and civilians (Vreven et al., 1995) can be used for diagnosis, but are even more helpful in assessing the impact of PTSD on the individual's life over time. These instruments are essential aids to developing a comprehensive, multi-dimensional treatment plan, and monitoring and modifying the plan over time.

The epidemiology of acute and chronic PTSD is shocking, and almost incredible when those with partial PTSD are included. About 30–50% of those exposed to a traumatic stress will develop an acute stress response disorder. Chronic PTSD, a lifetime diagnosis in some, develops in about 50% of those with acute PTSD (Breslau and Davis, 1992; Norris, 1992), and, like affective disorders, can be in partial or complete remission with recurrent exacerbations.

While much of the initial focus was on what type of trauma caused PTSD, it is still not known why approximately 50% of trauma-exposed individuals do not get PTSD. As in other psychiatric and many medical disorders, the model is a stress-diathesis one. For PTSD, this means that the factors to be considered which may protect or make individuals more vulnerable are pre-traumatic (biological predisposition, e.g. CNS responsivity, or conditionability, hypnotizability; development, exposure to previous trauma, coping skills, cultural background), peri-traumatic (subjective response to the traumatic event, helplessness, severity of trauma, type of trauma (human versus nature)) and post-traumatic (long-term disability, social support, coping skills).

Other Traumatic Stress Response Disorders

Other less well defined syndromes and courses of illness are more complex, and may be related to other variables such as genetic or developmental predisposition, nature of the trauma, age when traumatized, previous trauma or psychiatric history, and what happened after the trauma.

The spectrum of traumatic stress response disorders may include acute stress response, acute PTSD, chronic PTSD, multiple trauma response disorders, personality disorders related to chronic/early trauma such as borderline personality disorder/multiple personality disorder or complex PTSD (Herman, 1992), and disorders of extreme stress, not otherwise classified.

Comorbidity

One of the reasons that PTSD was so difficult to recognize is that it rarely occurs in pure form, and is often accompanied by other comorbid disorders. This distinction among diagnoses may be a somewhat artificial division into other syndromes or diagnoses than can result from traumatic stress versus the interaction of PTSD with other independent disorders. While this distinction may be difficult or impossible to make with current knowledge, the clinical application is to find and treat traumatic stress sequelae in any patient.

1. Are secondary diagnoses (substance abuse, anxiety disorders, mood disorders (especially depression) part of the spectrum? Extensive work by Yehuda et al. (1991) suggests that the depression seen in PTSD is different from primary unipolar depression.

2. Exacerbation of other psychopathology. While traumatic stress is not thought to cause psychosis, patients with a psychotic disorder with traumatic stress disorder comorbidity may have a more severe course of illness and be less responsive to standard treatment for psychosis.

CURRENT ASSESSMENT AND FORMULATION

Formulation is a comprehensive arrangement of the information collected within a defined theoretical framework. Psychiatry in general, and in the area of traumatic stress response disorders in particular, needs to pay close attention to this foundation of evaluation and treatment because the theoretical models are still under development, and the integration of biological, psychological and social domains is complex. The relationship among many of these clinical variables within and across domains remains controversial.

The guiding principles for the overall assessment of an individual who presents for evaluation of a traumatic stress response disorder are in general similar to those established for the evaluation for any psychiatric disorder in terms of evaluating signs and symptoms, obtaining a history, and developing a treatment plan. The general principles will be mentioned; areas requiring particular attention for PTSD will be developed further. The section is divided into traditional clinical assessment and potential assessments that are currently being evaluated in research.

Traditional Assessment

Chief complaint

Specific intrusive symptoms or referral can establish the direction more easily than less specific complaints. The key here is to always be sensitive to the possibility of a traumatic stress response disorder as the underlying problem without prompting for the diagnosis to the extent that one may be leading the witness down the slippery slope of false memory syndrome. As always, a quote is important in focusing the clinician on the patient's, rather than the clinician's agenda, and attention must be paid to secondary gain, either conscious or unconscious.

History

This is probably the most complicated area in the assessment of traumatic stress response disorders, whether evaluating the history of chronic childhood abuse or the past history of an adult survivor of a single incident of trauma. There are two corresponding major issues. A component of the traumatic stress response is dissociation and amnesia, which can be adaptive, but which make historically accurate, rather than psychologically relevant, recall difficult. It is easy to confuse the vague dissatisfaction with life presented by an individual with a personality or adjustment disorder with the fragmented, sensory-based traumatic memories that are the nidus of intrusive memories or dreams and the focus of psychotherapy for traumatic stress response disorders. The second controversy is the tension between pre-trauma vulnerability versus the impact of the trauma itself, especially in forensic evaluations where the extent to which the severity of a patient's symptoms are due to pre-existing vulnerability factors is an important consideration in litigation. Regardless of these controversies, a better understanding of the individual's history can only help to put the trauma in particular perspective and help to evaluate strengths and weaknesses that mediate between the trauma and the individual's symptoms, and aid in the psychotherapeutic work. A history of mixed cognitive-affective symptoms, variable treatment response (initially very good then very poor), chaotic lifestyle, i.e. similar to or meeting criteria for borderline personality disorder, should always alert the clinician to consider a traumatic stress response disorder, but proceed carefully! This means take a careful history, probe responses and vague memories that could develop into clearer memories of abuse, but *do not* jump to conclusions.

The documentation of impaired function in the history is increasingly important for the diagnosis, to justify treatment and possibly for disability and liability purposes. Evaluating function in social, family, work and leisure domains helps to determine the extent and consistency of impaired function.

Physical examination

The usual thorough medical evaluation that is part of the initial diagnostic work-up in any psychiatric disorder is needed. Apart from some rare brain tumours, a medical disorder is not likely to cause cardinal symptoms of intrusive recollection, but it could exacerbate pre-existing PTSD. Physically traumatized patients, especially those abused in childhood, may have injuries which interfere with function. Hippocampus neurones are particularly vulnerable, so physically traumatized patients may be at higher risk of temporal lobe epilepsy because of head injuries.

Mental status

A structured mental status examination is an essential part of any medical evaluation. Neuropsychological testing is indicated when problems of concentration, memory and intellect are suspected. Survivors of traumatic stress (especially childhood chronic abuse), however, as mentioned above, are likely to have vague, fragmented, sensory-based memories. The therapist must be extremely careful in proceeding to evaluate these memories in such individuals, as discussed above.

Potential Assessments

Understanding of the psychological meaning and effect of the traumatic experience(s) is the cornerstone of treatment and becomes more clear over time because of the initial reluctance to discuss the event and the difficulty in actually remembering the details. The range of traumatic experiences is covered by a number of new rating scales in the literature. A lifetime history is essential because the impact of the current or presenting trauma will be influenced by past trauma. The importance of having trauma history develop from the patient with a minimum of therapist definition is underlined by recent concerns of false memories in lawsuits; we are probably travelling the path that Freud took. Other aspects of the patient's psychological abilities must also be assessed to decide which psychotherapeutic approach (or combination) to take.

The patient's current level of social, family and vocational function needs to be evaluated to determine to what level the patient might return (rehabilitation) or aim for (habilitation), depending on the person's skills and aptitudes. For example, how isolated has the patient become because of the nature of the trauma (human perpetrators, lack of support of others) or the social isolation associated with the syndrome?

While this collection of information will be put together in a formulation which will point to specific combinations of treatment modalities, it is also important to remember that one's theoretical perspective will guide which information to collect and how it is understood.

TREATMENT

The biopsychosocial model still appears to be the best overall construct for organizing data within and across these three domains. Our best treatment algorithm is based on the biopsychosocial formulation developed above, with some caveats. Just because an aetiology is biological, psychological or sociological, it does not follow that the treatment has to be in the same domain. The objective is to develop a specific treatment plan for each individual patient, including specifying biological, psychological and social elements, how they are to be combined, and how efficacy will be evaluated for the purpose of deciding how and when to add, continue and/or stop various elements of treatment. Treatment is based on a combination of theoretical and empirical perspectives. That is, we develop theories based on preclinical research and clinical experience, then, ideally, test out these theories by examining how well our patient's story (collected in as unbiased a fashion as possible, of course!) fits the theory. Obviously, one problem is that the theory can drive the questions which can drive the answers; this is especially a concern in traumatic stress response disorders with the issue of false memory syndrome. Perhaps the most helpful recent perspective is the notion of continuous quality improvement. That is, we develop both a formulation and a treatment plan, but continuously question both, saying 'How can this be improved?'.

Biological

The pharmacological treatment described below assumes that any other medical disorders have been appropriately treated. Pharmacotherapy is perhaps the primary intervention that comes to mind when biological treatment is considered, and is based on formulations of abnormal neurotransmitter metabolism in PTSD (Friedman, 1988; Sutherland and Davidson, 1994). Neurotransmitter formulations include changes in norepinephrine (noradrenaline) (Anisman and Sklar, 1979), the neurotransmitter of the locus coruleus and other nuclei that are a major component of the vigilance/alarm system (for comprehensive review see Murburg, 1994). Serotonin transmission, however, which may play a part in learning and anxiety (Kandel, 1983) and also seems to be associated with impulsive, aggressive behaviour (Linnoila et al., 1983; Coccaro et al., 1989), might be abnormal in PTSD. This may be the reason that only anti-depressants with a serotonin effect (selective serotonin reuptake inhibitors (SSRIs), amitriptyline, imipramine, monoamine oxidase inhibitors (MAOIs)) have been reported to work, while desipramine, which primarily affects norepinephrine, was reported to be ineffective. Both norepinephrine and serotonin influence neuronal activity in many areas of the brain, including the brainstem, limbic system and cortex, so abnormalities in neurotransmission at one or many sites may be associated with symptoms. One possibility is that the SSRIs optimize serotonin transmission in the prefrontal cortex, which may play an important role in mediating the individual's interaction with the environment, especially the interpersonal environment. This could explain the efficacy of the SSRIs in panic, obsessive–compulsive disorder (OCD) and depression as well as PTSD. Other possibilities are that alterations in dopamine (Zacharko, 1994) and other neuroregulator systems such as the endorphins may be involved (van der Kolk et al., 1985). Rather than simple increases or decreases in neurotransmitter levels or transmission, however, the problem may be one of dysregulation (von Bertalanffy, 1968) in which these systems do not respond appropriately to external stimuli or memories, as has been described for depression (Siever and Davis, 1985).

The focus here is on the algorithm of selecting a particular medication, then evaluating the treatment response, then deciding to continue or modify treatment, all within the context of other treatment modules. For PTSD, clinical trials in the literature suggest that the minimum duration should be 8–12 weeks, but the medication must be then continued until the symptoms disappear or plateau to decide whether or not the patient is a responder, partial responder or non-responder. As with major depressive disorder, effective pharmacotherapy should be for at least 6 months, although some patients may require lifetime maintenance medication.

Short-term benzodiazepine treatment is clinically considered to be effective for acute stress response disorders and for the anxiety, hyperarousal and sleep disruption of PTSD, but this is based on clinical experience rather than clinical trials. While clinical trials of alprazolam have shown efficacy in the treatment of PTSD (Dunner et al., 1985; Giller et al., 1990), results are discrepant about whether core symptoms of PTSD are significantly helped (Braun et al., 1990).

Antidepressants are the cornerstone of pharmacological treatment for PTSD. While the number of randomized clinical trials (RCTs) is around ten, the results are reasonably consistent with open trials. A summary of the RCTs with the tricyclic antidepressants (TCAs) and monoamine oxidase inhibitor phenelzine supports the efficacy of these compounds against PTSD symptoms, although the intrusive symptom cluster seems to respond better than the avoidant or arousal clusters (Southwick et al., 1994). The possible stronger efficacy of phenelzine is offset by concerns about hypertensive reactions in combination with certain medications or foods. More recently, open trials of the SSRIs have supported efficacy of these antidepressants in PTSD, more so for avoidant symptoms (McDougle et al., 1991; Nagy et al., 1993), although this has support from only one RCT (van der Kolk et al., 1994). For antidepressants, then, the algorithm is the same as for major depressive disorder: start with an SSRI, TCA or phenelzine, and evaluate efficacy and side-effects over at least 8–12 weeks until symptoms reach a plateau. If the patient is a partial responder or non-responder, augmentation therapy can be tried, although this approach has not been researched. The level of response contributes to the decision to try another class of antidepressant.

Mood stabilizers such as lithium (Kitchner and Greenstein, 1985; van der Kolk, 1983; Forster et al., 1995), and the anticonvulsants carbamazepine (Lipper et al., 1986; Wolf et al., 1988) and valproic acid (Szymanski and Olympia, 1991; Fesler, 1991) have been reported as helpful, especially for irritability and hyperarousal.

The adrenergic receptor drugs propranolol and clonidine have been reported to be helpful in some open clinical trials, but have not achieved widespread clinical use. They may be more helpful in children (Perry, 1994).

Antipsychotics have a bad reputation in the treatment of PTSD, likely because inpatients with severe intrusive symptoms, hyperarousal and/or irritability were diagnosed with schizophrenia and treated with long-term, high-dose antipsychotic medication, which may have contributed to avoidant and numbing symptoms. Low-dose, intermittent use of antipsychotics, however, for intrusive symptoms that become delusional in severity or behavioural control are helpful.

Buspirone has been reported to be effective in PTSD in case reports (Fichtner and Crayton, 1994).

Patients are often treated with an antidepressant plus some combination of these other categories of psychotropic medications. In such cases, polypharmacy may be helpful if different drugs are treating different symptoms or acting together, but polypharmacy by simple accretion (i.e., not considering what can be discontinued as well as added) should be avoided.

Another class of biological formulations of PTSD involves the brain function underlying orienting and alarm, and the basis for conditioning. These, however, are not well understood in psychiatry in general, although psychophysiological studies in PTSD have supported some theories that have behavioural treatment implications (Shalev, 1996).

Psychological

The range of available psychological treatments has been clinically applied to PTSD. Treatments based on conditioning theory are perhaps closest to the biological formulations of PTSD, but stand on their own as psychological constructs, i.e. do not require an understanding of brain mechanisms. The actual psychotherapy practised often combines elements from many theoretical perspectives such as the cognitive/behavioural (Roth et al., 1996), psychodynamic (Marmar et al., 1993) and constructivist (McCann and Pearlman, 1990) schools of thought. Rapid eye movement desensitization (Shapiro, 1995) is currently under evaluation. Some principles from these perspectives can be adapted for patients who may not be able to do such intensive psychotherapeutic work. We have had some success with an education-oriented, open-enrolment group focused on 'survival skills' for abuse-survivor inpatients with self-damaging behaviour where the focus is on understanding the contribution of abuse memories and effect on the dangerous behaviour, and using cognitive skills like relaxation, self-soothing, distraction and reframing to reduce self-mutilation or suicidal behaviour (Starr and Giller, 1993).

From a research perspective, the strongest treatment effect in PTSD has been shown for cognitive-behavioural (CBT) approaches (Solomon et al., 1992). These, however, range from the cognitive restructuring concept to almost pure behavioural treatments. Behaviour treatments focus on re-exposure of the patient to reminders of the trauma to extinguish the conditioned response thought to underly the symptoms of PTSD. Such exposure can range from the gradual (desensitization) to the extensive (flooding).

Cognitive therapy focuses on the effect of the traumatic experience on the individual's thoughts and assumptions about himself and the world, attempting to reduce thoughts of inadequacy and a pre-occupation with danger. In contrast to the decision algorithm for pharmacotherapy, which focuses on symptoms and somewhat on acute stress response versus PTSD, the CBT focus may depend on chronicity and specificity of the trauma, and also some patient characteristics, such as the ability to tolerate exposure, and the level of cognitive skills. One comprehensive description of the important elements of therapy (Roth et al., 1996) includes recovery and authentication of traumatic memories, controlling and contextualizing the effect associated with these memories, reframing of the traumatic experience, mastery of the abuse dynamics that contribute to current behaviour, the establishment of positive attachments to people and improving safety and coping strategies.

The analytical perspective of PTSD recognizes that damage has been done to the psychological organization and processing capabilities of the individual (Freud, 1920; van der Kolk and van der Hart, 1989; Krystal, 1988), and that consequently psychotherapy is not simply resolving unconscious conflicts. It is now recognized that the complexity of the therapeutic process involves elements of desensitization as well as cognitive and affective processing of the traumatic memories (Marmar et al., 1993).

Social

Psychiatry has usually included the social aspect of neuropsychiatric disorders, not only in considering psychosocial precipitants but also the social effects of the disorder, and the need for patients to achieve social rehabilitation or habilitation. This aspect of treatment is especially important for traumatic stress response disorders, and can be part of the psychological work (Herman, 1992) as well as simply getting the person back into social function.

Active social involvement in groups and political activity, dealing with helplessness, is an important component in recovering from trauma (Herman, 1992; Raphael, 1996). Another major social issue is the legal question about liability for PTSD resulting from a traumatic event, where a judgement must be made about the relationship between a particular event and PTSD symptoms.

POTENTIAL ADVANCES IN ASSESSMENT AND TREATMENT

The above traditional structure for evaluation and treatment provides a great deal of essential information, but is supplemented by extensive laboratory tests and procedures in many areas of medicine. Psychiatry remains unique in lacking biological measures of the pathophysiology of disorders, which also, of course, means that diagnoses are syndrome-based. Psychiatry, while searching for magic markers, has not developed biological assessments to aid in diagnosis of particular disorders or syndromes, or even to measure the hypothesized abnormalities in neurotransmitter function that psychotropic drugs normalize. Biological abnormalities reported in PTSD include psychophysiological documentation of increased responsivity to reminders of the trauma (Shalev, 1996), alterations in catecholamine (Giller, 1990; Murburg, 1994) and cortisol (Yehuda et al., 1991) metabolism, and initial reports of reduced hippocampal volume in some patients with PTSD (Bremner et al., 1995). These findings provide the possibility of biological testing in PTSD to establish the diagnosis and to monitor treatment effects over time. Even more speculatively, hippocampal volume reduction may be secondary to the course of illness of PTSD, and might be preventable with treatment.

Testing strength still lies in the psychological domain, where neuropsychological testing can measure psychologically defined parameters of brain function, but while some understanding exists of brain areas involved in many neuropsychologically defined functions, we still lack a fundamental understanding and basic model of how networks combine to generate function, much less how specific regional neurotransmitter systems contribute to such function.

That said, PTSD does provide an exciting opportunity for integrating different concepts/domains of brain functions.

CONCLUSIONS

The understanding of traumatic stress response disorders has increased markedly over the past 15 years, expanding from a core of experienced clinicians who treated patients for years before the term 'post-traumatic stress disorder' was adopted.

Part of that understanding, however, was rediscovering information (van der Kolk and van der Hart, 1989) that had been buried by controversy and overshadowed by advances in the neurosciences. Preventing concepts of traumatic stress from generalizing to all stress and being extremely careful about traumatic memory work is important to avoid repeating the polarization that contributed to the eclipse of the importance of traumatic stress in the past century.

On the other hand, assessment and treatment of the traumatic stress response disorders holds the promise of serving as a model for the use of biological measures in the clinic, selection of alternative treatments in each of the biological, psychological and social domains, and the combination of such treatment modules into an integrated treatment plan that changes over time depending on the needs of the patient.

References

Anisman, H.L., Sklar, L.S. (1979) Catecholamine depletion in mice upon exposure to stress: mediation of the escape deficits produced by inescapable shock. *Journal of Comprehensive Psysiological Psychology* **93**: 610–625.

Blake, D.D., Weathers, F.W., Nagy, L.M. et al. (1990) A clinician rating scale for assessing current and lifetime PTSD: the CAPS-1. *Behavior Therapist* **13**: 187–188.

Braun, P., Greenberg, D., Dasberg, H., Lerer, B. (1990) Core symptoms of post traumatic stress disorder unimproved by alprazolam treatment. *Journal of Clinical Psychiatry* **51**: 236–238.

Bremner, J.D., Randall, P., Scott, T.M. et al. (1995) MRI-based measurement of hippocampal volume in patients with combat-related PTSD. *American Journal of Psychiatry* **152**: 973–981.

Breslau, N., Davis, G.C. (1992) PTSD in an urban population of young adults: risk factors for chronicity. *American Journal of Psychiatry* **149**: 671–675.

Coccaro, E.F., Siever, L.J., Klar, H.M. et al. (1989) Serotonergic studies in patients with affective and personality disorders. *Archives of General Psychiatry* **46**: 587–599.

Dunner, F.J., Edwards, W.P., Copeland, P.C. (1985) Clinical efficacy of alprazolam in PTSD patients. Abstracts: New Research, APA, 138th Annual Meeting, Los Angeles, CA.

Fesler, A.F. (1991) Valproate in combat-related PTSD. *Journal of Clinical Psychiatry* **52**: 361–364.

Fichtner, C.G., Crayton, J.W. (1994) Buspirone in combat-related posttraumatic stress disorder. *Journal of Clinical Psychopharmacology* **14**: 79–81.

Forster, P.L., Schoenfeld, F.B., Marmar, C.R., Lang, A.J. (1995) Lithium for irritability in PTSD. *Journal of Traumatic Stress* **8**: 143–149.

Freud, S. (1920/1957) *Beyond the Pleasure Principle*, Vol. 18, p. 64. London: Hogarth Press.

Friedman, M.J. (1988) Toward rational pharmacotherapy for PTSD. *American Journal of Psychiatry* **145**: 281–285.

Giller, E.L. (ed.) (1990) *Biological Assessment and Treatment of Post-traumatic Stress Disorder*. Washington DC: APA Press.

Giller, E.L. Jr, Kosten, R.T., Yehuda, R. et al. (1990). Psychoendocrinology and pharmacotherapy of PTSD. *Clinical Neuropharmacology* **13** (Suppl 2): 329–330.

Helprin, M. (1987) *A Soldier of the Great War*. Harcourt Brace & Co.

Herman, J. (1992) *Trauma and Recovery*. New York: Basic Books.

Kandel, E.R. (1983) From metapsychology to molecular biology: explorations into the nature of anxiety. *American Journal of Psychiatry* **140**: 1277–1293.

Kardiner, A., Spiegel, H. (1947) *War Stress and Neurotic Illness*. New York: Paul B. Hoeber.

Keane, T.M., Caddell, J.M., Taylor, K.L. (1988) Mississippi Scale for combat-related PTSD. *Journal of Consulting and Clinical Psychology* **56**: 85–90.

Kitchner, I., Greenstein, R. (1985) Low dose lithium carbonate in the treatment of PTSD. *Military Medicine* **150**: 378–381.

Krystal, H. (1988) *Integration and Self-Healing*. Hillsdale, NJ: The Analytic Press.

Linnoila, M., Virkunen, M., Scheinin, M. et al. (1983) Low CSF 5-HIAA concentration differentiates impulsive from nonimpulsive violent behavior. *Life Science* **33**: 2609–2614.

Lipper, S., Davidson, J.R.T., Grady, T.A. et al. (1986) Preliminary study of carbamazepine in post traumatic stress disorder. *Psychosomatics* **27**: 849–854.

Marmar, C.R., Foy, D., Kagan, B. et al. (1993) An integrated approach for treating posttraumatic stress. In Pynoos, R. (ed.) *Posstraumatic Stress Disorder*, pp. 239–272. APA Review of Psychiatry, Washington DC: APA Press.

McCann, I.L., Pearlman, L.A. (1990) *Psychological Trauma and the Adult Survivor*. New York: Brunner/Mazel.

McDougle, C.J., Southwick, S.M., Charney, D.S., St James, R.L. (1991) An open trial of fluoxetine in the treatment of posttraumatic stress disorder (letter). *Journal of Clinical Psychopharmacology* **11**: 325–327.

Murburg, M.M. (ed.) (1994) *Catecholamine Function in Posttraumatic Stress Disorder*. Washington DC: American Psychiatric Press.

Nagy, L.M., Morgan, C.A., Southwick, S.M., Charney, D.S. (1993) Open prospective trial of fluoxetine for posttraumatic stress disorder. *Journal of Clinical Psychopharmacology* **13**: 107–113.

Norris, F. (1992) Epidemiology of trauma: frequency and impact of different potentially traumatic events on different gender groups. *Journal of Consulting and Clinical Psychology* **60**: 409–418.

Perry, B.D. (1994) Neurobiological sequelae of childhood trauma: PTSD in children. In Murburg, M.M. (ed.) *Catecholamine Function in Posttraumatic Stress Disorder*, pp. 233–255. Washington DC: American Psychiatric Press.

Raphael B. (1996) Social re-integration and political action. In: Giller E.L., Weisaeth, L. (eds) *Post-Traumatic Stress Disorder*, vol. 2, no. 2, pp. 329–357. Baillière's Clinical Psychiatry. London: Baillière Tindall.

Remarque, E.M. (1929) *All Quiet on the Western Front*. New York: Little, Brown & Co.

Roth, S., De Rosa, R.R., Turner, K. (1996) Cognitive-behavioral intervention for PTSD. In Giller, E.L., Weisaeth, L. (eds) *Post-Traumatic Stress Disorder*, pp. 281–296. Baillière's Clinical Psychiatry. London: Baillière Tindall.

Shay, J. (1994) *Achilles in Vietnam*. New York: Atheneum.

Shalev, A. (1996) Psychophysiology of PTSD: clinical implications. In Giller, E.L., Weisaeth, L. (eds) *Post-Traumatic Stress Disorder*, pp. 263–279. Baillière's Clinical Psychiatry. London: Baillière Tindall.

Shapiro, F. (1995) *Eye Movement Desensitization and Reprocessing*. New York: Guildford Press.

Siever, L.J., Davis, K.L. (1985) Overview: toward a dysregulation hypothesis of depression. *American Journal of Psychiatry* **142**: 1017–1031.

Solomon, S.D., Gerrity, E.T., Muff, A.M. (1992) Efficacy of treatments for post traumatic stress disorder; an empirical review. *Journal of the American Medical Association* **268**: 633–638.

Southwick, S., Yehuda, R., Giller, E.L., Charney, D.S. (1994) Use of tricyclics and monoamine oxidase inhibitors in the treatment of PTSD: a quantitative review. In M. Murburg (ed.) *Catecholamine function in Posttraumatic Stress Disorder*, pp. 293–305. Washington DC: American Psychiatric Press.

Starr, C., Giller, E.L. (1993) Survival skills training group therapy for abuse survivors with self-injurious behaviour. International Society for Traumatic Stress Studies Proceedings (Abstract).

Sutherland, S.M., Davidson, J.R.T. (1994) Pharmacotherapy for PTSD. *Psychiatric Clinics of North America* **17**: 409–421.

Szymanski, H.V., Olympia, J. (1991) Divalproex in posttraumatic stress disorder. *American Journal of Psychiatry* **148**: 1086–1087.

van der Kolk, B.A. (1983) Psychopharmacological issues in PTSD. *Hospital and Community Psychiatry* **34**: 683–691.

van der Kolk, B.A., Greenberg, A.M., Boyd, H., Krystal, J.H. (1985) Inescapable shock, neurotransmitters and addiction to trauma: toward a psychobiology of PTSD. *Biological Psychiatry* **20**: 314–325.

van der Kolk, B.A., Dreyfuss, D., Michaels, M. et al. (1994) Fluoxetine in PTSD. *Journal of Clinical Psychiatry* **55**: 517–522.

van der Kolk, B.A., van der Hart, O. (1989) Pierre Janet and the breakdown of adaptation in psychological trauma. *American Journal of Psychiatry* **146**: 1530–1540.

von Bertalanffy, L. (1968) *General System Theory*. New York: George Braziller.

Vreven, D.L., Gudanowski, D.M., King, L.A., King, D.W. (1995) The civilian version of the Mississippi PTSD scale: a psychometric evaluation. *Journal of Traumatic Stress* **8**: 91–109.

Wolf, M.E., Alavi, A. Mosnaim, A.D. (1988) Posttraumatic stress disorder in Vietnam veterans. *Biological Psychiatry* **23**: 642–644.

Yehuda, R., Giller, E.L., Southwick, S.M., Lowy, M.T., Mason, J.W. (1991) Hypothalamic-pituitary-adrenal dysfunction in PTSD. *Biological Psychiatry* **30**: 1031–1048.

Zacharko, R.M. (1994) Stressors, the mesocorticolimbic system and anhedonia: implications for PTSD. In Murburg, M. (ed.) *Catecholamine Function in Posttraumatic Stress Disorder*, pp. 99–130, Washington DC: American Pyschiatric Press.

2

Chronic Fatigue Syndrome

Simon Wessely

BACKGROUND

The problems of the patient with profound physical and mental fatigue that defies simple medical explanation have been the subject of considerable professional and public interest for the last ten years or so. Many such patients have been diagnosed with labels such as myalgic encephalomyelitis (ME), postviral fatigue syndrome (PVFS) or chronic fatigue syndrome (CFS). Despite the interest, little is established about the condition, except that it is controversial.

Even the name is a source of dispute. ME is misleading, since encephalomyelitis describes a distinct, frequently lethal, pathological process, which is absent from this condition. More acceptable in professional circles is the second term, postviral fatigue syndrome. The concept is straightforward – a fatiguing illness that follows a viral infection. However, in practice substantial difficulties exist even with this term (see below). For the rest of this review I shall follow the international consensus and use the term chronic fatigue syndrome (CFS), a label that is at least both accurate, short and free from unproven aetiological assumptions.

Whatever we choose to call them, it is frequently stated that such illnesses began with the now infamous outbreak of illness at the Royal Free Hospital in 1955, and it is from there that the term ME originates (Medical Staff, 1955). The often bitter controversy that seems to be an integral part of these illnesses can also be traced to that outbreak, since first epidemiologists, and later psychiatrists, suggested that the outbreak was caused not by an infectious agent, but by transmitted emotional distress, so called 'mass hysteria' (McEvedy and Beard, 1970). The truth will never be known, but such arguments have little relevance now. The epidemic at the Royal Free Hospital (and those associated with it), was an acute, paralytic, contagious illness with abnormal neurological signs. The current problem facing doctors is a chronic, fatiguing, non-contagious illness, in which neurological signs are absent. Much harm has resulted from these two processes being grouped under the same label of ME.

Instead, more attention is now being devoted to the illness that represents a more likely origin for modern ME/CFS, neurasthenia. The parallels, not just in terms of symptoms, but also of social class, aetiology, relationship to infections, links with psychological disorders, and, not the least, the ability to cause intense disagreements among doctors, are striking. These are discussed in greater detail elsewhere (Abbey and Garfinkel, 1991; Wessely, 1991).

EPIDEMIOLOGY

Case Definition

The rise of CFS during the 1980s can be traced to the coincidence of new clinical and research observations, largely concerning possible links with infective agents and immune dysfunction (see below), the changing nature of the relationship of doctor and patient (Shorter, 1992), and consumer pressure. The consequence was immediate confusion about its definition and nosological status. Most observers, usually working in specialist centres, noted certain characteristics of clinical samples. These included an over-representation of females, and of higher socio-economic groups. Strong physical attribution and intense disease conviction were the norm (Wessely and Powell, 1989; Hickie et al., 1990; Schweitzer et al., 1994), whilst certain professions, such as doctors and teachers, seem to be particularly at risk. In contrast, ethnic minorities were rarely encountered.

In 1988, David and colleagues (David et al., 1988) argued that the lack of information on the prevalence, nature and aetiology of CFS could be traced to the lack of epidemiological data and neglect of epidemiological principles in many of the published studies. Annual prevalence estimates then varied from 3 to 2800 per 100 000. Since then progress has been made in some areas, in particular the realization of the need for uniform case definitions, but the neglect of epidemiological principles, such as selection bias and confounding, continues to cause difficulties (Richman et al., 1994). Considerable variation in diagnostic practice remains.

At present, four operational case definitions have been presented (Table 2.1). One started with the efforts of American infectious disease and immunology specialists (Holmes et al., 1988), and has been refined on two occasions (Schluederberg et al., 1992; Fukuda et al., 1994). The second comes from an Australian group (Lloyd et al., 1990), and the third from a British consensus conference (Sharpe et al., 1991). These definitions are listed below. There are a number of similarities, such as the requirement for substantial functional impairment in addition to the complaint of fatigue (although all are vague on how this should be measured). Differences are also apparent. For example, the American criteria attach particular significance to certain somatic symptoms such as sore throats, painful muscles and lymph nodes, and, although the requirement for multiple symptoms has been modified in the latest revision, four symptoms chosen from a list of eight are still required (Fukuda et al., 1994). The choice of symptoms reflects one school of thought that holds that an infective and/or immune process underlies CFS. In contrast, the British definition does not emphasize somatic symptoms, instead insisting on both physical and mental fatigue and fatigability.

Epidemiology of Chronic Fatigue

Before considering the epidemiology of CFS, it is first necessary to consider what is known about the chief symptom, chronic fatigue. Lewis and Wessely (1992) reviewed 15 community and 10 primary care studies. They concluded that fatigue is one of the commonest symptoms encountered in the community – it is, as another reviewer noted, 'the normal chaff of living' (Ridsdale, 1989). In a subsequent British community survey, 38% of the sample reported substantial fatigue, which had been present for over six months in 18% (Cox et al., 1987). In Germany, 26.2% of a population survey in Mannheim complained of 'states of fatigue and exhaustion' over a seven-day period (Schepank, 1987). Similar figures are encountered in other Western countries (Lewis and Wessely, 1992).

Most fatigued people neither consider themselves ill, nor consult a doctor (Zola, 1966; Morrell and Wale, 1976). Despite that, fatigue remains a common symptom encountered in both primary and secondary care. A point prevalence of 21% for fatigue of six months duration, associated with other somatic symptoms such as sore throat,

Table 2.1 Case definitions for chronic fatigue syndrome

	CDC – 1988	CDC – 1994	Australian	UK
Minimum duration (months)	6	6	6	6
Functional impairment	50% decrease in activity	Substantial	Substantial	Disabling
Cognitive or neuro-psychiatric symptoms	May be present	May be present	Required	Mental fatigue required
Other symptoms	6 or 8 required	4 required	Not specified	Not specified
New onset	Required	Required	Not required	Required
Medical exclusions	Extensive list of known physical causes	Clinically important	Known physical causes	Known physical causes
Psychiatric exclusions	Psychosis, bipolar disorder, substance abuse	Melancholic depression, substance abuse, bipolar disorders, psychosis, eating disorder	Psychosis, bipolar disorder, substance abuse, eating disorder	Psychosis, bipolar disorder, eating disorder, organic brain disease

myalgia and headache, was recorded in an American ambulatory care survey (Buchwald et al., 1987). Thirty-two percent of those attending an Israeli general practice reported at least one asthenic symptom (Shahar and Lederer, 1990). Slightly lower prevalence is reported in British primary care, where 10% will admit to chronic fatigue (David et al., 1990), and in Canada, where 14% of new attenders complained of fatigue (Cathebras et al., 1992). It was the principal reason for consultation in 7% of new attenders in primary care in both France and Canada (Cathebras et al., 1992; Fuhrer and Wessely, 1995).

Relevant prevalence data can also be obtained from studies using the ICD-10 criteria for neurasthenia, which has considerable overlap with CFS – 97% of those attending a multidisciplinary CFS clinic in Wales also fulfilled criteria for neurasthenia (Farmer et al., 1995). In the Zurich longitudinal survey, Merikangas and Angst (1994) reported prevalence of 6% for men and 10% for women. The recent multinational WHO study of mental disorder in primary care reported a prevalence of ICD-10 neurasthenia of 5.5% (Ormel et al., 1994). In the longitudinal study on the Swedish island of Lundby, the lifetime prevalence of fatigue syndrome (defined similarly to neurasthenia as excessive fatigue in the absence of clear-cut features of anxiety or depression) was 33% for women and 21% for men (Hagnell et al., 1993). Intriguingly, the prevalence appeared to be increasing over time.

Whatever the label, all agree that physical investigations are rarely helpful, except in certain groups such as the elderly (Lane et al., 1990; Valdini et al., 1989; Ridsdale et al., 1993).

Turning to medical outpatients, one third of those attending two American ambulatory medical clinics reported fatigue (Kroenke et al., 1990; Bates et al., 1993) making it the commonest overall symptom, and it was the main reason for presentation in 8% (Kroenke et al., 1990). Routine investigations failed to identify a cause for nearly all these subjects (Kroenke et al., 1990; Kroenke and Mangelsdorff, 1989). In response, Komaroff (1990) wrote an editorial entitled '"Minor" illness symptoms: the magnitude of their burden and of our ignorance'.

Epidemiological Data on the Prevalence of CFS

Chronic fatigue is thus common, but what about CFS? On the basis of laboratory request forms, Ho-Yen (1988) estimated the prevalence in the west of Scotland as 51 per 100 000. The first attempt at a population-based study using an operational case definition came from Lloyd and colleagues in Australia (Lloyd et al., 1990). Cases were identified using general practitioners as key informants. A point prevalence of 37 per 100 000 was recorded. However, only 25% of those physicians approached agreed to participate. Ho-Yen and McNamara (Ho-Yen, 1991) achieved a better response rate in their survey of Scottish general practitioners. They estimated a prevalence of 130 per 100 000, but recognition of CFS varied. Professional workers remained over-represented, although this could still reflect differences in labelling. CFS consumed considerable amounts of medical time.

The Center for Disease Control and Prevention (CDC) estimated the prevalence of CFS based on surveillance of selected physicians in four US cities (Gunn et al., 1993). The observed prevalence of CFS was lower than the Australian figures – between 2 and 7 per 100 000. There was a female excess, and a high rate of psychiatric morbidity. Like the other studies, this was a further example of a

key informant/sentinel physician design, and thus reports administrative rather than true prevalence.

This and the previously mentioned studies suggest that CFS is not
a common problem. Recent studies with systematic case ascertainment report a different picture. Bates et al. (1993) surveyed an
American ambulatory care clinic at an academic teaching hospital.
In keeping with the literature, 27% of those attending a primary
care clinic had substantial fatigue lasting more than six months and
interfering with daily life. The point prevalence of CFS according to
the various definitions was 0.3% (CDC-1988), 0.4% (UK) and 1.0%
(Australian) respectively, and 0.9% of an occupational sample fulfilled
CFS criteria (Shefer et al., 1994). A questionnaire-based study of
subjects registered with a single Scottish general practice (Lawrie
and Pelosi, 1995) reported a point prevalence of 0.6% (95% confidence limits 0.2–1.5) according to the UK criteria, but this was based
on only four cases. We found even higher prevalences in a six-month
follow-up study of 2376 subjects aged between 18 and 45 seen in five
general practices across the south of England (Wessely et al., in
press). The point prevalence of CFS using the 1994 CDC criteria
was 2.6% (95%, c.i. 1.7–3.4%), falling to 0.5% (95%, c.i. 0.1–0.3%) if
comorbid psychological disorders were excluded.

These primary care figures are an order of magnitude greater than
those obtained in the first wave of primary care and community
surveys. Why? The answer is that nearly all those who fulfilled operational criteria for CFS were not labelled as such by either themselves
or their general practitioners, and thus would not be identified in a key
informant survey, or a tertiary setting (Wessely, 1995). Among the vast
numbers of subjects with excessive fatigue, only 1% believed themselves to be suffering from CFS (Pawlikowska et al., 1994). Amongst
the smaller numbers who fulfilled criteria for CFS, only 12% used this
or a related term to describe their illness (Euba et al., 1996). Few of
those who could be classified as CFS are labelled as CFS. This also
highlights the powerful role of selection bias in previous studies, which
are almost all based on tertiary care samples of patients who have
frequently made their own diagnosis before seeking specialist help, and
are almost certainly an atypical and unrepresentative sample of CFS
cases (Richman et al., 1994; Euba et al., 1996).

The Nosological Status of CFS: Dimension versus Category

Despite the current interest in CFS, both by the public and professions, the nosological status of the disorder remains uncertain. Is it

an independent entity, or alternatively does CFS simply reflect an arbitrarily defined end of a spectrum of severity? To date no study has reported that CFS can be distinguished from CF by any particular laboratory, demographic or psychiatric variable (Lane et al., 1991; Swanink et al., 1995). Is there a particular symptom profile that serves to distinguish CFS?

The answer seems to be no. Several studies have found a strong correlation between the experience of somatic and psychological symptoms. This relationship was identical for both symptoms included in the current definition of CFS and those excluded, which is not surprising since there was a close relationship between the two sets of symptoms anyway (Wessely et al., 1996a). There is no epidemiological justification for stating that certain symptoms are characteristic of CFS (and hence form part of the case definition) solely because they resemble those of an infective or immunological disorder held to underlie CFS. Most symptoms may instead reflect the joint experience of somatic and psychological distress (Lane et al., 1991; Simon and VonKorff, 1991; Kroenke et al., 1994).

There is already compelling evidence that fatigue is dimensionally and not categorically distributed. A survey of general practice attenders in south London found that the number of fatigue items endorsed was best described along a continuous distribution (David et al., 1990), whilst an American study of an internal medicine practice found that all the symptoms that make up the CFS criteria were commoner in those with unexplained fatigue, and not just CFS (Chester, 1994). A population study also showed a continuous distribution of fatigue symptoms and severity (Pawlikowska et al., 1994). Another population-based study, this time from the United States, grouped together ten items on tiredness, weakness, slow recovery from viral infections and need to rest, termed 'asthenia'. Once again, plotting the number of items endorsed against the number of persons with each score yielded a continuous distribution (Lewis and Wessely, 1992).

Our group found little evidence that the other variables that make up the current concepts of CFS can be used to impose a clear cut-off, separating those with severe fatigue from those with CFS (Wessely et al., 1996a). Only post-exertional malaise, muscle weakness and myalgia were significantly more likely to be observed in CFS than in chronic fatigue or idiopathic chronic fatigue. None of the other 35 symptoms distinguished CF, ICF or CFS, nor did the presence or absence of psychological disorder.

The stated desire of all the current CFS case definitions is to attempt to isolate a 'pure' syndrome, distinct from other medical or psychiatric categories. We and others have argued that the current CFS case definitions instead achieve the opposite of that intended (Hickie et al., 1995). By insisting on a minimum symptom require- ment, these definitions actively select subjects at increased risk of psychiatric disorder (Lane et al., 1991; Katon and Russo, 1992; Wessely et al., 1996). It if is intended to produce case definitions of CFS that distinguish the syndrome from existing categories of psychi- atric disorder, it would be more logical to insist on maximum rather than minimum symptom criteria.

A convincing case for heterogeneity in CFS has already been made (Swartz, 1988). Current definitions of CFS represent an arbitrary imposition where there may be no natural division. Case definitions are obligatory for many types of research into the problems of chron- ically fatigued patients, including treatment, outcome and service development. However, at present, all such definitions must not be taken as verification of a specific nosological entity. No one has provided sound evidence from a population-based study of a discrete syndrome of excessive fatigue, called CFS or anything else.

The situation is thus analogous to the nature of hypertension. During the 1960s there was a famous debate between Platt and Pickering on the nature of high blood pressure, with the former main- taining that a discrete disease ('hypertension') existed, the latter that there was a continuous distribution of blood pressure across the community. It is now concluded that the evidence supports the dimensional view, and that no discrete disease called 'high blood pressure' exists.

Continuing the analogy with hypertension, it is true that, in specialist practice, cardiologists are always alert to the possibility of renal artery stenosis or phaeochromocytoma, although their public health impact is slight. Similarly, discrete diseases associated with severe fatigue also exist, some known, and no doubt others yet to be identified. Nevertheless, the epidemiology of fatigue serves to put such diagnoses as CFS into a population perspective.

Even if chronic fatigue is a dimensional variable that cannot be easily separated from the normal sensation and experience of tired- ness, it still requires understanding and treatment. Hypertension, even if labelled 'essential', is not benign. So it is with CFS. Because one cannot detect a clear-cut division between 'normal' fatigue and the devastating illness so vividly detailed in the numerous first- person accounts of CFS sufferers, this no more invalidates the latter than the dimensional view of blood pressure invalidates the medical importance of severe hypertension. Community cases of CFS have levels of functional impairment greatly in excess of that found for all comparative chronic conditions such as ischaemic heart disease, arthritis or chronic bronchitis (Wessely et al., in press).

AETIOLOGY

An Infective Disorder?

There can be no doubt that at present the majority of those seen in specialist clinics trace their illness to the aftermath of a viral infection. However, such factors as the frequency of common viral infections, recall bias and search after meaning reminds us that a little more evidence is required before accepting that the cause of 'postviral fatigue' is indeed one or many viruses.

It has been strongly argued that one, and for some the principal, cause of CFS is persistent infection by Coxsackie virus. These claims began with a series of reports linking epidemic and sporadic cases of ME, usually in Scotland, to high static antibody titres to the Coxsackie virus. However, doubts set in on the interpretation of such studies, and although the introduction of an IgM test for Coxsackie promised more, recent case-control studies showed equivalent exposure in both cases and controls (Miller et al., 1991; Gow et al., 1994; Swanink et al., 1994). The enterovirus family was again implicated when a team at St Mary's Hospital identified a group specific antigen, the VP-1 antigen, in half of a selected sample of CFS cases, and no controls, and suggested viral persistence (as opposed to exposure) in the condition (Yousef et al., 1988). Public and media interest in the new test was intense, but further work showed that it was neither sensitive nor specific (Lynch and Seth, 1989; Halpin and Wessely, 1989) and a recent blinded study found equal levels of the antigen in both cases and controls (Swanink et al., 1994).

The next piece of evidence implicating enteroviruses in CFS came from two studies using new molecular techniques to find direct evidence of enteroviral involvement. In situ hybridization was used to demonstrate enteroviral RNA in 24% of muscle biopsies from a selected sample of CFS cases (Archard et al., 1988), whilst a study using the polymerase chain reaction (PCR) found evidence of enteroviral genome in 53% of cases from the same clinical centre, but only 15% of older surgical controls (Gow et al., 1991). However, these findings have not been replicated (McArdle et al., 1996), even by the original group (Gow et al., 1994), who concluded that CFS was not 'dependent on persistent viral infection of muscle'. The Dutch group also used the PCR test, this time on stool samples, and found no cases of enteroviral persistence. They concluded that the 'persistence of enteroviruses is unlikely to play a role in the development of CFS' (Swanink et al., 1994). However, just when the enterovirus hypothesis of CFS seemed to be on its last legs, it has been resurrected by a recent blinded study that detected enteroviral specific sequences in substantially more CFS patients than healthy controls, and was even increased compared to a second control group with acute viral infections (Clements et al., 1995).

Other agents have also been proposed. An American group made claims for a retroviral involvement in CFS, but subsequent groups were unable to confirm these findings. Human herpes virus-6 (HHV-6) is another candidate proposed for the infective basis of CFS. HHV-6 infection is ubiquitous, rendering interpretation of serological studies difficult. A recent review concluded that whereas it was an unlikely aetiological candidate, secondary reactivation by some other mechanism or stress might contribute to symptoms (Hay and Jenkins, 1994).

Although there is clinical evidence linking chronic fatigue with several infective agents, such as toxoplasmosis, Q fever or viral hepatitis (Berelowitz et al., 1995), at present the infective agent for which the best evidence exists for a post-infectious syndrome is the Epstein–Barr virus (EBV), the virus that causes glandular fever. It was reports of an association between CFS and EBV that triggered the current revival of interest in CFS in the United States. These original studies are now seen as flawed (Straus, 1988; Fekety, 1994), and there is no evidence for reactivation of EBV in CFS (Swanink et al., 1994). In the USA interest in the EBV virus has waned. However, researchers at St Bartholomew's Hospital, led by Peter White, have completed the first prospective cohort study of the outcome of EBV. In a meticulously designed and executed study, they provided firm evidence that EBV is associated with a post-infection fatigue syndrome that is both more frequent than, and can be distinguished from, anxiety and depressive illnesses (White et al., 1995; White et al., submitted). Unlike depressive illnesses arising after EBV, the post-infectious syndrome was not associated with concurrent measures of life events (Bruce-Jones et al., 1994).

Nevertheless, even after EBV, prolonged fatigue is the exception rather than the rule. Of 337 cases presenting to a student health centre, only 1.5% developed prolonged fatigue (Chang and Bittner, 1991), and the median duration of fatigue is only 12 weeks (White et al., submitted). Furthermore, precisely why EBV should be associated with a fatigue syndrome remains unclear.

Cope and colleagues made the first attempt to bring these various strands together in a study of the outcome of viral infection in primary care (Cope et al., 1994). They reported a modestly increased rate of fatigue in subjects six months after presenting to the GP with a symptomatic 'viral' infection, but this is open to doubt because of the inadequate control group. A prospective study using contemporary controls found no difference in chronic fatigue between those presenting with a clinical infection and those presenting with a range of other problems (Wessely et al., 1995). The same study also reported a strong association between measures of fatigue and psychological vulnerability completed *before* presenting to the general practitioner with a viral infection, and fatigue assessed six months later. Cope and colleagues also analysed the predictors of fatigue in their postviral group. They found that somatic attributional style, less definite diagnosis by the GP, and the provision of a sick note, were the only significant predictors of chronic fatigue (Cope et al., 1994).

We can now bring these strands together. The list below includes those factors for which there is sufficient evidence from well conducted longitudinal factors to suggest a relationship with fatigue after infection. It will be seen that a variety of factors – infective, physiological and psychological – are involved:

- Epstein–Barr virus infection;
- premorbid psychological disorder;
- somatic attributional style;
- encephalitis;
- physical deconditioning.

A Neuromuscular Disorder?

Given that fatigue and myalgia are so central to CFS it is understandable that several authors have suggested that a disorder of muscle function underlies the condition. The literature contains several papers with evidence of biochemical, functional and structural abnormalities of muscle. However, the evidence for a neuromuscular origin to the symptoms of CFS is far from convincing. First, most agree that physical *and* mental fatigue and fatigability are at the heart of CFS, and cannot be accounted for by any known mechanism of muscular function. The neuropsychiatric symptoms of CFS, such as poor concentration, short term memory impairment and so on, are not those of peripheral neuromuscular disorders (Wessely and Powell, 1989; Wood et al., 1991).

Some evidence has been presented of abnormalities in muscle structure, or on neurophysiological testing, such as single fibre EMG. However, these studies have largely either not been replicated, or could be explained as the consequences of inactivity, a *sine qua non* of the diagnosis of CFS (e.g. Wagenmakers et al., 1988; Roberts and Byrne, 1994). Instead, more attention should be paid to studies of actual neuromuscular function (as opposed to structure). There is a surprising degree of consensus, especially for a subject as diverse as CFS. Meticulously conducted studies of dynamic muscle function have failed to show any evidence of peripheral neuromuscular dysfunction. These include subjects with CFS as defined in the UK (Stokes et al., 1988; Riley et al., 1990), subjects with immune dysfunction as seen in Australia (Lloyd et al., 1988, 1991), with CFS as defined in the USA (Kent-Braun et al., 1993; Sisto et al., 1996), and with post-Epstein–Barr virus fatigue syndrome (Rutherford and White, 1991). There is also no objective evidence of a delayed appearance of abnormal post-exertional muscle fatigability (Lloyd et al., 1988; Gibson et al., 1993; Sisto et al., 1996). Instead, it seems likely that any changes in CFS are more likely to be the consequence, and not the cause, of fatigue and inactivity. Some, but not all, groups have also reported a disorder of the perception of effort – CFS patients rate themselves as more fatigued than they are physiologically, and thus cease work at an earlier stage than indicated by the state of their muscles.

Some differences have emerged. All agree that the fatigue in CFS is usually centrally mediated. However, whereas some have found totally normal recruitment, activation and function (Lloyd et al., 1988, 1991; Rutherford and White, 1991), others report that central activation is impaired (e.g. Stokes et al., 1988; Kent-Braun et al., 1993). There are a number of explanations, including impaired motivation, the effect of pain and so on. Whether or not the symptoms are similar to the central symptoms encountered in multiple sclerosis, as has been claimed (Deluca et al., 1993) also remains to be seen, but is already disputed (Djaldetti et al., 1996; Vercoulen et al., 1996a). The important message is that 'on physiological and pathological grounds it is clear that CFS is not a myopathy' (Edwards et al., 1993). These observations are of direct clinical relevance, since the implication is that patients can be strongly reassured that physical activity is unlikely to be harmful, provided that it takes place within the limits of the subject's current physical status.

Considerable excitement has been generated by recent claims that a failure of cardiovascular regulation underlies CFS. A group at Johns Hopkins in Baltimore claim that neurally mediated hypotension, also known as vasovagal syncope, is associated with prolonged fatigue (Bou-Holaigah et al., 1995). The term describes an abnormal cardiovascular reflex causing subjects to develop severe dizziness or even syncope (fainting) in response to orthostatic stress. The team first noted that a group of adolescents with vasovagal faints had similar symptoms to those of CFS, and second that vasovagal faints could be induced in CFS patients. The authors then gave some patients treatments that have been used for vasovagal fainting, such as fludrocortisone, to increase blood volume. Uncontrolled data were encouraging, and the authors are now carrying out a controlled clinical trial. Before it is possible to accept autonomic dysfunction as a primary cause of CFS (rather than a secondary contributor to symptoms) it is essential that two important confounders are addressed. One is the role of inactivity. Physical inactivity is a well known cause of postural hypotension, dizziness on standing and blood pressure instability (Saltin et al., 1968). The other is the role of anxiety and panic. Sympathetic dysfunction in response to stress has been found in CFS, similar to that observed in anxiety disorders (Pagani et al., 1994).

An Immunological or Allergic Disorder?

In the USA it is widely believed that CFS represents an immunological disorder, partly because the symptoms reported by sufferers (sore throats, swollen glands, allergies) seem reminiscent of some immune dysfunction (although actually these symptoms are far from specific to CFS). There has been a great deal of research using the tools of modern immunology, and, although evidence has been presented of alterations in various immune parameters, it is difficult to place these in perspective.

A number of abnormalities have been noted, chief amongst which are impairment of natural killer cell activity, and of T cell subsets. In particular, three groups have noted a reduced ratio of CD4/CD45 RA T cells (Straus et al., 1993). It has been argued that this represents the response of the immune system to chronic antigen stimulation. However, there is a great deal of overlap between cases and controls, and no relationship to clinical status. A similar finding has been reported in major depression (Maes et al., 1992), although there are also differences between the immune findings in CFS and in less severe depressive conditions (Lloyd et al., 1994). Even if immune parameters are abnormal in a subgroup, no one has ever presented data on actual immune impairment. Immune dysfunction has also been reported, but to a lesser extent, in chronically fatigued adults who do not meet CFS criteria, suggesting that immune dysfunction also lies on a continuum and is affected by behavioural status (Masuda et al., 1994). The links between psychiatry, stress and the immune disorder are far from established, but it is clear that psychological status has an impact on immune function.

The most recent and detailed reviews have therefore concluded that it is currently impossible to determine the significance of the observed changes in immunological status in CFS. One authority suggests that these changes are those of a hyperactive immune system secondary to viral infection (Levy, 1994), whilst another writes, 'The possibility that the immunological findings in CFS are also found in more classic psychological diseases remains very much alive ... perhaps secondary to subtle endocrine changes, character-istic of certain abnormal psychological states' (Strober, 1994). The next generation of studies of immune dysfunction and CFS must certainly consider the possibility that observed changes are secondary to the alterations in HPA function described elsewhere (see above).

A possible role for atopic vulnerability is plausible in CFS, with one case control study reporting increased lifetime histories of atopic disorder in a selected sample of CFS cases (Straus et al., 1988), but not another (MacDonald et al., 1996). However, no evidence has been presented of any link with less conventional allergic diseases. In particular, despite the frequent assertion in the popular literature of a link between CFS and ill-defined conditions such as multiple chemical sensitivity, food allergy or total allergy syndrome, any such links may be via an underlying predisposition to somatization (Manu et al., 1993).

A Psychiatric Disorder?

Prevalence of psychiatric disorder

Numerous studies have been published concerning the role of psychi-atric disorder in CFS, of which at least 13 use direct interviews (David, 1991; Clark and Katon, 1994). A variety of instruments and operational criteria have been used, but the results are reasonably consistent. Approximately half of those seen in specialist care with a diagnosis of one or other form of CFS fulfil criteria for affective disorder, even with fatigue removed from the criteria for mood disorder. The majority of studies find that a further quarter fulfil criteria for other psychiatric disorders, chief amongst which are anxiety and somatization disorders. Nearly all also agree that between one quarter and one third do not fulfil any criteria. The figures for the comorbidity of neurasthenia and psychiatric disorders are also congruent with these findings – in the multinational WHO study of mental disorder in primary care (Ormel et al., 1994) ICD-10 neurasthenia showed 71% psychiatric comorbidity.

Affective disorder is thus linked with CFS, but the association is not a simple one. First, the pattern of mood disorder is not always that with which psychiatrists are most familiar, and there is a suggestion that the atypical depressive disorders (in which there is increased sleep and appetite rather than the more customary decrease) may be particularly relevant. Assessing the phenomenology of depressive illness in CFS subjects is also not always straightforward – considerable difficulties can arise in distinguishing anhedonia from an inability to perform previously enjoyable activities.

Anxiety disorders are also common (Fischler et al., 1996a), but often overlooked, partly because of the difficulties in determining whether or not avoidance is related to phobic processess, or neuromuscular weakness, and partly because of the hierarchical nature of psychiatric diagnostic classifications that place mood above anxiety disorders. The latest neuroendocrine findings place CFS closer to post-traumatic stress disorder than depression, and the latest treatment studies, which are more supportive of behaviour interventions than antidepressants (see below), suggest that a reappraisal of the previous tendency to emphasize the links between CFS and mood rather than anxiety disorders is due.

Hyperventilation can play an important role in some patients. There have been claims that hyperventilation was found in all CFS patients (Rosen et al., 1990). Like any unitary explanation of CFS, this seems implausible, but a systematic study did suggest that between 10% and 25% of patients may have evidence of hyperventilation (Saisch et al., 1994).

Somatization disorder presents another difficult problem. Patients with long histories of multiple somatic symptoms, stretching back to adolescence, are common in CFS clinics, as they are across general medicine (Van Hemert et al., 1993). They may have previous episodes of unexplained abdominal pain, food allergies, chemical sensitivities, unresolved gynaecological problems, funny turns and so on. Some may fulfil criteria for somatization disorder (Briquet's syndrome).

To a certain extent, this overlap between CFS and somatization disorder (SD) is predictable, since the definitions of both CFS and somatization disorder require multiple symptoms (Johnson et al., 1996a). When Lane and colleagues compared those with CFS with chronically fatigued patients who did not fulfil the criteria for CFS, one of the chief differences between them was that the former were more likely to fulfil criteria for somatization disorder (Lane et al., 1991). They concluded that the multiple symptom criteria for CFS actively select for somatization disorder. When another group of researchers excluded those symptoms common to the definitions of CFS and SD, the prevalence of SD fell, but was still substantially elevated at 20% (Katon et al., 1991). Bear in mind that the expected prevalence of somatization disorder in community samples is of the order of 0.03% to 0.3% (Escobar et al., 1987).

Patients who fulfil criteria for somatization disorder have some of the highest disabilities encountered in medical practice. These patients have greater functional impairment, longer illness durations and more symptoms than CFS cases without multiple symptoms (Hickie et al., 1995). Current definitions of CFS exclude such patients, although they may paradoxically be the group that clings most firmly to the label. They are also the group more likely to be found in specialist CFS settings – somatization disorder is uncommon in samples of chronically fatigued patients identified in general practice – with a prevalence of 0.6% in the ECA sample (Walker et al., 1993). No cases were found in two UK community samples (McDonald et al., 1993; Wessely et al., in press).

Explanations

If psychiatric disorders are common, what are the possible explanations? One is artefactual – the criteria used to diagnose common psychological disorders overlap with those for the diagnosis of CFS. High rates of psychiatric disorders in CFS are thus inevitable, and do not themselves imply causality. As Kendell (1991) has written in the context of CFS, 'the statement that someone has a depressive illness is merely a statement about their symptoms. It has no causal implications'.

The next explanation is that these are simply misdiagnosed cases of depression or anxiety (e.g. Greenberg, 1990). This must be true for some, and there are many subjects for whom the standard psychiatric classification, explanations and treatments are adequate to the situation. In its severe form, the symptoms of CFS and those of major depression are hard to distinguish (Levine et al., 1989), and it is also known that depressive disorder alone is associated with severe functional impairment (Wells et al., 1989).

However, this unitary explanation flounders a little on the reasons outlined in the previous paragraph, since, with the occasional exception, it implies an implicit hierarchy of symptomatic classification. It also ignores the fact that in many there is insufficient evidence to justify a psychiatric diagnosis.

Could the observed psychological disorder simply be a reaction to physical illness? This explanation is the least appealing, since first there is as yet no definitive evidence of a specific physical pathology, and second, studies that use medical controls find rates of psychiatric disorder in the CFS cases that are invariably in excess of those in the control, often substantially so (Wessely and Powell, 1989; Wood et al., 1991; Katon et al., 1991; Pepper et al., 1993; Johnson et al., 1996b). Alternatively, could it be due to selection bias? This is one explanation for the finding that both irritable bowel syndrome and fibromyalgia are associated with psychiatric disorder in specialist, but not primary, care (Aaron et al., 1996; Smith et al., 1990). However, this seems unlikely in CFS, since a similar proportion seen in primary care with chronic fatigue or chronic fatigue syndrome also fulfil criteria for psychiatric disorder (McDonald et al., 1993; Cope et al., 1996; Wessely et al., 1996a), although in many other ways the samples are different (see above).

The final explanation suggests that CFS and psychiatric disorder arise from a common pathology. This argument must therefore involve some common neurobiological dysfunction. It is an appealing suggestion, for which there is some experimental support. This will be discussed in the next section.

A Neurobiological Disorder?

Models linking CFS with muscular dysfunction no longer find much favour. That interest has largely been transferred to studies of possible central nervous or neuroendocrine disorder. This is a welcome development, since, unlike muscular studies, this paradigm is closer to the clinical features of the condition. It is intriguing that a similar shift from peripheral to central models also occurred during the Victorian involvement with neurasthenia.

The first line of evidence comes from studies of neuroendocrine function. Several lines of inquiry have centred on neuroendocrine aspects of CFS. First, there is the relationship between mood disorder, with its well documented abnormalities in neuroendocrine function. Second, some have pointed out the similarities between CFS and glucocorticoid deficiency. Several fatigue (including post-exertional fatigue), myalgia, arthralgia, mood and sleep disturbances occur in both. Abnormalities of the hypothalamic-pituitary adrenal axis (HPA) have recently been described in a series of 30 patients with CFS compared to 72 normal controls (Demitrack et al., 1991). The patients had lower urinary excretion rates of free cortisol and reduced evening plasma cortisol concentrates in conjunction with an elevated plasma adrenocorticotrophin releasing hormone (ACTH). The adrenal cortex was hypersensitive to low doses of ACTH, with a blunted ceiling response. ACTH responses to corticotrophin releasing hormone (CRH) were attenuated, despite low ambient cortisol levels (which therefore cannot be exerting an inhibitory feedback effect). The impaired HPA function cannot be due to primary adrenal insufficiency because ACTH responsiveness is preserved, and pituitary insufficiency is unlikely because of the elevated ACTH concentrations: the findings are thus most compatible with impaired function at the level of the hypothalamus, which is compromising CRH synthesis/secretion. Demitrack and colleagues excluded adrenal dysfunction in their subjects, although a small study from our group still leaves this possibility open (Bearn et al., 1995). Meanwhile, in the related condition of fibromyalgia, Crofford and colleagues also reported low 24 hour urinary cortisol, but a different pattern of response to CRH challenge (Crofford et al., 1994).

It can thus be argued that in a subgroup of CFS (those without evidence of major depression) a pattern can be discerned of an underactive HPA system, which should be contrasted with the overactive pattern classic of severe depression. Indeed, one can speculate that CFS and depression lie along a continuum of serotonin activity in the central nervous system, reflected in differing patterns of HPA activity, and finally in differing patterns of exhaustion versus agitation, insomnia versus hypersomnia and so on (Bearn and Wessely, 1994). Furthermore, as a recent study was able to reproduce the neuroendocrine profile of CFS in a group of healthy night-shift workers, the possibility that such changes are the consequences, and not the causes, of the pattern of symptoms found in CFS remains very much open (Lesse et al., 1996).

Another role for neuroendocrine studies is to gain information on central neurotransmitter function – the 'window on the brain' paradigm. Studies using agents that act at the 5HT receptor have shown that 5HT neurotransmission is increased relative to not only normal, but also depressed controls (Bakheit et al., 1992). Cleare and colleagues measured the prolactin response to D-fenfluramine, a selective 5HT releasing agent. The prolactin response was highest in the CFS patients, lowest in the depressed subjects (as expected), and intermediate in the controls (Cleare et al., 1995). The tentative conclusion is that those CFS patients without concurrent depression show evidence of reduced HPA axis activity and increased 5HT function, the mirror image of major depression. This might either explain (or be the result of) the clinical observation that CFS is characterized by hypersomnia and preserved appetite, in contrast to classic major depression.

Perhaps the most attractive model of CFS yet proposed is that by Demitrack and colleagues, who have integrated the findings of hypocortisolaemia, hypersomnia and immune activation in an attractive, albeit preliminary, disease model (Demitrack and Greden, 1991). For them, CFS represents the 'occurrence of final common biological pathology that may be precipitated by a variety of infectious or non-infectious pathophysiological antecedents' (Demitrack and Greden, 1991). It is now plausible to argue that this pathway involves at some stage a disturbance of neuroendocrine and neurotransmitter function, but the direction of causality remains unknown.

The next piece in the jigsaw is provided by neuropsychological studies. To date there have been at least 15 of varying degrees of methodological sophistication. By now the reader will not be surprised by the next statement – results and confusing and conflicting. There is no doubt that patients experience substantial complaints of cognitive dysfunction (clinical evidence that by itself makes a neuro-muscular origin to symptoms unlikely). Pierre Janet recognized the same when he wrote that 'Tiredness and a horrible sense of fatigue is caused in psychasthenics by the least series of physical or psychological effort ... fatigue rapidly affects sensations and perceptions, intellect and movement' (Janet, 1919). Modern neuropsychological testing has revealed few further insights beyond his observations (Moss-Morris et al., 1996; Wearden and Appleby, 1996).

A few cautions are relevant. First, neuropsychological tests are not as objective as their advocates often suggest, and are critically dependent upon such variables as co-operation and expectation. Second, despite the occasional claim to the contrary, they do not provide any evidence of a specific aetiology – they are functional in the true meaning of the word. Third, the confounding effects of depression and anxiety, with their known effects on cognitive function, must also be addressed.

The most meticulous studies have provided the least impressive results. Jordan Grafman and his colleagues at National Institute of Health used an exhaustive two-day test procedure (Grafman et al., 1993). They reported a consistent, and strong, correlation between the severity of mood disturbance and the number and severity of memory complaints. The same authors then administered a variety of neuropsychological tests over two days to a subgroup of 20 patients. General intellectual performance was normal. Measures of reaction time, other timed tasks, planning, problem solving, digit span and extensive tests of semantic and verbal memory were normal. Specific deficits were noted only on tests of complex visual reproduction. Unusually, patients performed worse in cued situations, also noted elsewhere. Graftman and colleagues concluded that neuropsychological deficits in CFS are relatively modest in contrast to the severity of the subject's complaints (Grafman et al., 1993; see also Ray et al., 1993). Deluca and colleagues failed to find any evidence of memory impairment, but did report problems in selective attention (Deluca et al., 1995). Several groups have noted correlations between performance and ratings of psychopathology, and some have failed to distinguish between depression and CFS (e.g. Schmaling et al., 1994). However, other well-designed studies find an overlap between neuropsychological performance and psychopathology, but not one which accounts for all the features of cognitive dysfunction (McDonald et al., 1993; Deluca et al., 1995).

What seems to be emerging is a picture of a mismatch between the subject's own perception of cognitive disturbance, and the level of actual decrements in performance determined on testing (Schmaling et al., 1994). Although selective attention may be impaired (Joyce et al., 1996), formal deficits in memory appear increasingly unlikely. The complaints of poor memory and concentration are most likely to be related to the same processes observed in mood disorder, but the problems of selective attention are less likely to be the result of depression. CFS may be associated with a disorder of effortful cognition, rather than any actual deficits in recall, just as it is associated with an increased sense of motor effort, rather than any objective deficits in neuromuscular function.

Perhaps the best publicized, but the least researched, area is that of neuroimaging. Studies using magnetic resonance techniques have concentrated on the appearance of punctate foci of high signal intensity (so called 'unexplained bright objects' (UBOs)). These have either been substantially increased, moderately increased or not increased at all compared to controls (Buchwald et al., 1992; Natelson et al., 1994; Cope et al., 1995).

It is also too early to judge the results of functional neuroimaging studies. There are a few published studies using functional neuro-imaging techniques such as single photon emission tomography (SPET) in CFS (Ichise et al., 1992; Schwartz et al., 1994; Mountz et al., 1995; Costa et al., 1995; Patterson et al., 1995; Fischler et al., 1996b). Some studies to date have used inconsistent case definitions, resting scans, poor-resolution SPET scanners and semi-quantitative methods to detect changes in regional cerebral blood flow (RCBF) (Cope and David, 1996). In one study (Schwartz et al., 1994) a substantially increased number of defects was seen in CFS subjects compared to normal controls. However, there was no difference in the number or situation of defects between CFS and depressed controls, all being confined to the frontal and temporal lobes. There were, however, differences in the patterns of radionucleotide uptake between depression and CFS. The authors note that the pathophysio-logical basis of these abnormalities cannot be determined by imaging (just as evidence of neuropsychological dysfunction does not indicate the cause of that dysfunction). On the basis of a comparison with AIDS patients, the authors suggest that CFS is associated with a chronic viral encephalitis, although this seems a premature claim. The most widely publicized study found that brainstem perfusion was significantly reduced in CFS subjects compared to controls, with depressed patients showing intermediate values (Costa et al., 1995). However, other groups do not report brainstem perfusion values because of the technical difficulties of imaging this small structure. Any interpretation of this finding must await its independent repli-cation (Cope and David, 1996). It is, however, most unlikely that this will be a test for ME, as so frequently claimed by the media.

Even in such a small literature, variations in results are already observable, and it is at present impossible to come to any firm con-clusions – 'findings are neither sufficiently sensitive nor specific to allow its use as a diagnostic tool, although it may have a role in understanding the pathophysiology of the disease (Patterson et al., 1995).

In summary, the neurobiological basis of CFS is ill understood, but is a valid and exciting line of inquiry. The search for such abnor-malities is not, of course, incompatible with the previously reviewed evidence of high rates of psychiatric disorder. The frequent news-paper headlines, such as 'Brainwaves suggest ME is physical illness, not a psychiatric condition', merely reflect the common ignorance of modern psychiatry (Mihill, 1992).

PROGNOSIS

The prognosis for chronic fatigue, even in primary care, is unsatisfactory. At one-year follow-up, only a third of fatigued patients seen in American ambulatory care (something which probably lies half way between UK primary and specialist care) had improved (Kroenke et al., 1988).

The prognosis for patients with the label of ME who reach specialist care is particularly worrying. Behan and Behan (1988), who have extensive experience of CFS in this country, wrote that 'most cases do not improve, give up their work and become permanent invalids, incapacitated by excessive fatigue and myalgia'. Sixty percent of those seen in a Seattle clinic were the same or worse two years later (Clark et al., 1995). Only 18% of those referred to a Belfast clinic improved (Hinds and McCluskey, 1993), and only 13% of those seen in an infectious disease clinic in Oxford considered themselves fully recovered two years later, although more had improved (Sharpe et al., 1992). Only 6% of subjects who had taken part in treatment studies in Australia had fully recovered at three years (Wilson et al., 1994a).

In the Oxford study, poor prognosis was independently associated with a belief in a viral cause for illness, membership of a self-help organization, current emotional disorder and alcohol avoidance. Particular attention must be given to a follow-up study performed by the Sydney group, who have been consistent and effective advocates of an immunological basis for CFS. In their follow-up study the strongest association of poor outcome in CFS was again the strength of belief in an exclusively physical cause for symptoms (Wilson et al., 1994a). Immunological variables played no role. No laboratory marker has been shown to play any role in predicting outcome, in contrast to the presence of psychiatric disorder, or the strength of the belief in a solely physical cause to symptoms (Sharpe et al., 1992; Wilson et al., 1994; Clarke et al., 1995; Vercoulen et al., 1996b).

We can now start to see a thread linking the different perspectives seen from primary and specialist care. Cases of chronic fatigue and the associated symptoms of CFS are by no means unusual in primary care. Most will be associated with psychological disorders.

Exhaustion after viral infections such as the Epstein–Barr virus is also common, and is probably not psychosocially determined. Most sufferers from either condition probably do not consider themselves to have ME, and there is no particular social class distribution.

On the other hand, patients with long illness histories, a label of ME and a strong conviction of physical illness may represent a different population. There remains a strong association with psychological disorder, and little evidence of a link with viral persistence. Higher social classes are over-represented. The prognosis seems poor.

ASSESSMENT

The differential diagnosis of chronic fatigue reads like a joint edition of the Oxford Textbooks of Medicine and Psychiatry. The psychiatric differential diagnosis has already been reviewed. Possible medical conditions that might be confused with CFS include the following:

- malignancy;
- neurological disorder, such as myasthenia, multiple sclerosis;
- thyroid disease;
- electrolyte imbalance (Addison's hypercalcaemia);
- chronic infection (tuberculosis, HIV, Lyme, giardiasis);
- autoimmune disease (rheumatoid, SLE);
- sleep apnoea.

In practice the position is more simple. In nearly all cases the diagnosis becomes clear after history, examination and simple investigations. Overall research suggests that in anyone with fatigue lasting more than six months, physical investigation is largely unhelpful (Kroenke et al., 1988; Valdini et al., 1989; Lane et al., 1990; Ridsdale et al., 1993). Although changes have been noted in various other parameters, such as antinuclear factor, immune complexes, cholesterol, immunoglobulin subsets and so on, these are encountered only in a minority, and are rarely substantial. Their significance is for researchers rather than clinicians (Bates et al., 1995). The following simple battery of tests remains a sensible compromise between under- and over-investigation:

- full blood count;
- ESR;

- liver function tests;
- urea and electrolytes:
- thyroid function tests;
- urine for protein, sugar.

The following tests are not routine, but may be indicated by the history:

- EBV serology;
- chest X-ray
- rheumatoid factor and ANF;
- Lyme disease serology;
- brucellosis titres;
- ACh antibody (for myasthenia);
- Q fever titres;
- CMV and toxoplasmosis titres;
- HIV.

Abnormalities on these tests need to be followed up as appropriate. *Any neurological sign* is not compatible with a diagnosis of CFS, and must be appropriately investigated.

The following tests are of *no clinical value* in the diagnosis of CFS, and are useful only for research, or to exclude alternative diagnoses (such as an MRI for multiple sclerosis):

- enterovirus tests, including IgG, IgM, VP-1;
- lymphocyte subsets;
- natural killer cell assays;
- CT, MRI or SPECT scans.

MANAGEMENT

Many doctors are understandably bewildered by the controversy surrounding CFS. There are those who claim, with passion, that it is an organic condition due to a virus for which there is regrettably no treatment. For others it is a form of depression, treated by antidepressants, whilst some state it doesn't exist at all. All too few of those who pronounce on the subject take a genuinely multifactorial approach, even those who proclaim themselves to be 'holistic'.

CFS patients have an illness. What, if any, disease underlies that illness remains to be seen. At present management is focused on the illness, and not any putative underlying disease. Perhaps this will change, and a future generation will obtain convincing evidence of an underlying disease process, and establish the means to reverse it. Until then, the mainstay of treatment for CFS revolves around management and rehabilitation. In this section I will outline a pragmatic approach to rehabilitation that is derived from the vast body of literature in chronic pain, since chronic fatigue and chronic pain share many similarities (Blakely et al., 1991). Although pharmacological interventions have an important role, it is unrealistic to expect that any 'magic bullet' will reverse what can be months, or even years, of disability. Not everyone agrees – a recent book on CFS devoted only six out of 75 chapters to treatment, all of which were concerned with agents acting on the immune system.

In our unit we have developed treatment approaches based on cognitive–behavioural principles (Figure 2.1) (Wessely et al., 1991; Wessely, 1996; Sharpe, 1996). Before describing this pragmatic approach, it is necessary to review the evidence and thinking underlying the model. At the heart is the message that whatever triggers CFS may not perpetuate it. For example, an ordinary viral infection may *precipitate* fatigue which, for the majority of the population, is resolved when a normal recovery is made. However, on rare occasions the presence of *perpetuating* factors (such as psychosocial stressors, rapid deconditioning, failure to rest adequately or concurrent depression) may delay or impede recovery. Fatigue then becomes chronic, persisting long after the departure of the original trigger and maintained by new variables. Some of these variables are discussed in more detail below.

1. *The effects of inactivity:* all of us know that rest is appropriate in the initial stages of a viral infection, and may indeed have a protective function. However, the prolonged rest and extreme inactivity which is common in CFS (reinforced by the advice given to sufferers) is less helpful. Rest relieves fatigue in the short term, but in the longer term it reduces activity tolerance, and has profound effects on cardiovascular and neuromuscular function, as well as thermoregulation (Sharpe and Bass, 1992). Inactivity not only increases the sensation of fatigue on exertion, but also reduces the desire to undertake activity (Zorbas and Matveyev, 1986). With the passage of time, more symptoms, and greater fatigue will continue to occur at progressively lower levels of exertion. Inactivity therefore sustains symptoms, and increases sensitivity to them.

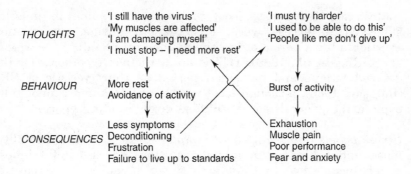

Figure 2.1 A cognitive–behavioural model for the perpetuation of disability in chronic fatigue syndrome (from Surawy et al., 1995).

2. *Inconsistent activity:* not every CFS sufferer is profoundly inactive – many strive to keep going, and to this end adopt a 'boom and bust' pattern, as do fibromyalgia patients (Nielson et al., 1992). Typically, excessive or prolonged rest is followed by a burst of activity, which, compared to the preceding level of inactivity, is often 'too much, too soon'. This pattern may also be reinforced by the sense of frustration often encountered in sufferers, and perhaps also by pre-existing personality and lifestyle factors such as perfectionism and high level of physical fitness. My impression, unsupported by any data, that many patients have personalities characterized by high internal standards, devotion to duty and perfectionism, make it hard for them to accept anything less than '100%'. Such expectations are frequently impossible to achieve in the setting of CFS and in the early stages of treatment, and are experienced by many patients as failure. In practice many patients have attempted sudden increases in activity, and find that they culminate in exhaustion, for which the inevitable response is further rest. This 'stop-start' pattern means that while extremes of disability are often avoided, sufferers are unable to build up a sustained level of recovery. This pattern often leads to the characteristic complaint of CFS sufferers, that any activity must be 'paid for' later by further pain and fatigue. Delayed fatigue and myalgia are well recognized physiological phenomena that occur between 24 and 48 hours after any exertion in excess of a person's current (and not previous) fitness (anonymous, 1987). The mechanism is due to the appearance of eccentric muscle

contractions leading to local muscle microtrauma in muscles subjected to excess work, occurring in anyone undertaking exertion after a period of inactivity (Jones et al., 1986; Newham, 1988; Klug et al., 1989). This is an attractive hypothesis for the delayed fatigue and myalgia reported as characteristic of CFS (Ramsay, 1986), although local muscle microtrauma cannot fully explain the generalized and diffuse myalgia often reported.

3. *Illness beliefs and fears about symptoms* can influence disability, mood and behaviour in any illness. In CFS, unhelpful illness beliefs include fear that any activity which causes an increase in fatigue is damaging or impossible; that 'doing too much' causes permanent muscle damage; and that CFS is irreversible or untreatable. Such catastrophic beliefs are both common in CFS patients, and are related to disability (Petrie et al., 1995). In the initial stages of CFS, such beliefs may fuel avoidance of activity, and are often powerfully reinforced by each successive aversive experience of activity-related fatigue, leading to increasing restrictions. Using avoidant strategies to cope with chronic fatigue was associated with worse disability (Antoni et al., 1994; Ray et al., 1995). A Dutch study reported a relationship between attributing fatigue to a physical cause and lack of physical activity, and between lack of physical activity and severity of fatigue, implying that in CFS it is the specific illness beliefs that determine the pattern of behavioural avoidance, and contribute to the experience of fatigue. Such a pattern was not found in controls with multiple sclerosis (Vercoulen et al., 1996a).

4. *Symptom focusing:* increased symptom focusing is also noted in CFS (Ray et al., 1995; Vercoulen et al., 1996a). Concern about the meaning and significance of symptoms (which are often interpreted as 'warning signals') is heightened by the unpredictable nature of CFS. Increased concern leads to heightened awareness, selective attention and 'body watching', which can then intensify both the experience and perceived frequency of symptoms, thereby confirming illness beliefs and reinforcing illness behaviour.

5. *Emotional consequences:* for some CFS patients, depression may be the primary cause of ill health, but for others, depression may arise during the illness, together with anxiety, frustration and simple boredom. Of whatever cause, depression and anxiety

are strongly associated with fatigue and muscle pain, impaired memory and concentration, and reduced activity. It has also been suggested that the aversive and apparently uncontrollable symptoms of fatigue and myalgia engender a state of 'learned helplessness' which can trigger or exacerbate mood disorder.

In summary, we and others have suggested that unitary models of CFS are an inadequate reflection of clinical reality, and instead that CFS may be better understood (and hence treated) by focusing on possible perpetuating factors, and the many ways in which they interact in self perpetuating vicious circles of fatigue, behaviour, beliefs and disability (Wessely et al., 1991; Sharpe and Chalder, 1994; Surawy et al., 1995).

How might treatment proceed in practice? The process of excluding other causes for chronic fatigue rarely takes much time. In contrast, engaging the sufferer in treatment can be a time-consuming process, but no part of the treatment process is as crucial. Any active intervention, be it graded activity, cognitive therapy or antidepressants, may be viewed with trepidation: either as a rigid exercise programme which will worsen the sufferer's condition, or, conversely, as little more than a thinly veiled way of telling them the problem is 'psychological' (and therefore not 'real') after all. Most will have had other, unsatisfactory encounters with health care practitioners, and therefore it is important that they feel listened to and taken seriously. The doctor should be explicit in conveying belief in the reality of both physical symptoms and psychological distress. The patients' own views on the nature of their illness and its management should be sought and discussed. Becoming enmeshed in a dichotomous 'psychological' versus 'physical' debate is to be avoided. The aim of management is not to replace one set of organic attributions with another set of psychological explanations. Not only would such explanations be unlikely to foster an effective therapeutic alliance, but also they would be as inaccurate as solely biological models. Instead, the doctor should open the discussion to a wider range of possibilities, and help the patient understand the multiple factors that contribute to ill health. It is vital to steer the patient towards accepting responsibility for getting well, but without conveying any sense of guilt for why the patient either became ill in the first place, or alternatively has not recovered so far.

The principal intention of treatment is to reduce functional disability, and hence increase activity. All treatments have the same intention, but in conventional approaches that is assumed to occur as the consequence of symptom relief. However, we have argued that in CFS, as in chronic pain, it is necessary to increase activity first, without waiting for symptoms to fully alleviate, since it is lack of activity that perpetuates the symptoms. Treatment enables increases in activity to be undertaken by allowing patients to reconsider any beliefs that might impede such progress, and then providing a safe framework for the activity increase to occur.

Following engagement, the next step is to offer a treatment rationale. Two explanations are shared with the patient (Wessely et al., 1991):

(a) the conventional view – 'you have a chronic illness in which viral persistence in your muscles is the cause of your symptoms. You must avoid all forms of physical and mental activity in order to prevent further damage. Any increase in symptoms must lead to further rest'.
(b) the alternative view – 'An acute infection has forced you to become inactive, and perhaps also triggered certain biochemical changes in your brain. As a result you experienced intense fatigue, ceased activity, and inevitably became unfit. You now experience symptoms whenever you attempt any activity, but, because of the fear of causing symptoms or a relapse, you never pursue these activities long enough to allow the symptoms to subside. These symptoms are real, but may not reflect continuing infection'.

Planning activity and choosing behavioural targets is the next step. Simply prescribing exercise can be counterproductive, and, if carried out to excess, may well cause precisely the type of myalgic symptoms that must be avoided. Targets may involve virtually no exercise at all – such as getting out of bed for a certain length of time, or going to the toilet unaided. The initial level of activity must be set sufficiently low to be attainable. It is often important to actually restrict activity, since many patients have become caught in a cycle of excessive rest followed by excessive activity on the few 'good days' that result – the 'boom and bust' pattern already mentioned.

As important as activity is the planning of rest. Immediate reductions in the amount of rest taken are rarely advised in the early stages. Instead, after a careful functional assessment, usually involving the keeping of a diary, the current pattern of rest is determined. This is averaged over a period of time – a week, for example, and the daily requirement determined. This is then built into the timetable. As with activity, the consequence is to make rest predetermined, and not in response to symptoms. The patient can be reassured that as the amount of rest remains the same, no physiological consequences will result. Instead, the goal of the early stages of treatment is to combat the experience of unpredictability of symptoms.

It is important to note that increasing activity can cause a temporary increase in symptoms, both by physiological mechanisms outlined above, and by understandable anxiety when carrying out a programme which others have said may be harmful, and which at first sight is contrary to previous experience. It is essential to emphasize that *gradual* increase in activity is not associated with harm, and that habituation will occur in time. One can anticipate that a gradually increased level of activity over several weeks causes a transient (inactivity associated), rather than a persistent, increase in muscle fatigue and pain (Sharpe and Chalder, 1994). The aim of treatment is to *avoid the handicapping stimulus-driven cycle* of CFS, in which symptoms are always a signal to rest, and *replace previous sensitization by tolerance*.

The key points in such treatment are:

- first stabilize activity and rest;
- make rest predictable by timetable, and not according to symptoms;
- develop a programme of predictable and regular activity;
- choose goals that are currently avoided, but are enjoyable;
- choose targets, not distances;
- warn about temporary symptom exacerbation;
- choose targets in the light of current fitness and activity levels, not past fitness or activity;
- prevent excess activity on 'good' days;
- prevent complete inactivity on 'bad' days;
- expect improvements to take weeks, not days;
- always encourage rehabilitation/management, and not 'cure'.

Difficulties in treatment are:

1. *From the patient*
   - untreated depression/anxiety/phobic disorders;
   - intense physical attributions;
   - doesn't accept treatment rationale.
2. *From the doctor*
   - targets too ambitious;
   - hostile or punitive attitudes;

- collusion between doctor and patient;
- premature introduction of fixed benefits/medical retirement.
3. *From others*
    - conflicting advice from others;
    - unresolved family factors;
    - unresolved work factors.

What explanation can be given to the patient – and what can the patient tell their own family and friends? This is an important point, since any improvement that might result from an intervention that is neither virologically nor immunologically based can be interpreted by the unsympathetic as proof that the problem was 'all in the mind' after all. One might compare the current situation with that of a road traffic accident victim, in which chasing the causative agent brings little or no benefit, but sustained attention to rehabilitation is the key to improvement. Whatever strategy is chosen, the principle behind therapy is to return to the patient the responsibility for their progress and treatment without conveying any guilt as to why they became ill in the first place.

Does it Work?

Early evidence for the efficacy of activity management programmes and/or cognitive behaviour therapy (CBT) came from the fibromyalgia literature, viewed by many as either synonymous, or overlapping with, CFS. Controlled trials of increased activity in fibromyalgia have shown that exercise retraining is beneficial on overall symptom scores, sleep and pain (Bennett, 1989; McCain et al., 1988; Klug et al., 1989), and this is not simply due to increased physical fitness. In fibromyalgia, unlike CFS, there seems to be no dissenting voice from the view that patients should be encouraged to cautiously interrupt the 'cycle of inactivity, fatigue, pain and inactivity' (Bennett, 1989), or that 'the safest and most effective approach seems to be the judicious use of amitriptyline, analgesic agents, an exercise program, and reassurance that fibromyalgia is not a crippling rheumatic disease or a degenerative neurologic illness' (Dinerman and Steere, 1992). There is now considerable enthusiasm for cognitive behavioural treatments in fibromyalgia, and although we await the definitive studies, early studies of varying methodological sophistication are encouraging (Nielsen et al., 1992; Goldenberg et al., 1994).

Most clinicians are now using similar approaches for the management of CFS, usually in a pragmatic commonsense fashion, based on a dislike of the therapeutic nihilism that can be associated with the diagnosis. Numerous papers include statements such as 'we have found that a regimented program of daily, increasingly vigorous exercise is effective in reintroducing dysfunctional patients to a more functional lifestyle' (Kyle and DeShazo, 1992). Graded exercise programmes are recommended for a variety of practical reasons (McCully et al., 1996). Fears that increased activity would cause muscle damage and/or 'relapse' have not been justified (Sisto et al., 1996). Two randomized controlled trials have been performed. In one the results were very encouraging (Fulcher et al., 1994), whilst in the other treatment completers had a good outcome, but problems were encoutered with compliance/acceptability (Wearden et al., submitted).

It is probable that, although theoretically graded exercise alone should be beneficial, and that, provided increases in activity are chosen with care and in the light of current fitness and capability, adverse effects should be minimal, a combination of the patient's previous experience ('I have tried that already, and it didn't work'), and the exhortations to rest that are so prevalent in the popular literature, simply assigning patients to a graded exercise programme is a 'high risk' strategy in terms of compliance. More sophisticated approaches may be needed. This can be straightforward – an example being Denman's use of a graded exercise programme with psychological counselling (Denman, 1990), or a more formal combined rehabilitation approach such as CBT outlined in the previous section.

The theoretical basis of CBT seems strong, but what is the practical evidence? In the first uncontrolled evaluation of CBT, Butler et al. (1991) treated 50 patients seen at the National Hospital for Neurology with severe, unexplained fatigue – all of whom would fulfil current criteria for CFS and were typical of the severe end of the CFS spectrum encountered in hospital care. Nearly all thought they had 'ME' and over half were members of a self-help group. Treatment was non-randomized and open. In addition to CBT, those fulfilling criteria for major depression were treated with dothiepin (Butler et al., 1991).

The principal obstacle was refusal, associated with the strength of physical attributions, and little else. However, of those who accepted, the results were encouraging: 23 (70%) of those starting therapy, described themselves as better, with changes maintained at three months. Using strict criteria, nine patients were symptom free at the end of treatment, and many were able to resume employment after prolonged absence. Treatment response was not influenced by duration of symptoms, but was associated with the strength of attribution of symptoms to an exclusively physical cause.

At four years, those who had responded to treatment were generally maintaining the gains. On the other hand, those who had refused treatment remained substantially impaired. There was also little evidence of spontaneous recovery in those who had done poorly in the treatment programme (Bonner et al., 1994). A second uncontrolled study was also encouraging (Cox and Findley, 1994b).

Two randomized controlled trials of CBT have been completed in the UK. One, in Oxford, in which the active treatment, following local tradition, has a distinctly cognitive flavour, used a waiting list/ 'usual treatment' control group. Active treatment placed particular emphasis on helping patients reappraise their illness beliefs, as well as increasing activity. Active treatment was effective, with considerable reductions in fatigue and disability (Sharpe et al., 1996). The treated group continued to improve during follow-up. A second trial took place at King's College Hospital. This time CBT had a more behavioural flavour, again in keeping with local tradition. Twelve sessions of CBT were compared to 12 sessions of relaxation therapy, as a control for the effects of therapist time, attention and encouragement. CBT was associated with significant improvements in fatigue and disability, and again this improvement became most apparent at the end of six month follow-up (Deale et al., 1996, in press).

These results should be contrasted with two negative studies. In the first, randomized controlled trial of CBT, six sessions of active treatment were no better than simple clinic attendance and reassurance (Lloyd et al., 1993). In the second, non-randomized trial, benefits were seen in measures of depression, but not fatigue or disability (Friedberg and Krupp, 1994). Several reasons exist for the failure of these interventions (Chalder et al., 1995). In the Australian study it is unclear precisely what, if any, behavioural intervention occurred, and there was no attempt to alter fundamental illness beliefs. The treatment rationale may have been compromised by the presence of an immunological trial involving regular injections of active or placebo immunotherapy. The rationale used for CBT in Oxford and London is based on the model that, although immune and/or infective factors may have been responsible for illness onset, other factors are responsible for symptom perpetuation. It would be hard to reconcile the two approaches being tested. The strong correlation between the patients' belief (albeit erroneous) at the end of the trial that they had received active immunotherapy and symptomatic improvement, suggests that the patient group found it similarly hard. The authors themselves wonder if the number of sessions was adequate (Wilson et al., 1994b). Finally, 'standard medical care', the comparison group, was itself reasonably effective.

In the second study (Friedberg and Krupp, 1994) the treatment model was very much based on enabling the patients to accept the limitations of illness without emotional distress, and thus neither challenged illness beliefs nor attempted any behavioural activation. The differences between the successful and unsuccessful studies relate to the different models of illness used – those that involved some form of gradual return to activity combined with some form of cognitive reattribution were successful, whilst those that did not offer adequate alternative explanations for symptom maintenance, or address illness and symptom beliefs, were less successful (Moss-Morris, 1996).

Cognitive behaviour therapy treatments have attracted much attention, probably reflecting the general popularity of such approaches in psychiatry overall, and their high research profile. A recent review on behalf of the NHS Research and Development Programme recommended CBT for the outpatient management of CFS (Best, 1996). A case series also reported promising results using CBT to manage extremely disabled patients, confined to bed or wheelchair, as hospital inpatients (Chalder et al., 1996). However, other approaches, especially family and systems models, will no doubt soon receive attention. In particular the family/systems model has great attraction in the management of the increasing numbers of children presenting with CFS (see below).

Pharmacological Approaches to CFS

There is no single established pharmacological management for CFS. The greatest professional interest is in antidepressant therapy. The rationale for its use in chronic fatigue is considerable (Wilson et al., 1994b), but at present most controlled studies are in the field of fibromyalgia (e.g. Carrette et al., 1986; Goldenberg et al., 1986). A systematic review in preparation will conclude that antidepressants are effective in the short-term management of pain and fatigue, but evidence for their long-term efficacy is still lacking.

In CFS the evidence has until recently come only from uncontrolled or open studies (Lynch et al., 1991; Goodnick and Sandoval, 1993), and a single case study (Gracious and Wisner, 1991). Current work on possible impairment in serotonergic pathways is used to justify the use of serotonin re-uptake inhibitors (SSRI) (Lane, 1994), and early studies were encouraging (Behan et al., 1994; Behan and Hannifah, 1995). It is therefore surprising that the first randomized controlled trial of an SSRI (fluoxetine) should have been resoundingly negative (Vercoulen et al., 1996c), although some indication of this result was given by a negative study of the same drug in fibromyalgia (Wolfe et al., 1994). The Dutch study also showed that fluoxetine was ineffective in CFS with comorbid depression, which remains a counter-intuitive finding (Vercoulen et al., 1996c). A further three randomized controlled trials of SSRIs are now underway in the United Kingdom and Australia which might shed further light.

Turning to the older antidepressants, there are some clinical reasons for avoiding drugs with a high sedative or anticholinergic profile (Wilson et al., 1994b), although we experienced few difficulties using dothiepin combined with CBT (Butler et al., 1991). Given the overlap between the symptoms of CFS and those of atypical depression, and the efficacy of monoamine oxidase inhibitors (MAOIs) in the latter (Liebowitz et al., 1988), a good case can also be made for trying them, confirmed by a small controlled trial (Natelson et al., 1996). A very preliminary observation also suggests some rationale for using moclobemide, a novel reversible MAOI agent (Wilson et al., 1994b).

Irrespective of the negative finding of the Dutch group using fluoxetine, antidepressants must still remain indicated for mood disorder, regardless of its origins. A more interesting question is the role of antidepressants in those without obvious evidence of affective disorder. A multicentre trial now underway in the United Kingdom using sertraline is currently addressing this question. Another question is the role of antidepressants in sleep disorder, an extremely common association of CFS, and thought by some to be of aetiological significance (Morriss et al., 1993). In conclusion, it is impossible at the moment to give any firm guidelines on the use and choice of antidepressants in CFS.

Moving away from antidepressants, a number of so-called specific treatments have been proposed to deal with the presumed underlying 'cause' of the abnormal fatigability. For example, given that recent formulations of CFS involve abnormal immunity, it was inevitable that immunoglobulins would be tried. One study found in their favour, and one against. Technical aspects of the study, and the problems of side-effects and cost had led the editorialists to conclude that immunoglobulin therapy is unjustified in CFS (Straus, 1990; anonymous, 1991). Less specific treatments are at present

extremely popular, in particular evening primrose oil and magnesium, both found efficacious in well-publicized clinical trials.
However, there is no convincing rationale for their use, and other
studies have been less favourable (McCluskey, 1993).

Perhaps the most common treatment modality used by CFS
patients are those encountered in the world of alternative medicine
(Dowson, 1993). It is the exceptional patient seeking treatment who
has not tried some combinations of vitamins, diets, nutritional
supplements and the like. There are several reasons. First, as in
any chronic disease, regression to the mean, also known as the
physician's friend, ensures that some will benefit. Second, these
approaches are in keeping with the contemporary *zeitgeist* surrounding CFS. Most self-help books effortlessly promote illness
models involving external environmental agents (allergy, amalgam,
candida, electromagnetic radiation, pollution, poor diet, viruses, and
so on) that owe more to 'green' ideas of health than any observable
evidence. In turn, these can lead to environmental and nutritional
interventions that probably owe their success to the congruence of
the illness model of patient and therapist. Third, all of these
approaches explicitly are based on an organic model of illness
(vitamin deficiency, virus, allergy and so on), in which the patient
avoids any stigma, however ill deserved, for his or her predicament.

Most of these approaches have not been systematically evaluated
(Dowson, 1993), whilst the results of those that have are not encouraging (Kaslow et al., 1989; Morris and Stare, 1993; Martin et al.,
1994).

I have already drawn attention to the historical continuities that
exist linking the various fatigue syndromes over the years. This is
equally true of treatment. The popular management of chronic
fatigue and exhaustion remains, as it always has, a balance between
a parody of the contemporary scientific terminology of the day, and
popular social concerns. It remains true that 'The mass media adver-
tising of cures for fatigue over the past century provides a remarkably
consistent theme during the midst of social change. Tonics, potions,
herbs, vitamins and an incredible array of other substances have
been advised as cures for pseudoanergic symptoms' (Karno and
Hoffman, 1974). When neurologist Charles Dana (1904) wrote that
'it is notorious the number of "cures" that exist for the neurasthenic'
he could equally well have been writing about CFS.

Advice on alternative therapies is thus guided more by personal
opinion than systematic evidence. It is our practice not to discourage
any treatment approach that passes a crude cost–benefit test. We

draw the line at treatments that involve drugs that carry an unjustified risk of side-effects, or that encourage further withdrawal from
the environment, which add, rather than relieve, the burden of
illness. In particular we cannot support treatments that involve
reduction in exposure to environmental stimulation (such as those
practised within the clinical ecology movement) which we suspect
are more likely to reinforce behavioural avoidance and sensitization
(Howard and Wessely, 1993).

Non-specific Aspects of Treatment

The key to successful management of CFS lies in what has been
called the 'non-specific' aspects of treatment, and in particular the
doctor–patient relationship. It is therefore appropriate to end the
section on management with some remarks made by Jerome Frank.
During his military service he observed the reaction of soldiers strug-
gling to overcome a mysterious infection (which later proved to be
schistosomiasis). Their clinical symptoms were dominated by fatigue
and weakness. Frank wrote that the most important factors in
recovery were faith in the physician, and the expectancy of recovery.
Overcoming the pathogenic agent was important, but equally important was 'maintaining the patient's confidence in the physician, and
encouraging his expectation of return to useful activity'. He also
noted that in all poorly understood diseases one should be alert to
the appearance of new rumours, which, if unchecked, could have a
detrimental effect on morale. However, 'when uncertainty exists it
is better to admit it' (Frank, 1946).

CHILDREN

The rise of ME in children is perhaps the most alarming addition
to an already overheated atmosphere. No systematic figures exist,
but anyone who works in this area will have become aware of
increasing numbers of children apparently suffering from CFS, and
often accompanied by dramatic morbidity and ill health. Cases now
exist of children confined to bed, or in a darkened room, for months
or, occasionally, years. The long-term consequences on physical,
psychological, social and educational development must be severe.
However, despite the recent upsurge in emotive media reports of
such cases, the professional literature is sparse on the subject. What

little research exists has a strong psychosocial flavour. It has been argued that CFS in children is associated with somatization (Garralda, 1992; Baetz-Greenwalt et al., 1993), depression (Smith et al., 1991; Walford et al., 1993; Giannopoulou and Marriott, 1994; Pelcovitz et al., 1995) or both (Carter et al., 1995).

As in adults, physical and virological investigations are unhelpful, with the exception of tests for infectious mononucleosis (Smith et al., 1991; Carter et al., 1995). No formal treatment studies exist, but the only successful reports in the literature follow the same principles of behavioural activation as used in adults (Feder et al., 1994; Wachsmuth and MacMillan 1991; Rikard-Bell and Waters, 1992; Vereker, 1992; Cox and Findley, 1994a; Sidebotham et al., 1994), often linked with a family therapy approach (Graham, 1990; Pipe and Wait, 1995). Involvement of the parents is, naturally, vital, since treatment failure may happen when the parents remain convinced that the child's illness has a solely organic basis and that active rehabilitation would be harmful (Vereker, 1992). Home tuition is to be discouraged where possible – in the largest series to date, if the children were no longer in school, immediate return to school was encouraged (Feder et al., 1994). Tuition at home should be reserved only for the most severely affected and should be for as short a time as possible, and always in close liaison with the school.

A recent paper reported the outcome of a case series of 50 children with severe chronic fatigue, most of whom recalled a triggering symptomatic infection. A programme beginning with careful assessment and engagement, followed by symptomatic relief, reduction of secondary gain, insisting on regular school attendance and the gradual resumption of activity despite ongoing fatigue resulted in a good outcome in 94% (Feder et al., 1994). Such findings are uncontrolled and based on selected cases, limiting the conclusions that can be drawn, but do contradict statements such as 'the average length of illness in teenagers lasts about four and a half years' (Franklin, 1995). Such sentiments can only add to the burden of affected children and their families.

American paediatricians recently wrote that dangers exist labelling children with a disease which 'has profound implications for their level of functioning in society, especially when the disease is not well defined in childhood and when there are no irrefutable laboratory markers for it' (Carter et al., 1993). Anyone contemplating the diagnosis in a child should be aware of the many difficulties that might follow, and should not do so without reflection (Lask and Dillon, 1990).

CFS, ME, SOCIETY AND THE DOCTOR

Mention has already been made of the passions surrounding the subject. It is indeed appropriate to do so, since this is one of the defining characteristics of the subject. Given the uncertainty and doubt that surrounds the subject, perhaps the most striking characteristic of the CFS literature, and sometimes the CFS patient, is the certainty they have in this grey and difficult area. Allied to that is the frequent assertion that medicine, or to be more specific, doctors, have failed them. Where has this arisen from?

The first, and most obvious, source of passion lies in the stigma that continues to be applied to disorders seen, whether rightly or wrongly, as of psychological or psychiatric origin. It is for this reason that so much emphasis is placed in the popular literature on social and cultural differences between CFS and psychiatric disorders – hence the constant use of stereotyped case histories of professional sufferers whose moral and physical stature is above suspicion. Such cases shed much light on the sociology of illness, and the stigma of psychiatric disorder (see Abbey and Garfinkel (1991) and Wessely (1994) for fuller discussion). Paradoxically such cases also confirm that other popular stereotype 'yuppie flu', so disliked by the sufferers. One supporter of CFS draws attention to the contradiction – it is necessary to steer the public and profession away from the stereotype of the neurotic woman in order to convince them of the legitimacy of the disease, but to do so one must portray sufferers as 'superachievers' (Feiden, 1990).

This must also be seen in the context of the changing nature of the relationship between doctor and patient that has occurred in recent years. Shorter (1992) has argued that the rise of media coverage of medicine, and the growth of the self-help movement, had led to a decline in medical authority (Shorter, 1992). In the popular literature, physicians are frequently described as 'heartless ignoramuses, blinkered in the cul-de-sac of mainline medicine' (Shorter, 1995). The CFS literature is thus another token of the general reaction against medical authority, paternalism and what is seen as the dangers of a narrow scientific approach to illness and healing.

Ironically the same literature is also characterized by a belief in the ultimate success of medical science in unlocking the enigma of CFS. Thus the medical literature is followed in great detail (all the self-help groups produce regular updates of medical research). Papers are analysed less on their merit but on how they help 'the cause' (Aronowitz, 1992). The CFS literature combines both a general suspicion of modern medicine (regarded as impersonal, reliant on tests and distant from the patient) with a belief that medicine possesses the answer, and that a test will be found. The relationship between CFS and the medical profession is paradoxical, since one can see both 'a vigorous attack on medical authority and the desire for its approval' (Aronowitz, 1992).

It is important for the clinician treating CFS to be aware of this popular literature, since it may influence patient attributions of illness, which can in turn be a major determinant of the form and prognosis of illness (see above). For example, most UK newspapers covered the claim that enteroviral persistence was a cause of postviral fatigue syndrome (Yousef et al., 1988), widely interpreted as a 'test for ME'. A newspaper greeted this announcement with the memorable headline 'Virus research doctors finally prove shirkers really are sick' (Hodgkinson, 1987) which tells us more about the sociology of chronic fatigue than any number of scholarly papers. The test provided considerable illness validation, and may have been instrumental in persuading many doctors that 'ME' was a nosological entity. It also assisted sufferers in combatting the threat of being labelled as having a psychiatric disorder – a fear which is by no means unrealistic. One sufferer was refused sickness insurance benefit because his policy excluded depression, of which he had a past history. His claim to be now suffering from ME was rejected, but he was informed that this decision would be changed if a test for ME were to be developed and he were to test positive (Stopp, 1993). The rejoicing that greets each premature claim for a 'test for ME' is thus not surprising. Equally unsurprising is the customary reluctance of patients to consider any psychological factors that might contribute to disability – this reluctance, to which attention has been drawn by too many writers to quote, is one of the most characteristic features of the CFS scene.

By persuading doctors to take sufferers seriously, and treat them with respect, the test did indeed have some benefit, even if it is now recognized as having little relationship to CFS (see above). However, other consequences were more detrimental. My experience, and that of colleagues, is that many sufferers regard such studies, usually inaccurately reported in the media (with the subtext 'ME is a real disease and is not psychiatric after all'), as confirming their belief that the only thing of benefit is rest, with all the adverse effects already outlined.

Related to the absence of laboratory verification of the principal complaint, and having a similar malign effect, is that patients with chronic fatigue do not look sick. A typical sufferer has written that

'My skin is clear and tanned. I don't have a plaster cast on a broken leg ... people say "you look so well"' (Berrett, 1991), and another identified 'looking healthy and strong' as a principal difficulty in dealings with doctors (Finlay, 1986). In chronic fatigue, like chronic pain (Basanzger, 1992), the absence of objective evidence is another barrier to the normal organization of relationships between sufferer and doctor. Both patients and doctors frequently attest to the fact that such relationships can be difficult – patients presenting with the label of ME are now regarded by doctors as likely to be non-compliant, to take up a lot of time, and to pose difficult management problems (Scott et al., 1995; Butler and Rollnick, 1996).

The rise of patient support organizations is also a mixed blessing. Their good intentions are not in question. They are one of most effective examples of a consumer lobby organization to date and provide a supportive service that is valued by their members. However, a controversial finding is that in two studies (Sharpe et al., 1992; Wearden et al., submitted), but not a third (Bonner et al., 1994), membership of a self-help group was associated with either poor prognosis or poor compliance with treatment. One interpretation is that membership is associated with longer illness duration and greater illness severity. Another is that membership of a self-help group is associated with certain beliefs and illness behaviours, such as a firm conviction about the physical nature of symptoms, a rejection of any role for psychological factors, a belief in the efficacy of rest and promotion of avoidance behaviours. One negative aspect to the current consumer activism is that one encounters on the fringes of the organizations a zealous intolerance of other views which neither helps their cause nor that of the sufferers, and antagonizes the medical profession whose support they so fervently desire.

Tony Cleare and myself concluded a recent review (Cleare and Wessely, 1996) with the observation that:

> *Perhaps the most potent cause of poor outcomes and mutual hostility between doctor and patient, which continues to be reported by sufferers in the media, and doctors in private, lies in a failure to understand each other's perspective. Doctors who attempt to dismiss the validity of patients illness experience by such phrases as "there's no such thing as ME", or "all you need is some exercise" contribute to the sense of alienation often felt by patients. On the other hand patients who continue to see any suggestion of psychological factors, such as depression, anxiety or stress, as accusations of malingering, also contribute to the mutual misunderstanding. With our fingers firmly crossed, we hope that both such unhelpful attitudes are on the decline.*

Anyone who watched a recent prime time television show devoted to the subject ('The Rantzen Report') may conclude that such pious hopes were premature.

It is these social issues that give CFS/ME its particular flavour and fascination, and make it so much more than just another cause of chronic ill health. For the psychiatrist, CFS/ME provides an uncomfortable reminder of the status of psychological medicine. CFS also provides a mirror through which to study attitudes to sickness, disease and disability in modern society.

References

Aaron, L.A., Bradley, L.A., Alarcon, G.S. et al. (1996) Psychiatric diagnoses in patients with fibromyalgia are related to health care-seeking behaviour rather than to illness. *Arthritis and Rheumatism* **39**: 436–445.

Abbey, S., Garfinkel, P. (1991) Neurasthenia and chronic fatigue syndrome: the role of culture in the making of a diagnosis. *American Journal of Psychiatry* **148**: 1638–1646.

Anonymous (1987) Aching muscles after exercise. *Lancet* **ii**: 1123–1125.

Anonymous (1991) Chronic fatigue syndrome: false avenues and dead ends. *Lancet* **337**: 331–332.

Antoni, M., Brickman, A., Lutgendorf, S. et al. (1994) Psychosocial correlates of illness burden in chronic fatigue syndrome. *Clinical Infectious Diseases* **18** (Suppl 1), S73–78.

Archard, L., Bowles, N., Behan, P., Bell, E., Doyle, D. (1988) Postviral fatigue syndrome; persistence of enterovirus in muscle and elevated creatine kinase. *Journal of the Royal Society of Medicine* **81**: 326–329.

Aronowitz, R. (1992) From myalgic encephalitis to yuppie flu: a history of chronic fatigue syndrome. In Rosenberg, C., Golden, J. (eds) *Framing Disease* pp. 155–181. New Brunswick: Rutgers University Press.

Baetz-Greenwalt, B., Jensen, U., Lee, A., Saracusa, C., Goldfarb, J. (1993). Chronic fatigue syndrome (CFS) in children and adolescents; a somatoform disorder often complicated by treatable organic disease. *Clinical Infectious Disease* **17**: 571.

Bakheit, A., Behan, P., Dinan, T., Gray, C., O'Keane, V. (1992). Possible upregulation of hypothalamic 5-hydroxytryptamine receptors in patients with postviral fatigue syndrome. *British Medical Journal* **304**: 1010–1012.

Basanzger, I. (1992) Deciphering chronic pain. *Sociology of Health and Illness* **14**: 181–215.

Bates, D., Schmitt, W., Lee, J., Kornish, R., Komaroff, A. (1993) Prevalence of fatigue and chronic fatigue syndrome in a primary care practice. *Archives of Internal Medicine* **153**: 2759–2765.

Bates, D., Buchwald, D., Lee, J. et al. (1995) Clinical laboratory test findings in patients with chronic fatigue syndrome. *Archives of Internal Medicine* **155**: 97–103.

Bearn, J., Wessely, S. (1994) Neurobiological aspects of the chronic fatigue syndrome. *European Journal of Clinical Investigation* **24**: 79–90.

Bearn, J., Allain, T., Coskeran, P. et al. (1995) Neuroendocrine responses to D-fenfluramine and insulin-induced hypoglycaemia in chronic fatigue syndrome. *Biological Psychiatry* **37**: 254–252.

Behan, P., Behan, W. (1988). Postviral fatigue syndrome. *Critical Reviews in Neurobiology* **4**: 157–179.

Behan, P., Hannifah, H. (1995) 5-HT reuptake inhibitors in CFS. *Rivista di Immunologia ed Immunofarmacologia* **15**: 66–69.

Behan, P., Hannifah, B., Doogan, D., Loudon, M. (1994). A pilot study of sertraline for the treatment of chronic fatigue syndrome. *Clinical Infectious Diseases* **18** (Suppl 1), S111.

Bennett, R. (1989) Physical fitness and muscle metabolism in fibromyalgia syndrome: an overview. *Journal of Rheumatology* **16** (Suppl 19), 28–29.

Berelowitz, G., Burgess, A., Thanabalasingham, T., Murray-Lyon, I., Wright, D. (1995) Post-hepatitis syndrome revisited. *Journal of Viral Hepatitis* **2**: 133–138.

Berrett, J. (1991) Condemned to live a lonely life. *Guardian*, 6 July.

Best, L. (1996) *Cognitive Behavioural Therapy in the Treatment of Chronic Fatigue Syndrome.* Southampton: Wessex Institute of Public Health Medicine.

Blakely, A., Howard, R., Sosich, R. et al. (1991) Psychological symptoms, personality and ways of coping in chronic fatigue syndrome. *Psychological Medicine* **21**: 347–362.

Bonner, D., Butler, S., Chalder, T., Ron, M., Wessely, S. (1994). A follow up study of chronic fatigue syndrome. *Journal of Neurology Neurosurgery and Psychiatry* **57**: 617–621.

Bou-Holaigah, I., Rowe, P., Kan, J., Calkins, H. (1995) The relationship between neurally mediated hypotension and the chronic fatigue syndrome. *Journal of the American Medical Association* **274**: 961–967.

Bruce-Jones, W., White, P., Thomas, J., Clare, A. (1994). The effect of social disadvantage on the fatigue syndrome, psychiatric disorders and physical recovery, following glandular fever. *Psychological Medicine* **24**: 651–659.

Buchwald, D., Sullivan, J., Komaroff, A. (1987) Frequency of 'chronic active Epstein–Barr virus infection' in a general medical practice. *Journal of the American Medical Association* **257**: 2303–2307.

Buchwald, D., Cheney, P., Peterson, D. et al. (1992) A chronic illness characterized by fatigue, neurologic and immunologic disorders, and active human herpes type 6 infection. *Annals of Internal Medicine* **116**: 103–116.

Butler, C., Rollnick, S. (1996) Missing the meaning and provoking resistance: a case of myalgic encephalomyelitis. *Family Practice* **13**: 106–109.

Butler, S., Chalder, T., Ron, M., Wessely, S. (1991) Cognitive behaviour therapy in chronic fatigue syndrome. *Journal of Neurology Neurosurgery and Psychiatry* **54**: 153–158.

Carrette, S., McGain, G., Bell, D., Fam, A. (1986) Evaluation of amitripty-line in primary fibrositis: a double-blind placebo controlled study. *Arthritis and Rheumatism* **29**: 655–659.

Carter, B., Edwards, J., Marshall, G. (1993) Chronic fatigue in children: illness or disease? *Pediatrics* **90**: 163.

Carter, B., Edwards, J., Kronenberger, W., Michalczyk, L., Marshall, G. (1995). Case control study of chronic fatigue in pediatric patients. *Pediatrics* **95**: 179–186.

Cathebras, P., Robbins, J., Kirmayer, L., Hayton, B. (1992) Fatigue in primary care: prevalence, psychiatric comorbidity, illness behaviour and outcome. *Journal of General Internal Medicine* **7**: 276–286.

Chalder, T., Deale, A., Wessely, S. et al. (1995) Cognitive behavior therapy for chronic fatigue syndrome. *American Journal of Medicine* **98**: 419–422.

Chalder, T., Butler, S., Wessely, S. (1996) In patient treatment of chronic fatigue syndrome. *Behavioural Psychotherapy*, in press.

Chang, R., Bittner, W. (1991) Chronic fatigue syndrome. *Journal of the American Medical Association* **265**: 337.

Chester, A. (1994) The prevalence of chronic fatigue syndrome symptoms in other forms of unexplained fatigue. In *American Association for Chronic Fatigue Syndrome Research Conference*, Fort Lauderdale, Florida, 7–9 October.

Clark, M., Katon, W. (1994) The relevance of psychiatric research on soma-tization to the concept of chronic fatigue syndrome. In Straus, S. (ed.) *Chronic Fatigue Syndrome*, pp. 329–349. New York: Dekker.

Clark, M., Katon, W., Russo, J. et al. (1995) Chronic fatigue; risk factors for symptom persistence in a 2.5-year follow up study. *American Journal of Medicine* **98**: 187–195.

Cleare, A., Wessely, S. (1996) Chronic fatigue syndrome: an update. *Postgraduate Update* **52**: 61–69.

Cleare, A., Bearn, J., Allain, T. et al. (1995) Contrasting neuroendocrine responses in depression and chronic fatigue syndrome. *Journal of Affective Disorders* **35**: 283–289.

Clements, G., McGarry, F., Nairn, C., Galbraith, D. (1995). Detection of enterovirus-specific RNA in serum: the relationship to chronic fatigue. *Journal of Medical Virology* **45**: 156–161.

Cope, H., David, A (1996) Neuroimaging in chronic fatigue syndrome. *Journal of Neurology Neurosurgery and Psychiatry* **60**: 471–473.

Cope, H., David, A., Pelosi, A., Mann, A. (1994) Predictors of chronic 'post viral' fatigue. *Lancet* **344**: 864–868.

Cope, H., Pernet, A., Kendall, B., David, A. (1995) Cognitive functioning and magnetic resonance imaging in chronic fatigue. *British Journal of Psychiatry* **167**: 86–94.

Cope, H., Mann, A., Pelosi, A., David, A. (1996) Psychosocial risk factors for chronic fatigue and chronic fatigue syndrome following presumed viral infection: a case control study. *Psychological Medicine* **26**: 1197–1209.

Costa, D., Tannock, C., Brostoff, J. (1995) Brainstem perfusion is impaired in patients with myalgic encephalomyelitis/chronic fatigue syndrome. *Quarterly Journal of Medicine* **88**: 767–773.

Cox, D., Findley, L. (1994a) Chronic fatigue syndrome in adolescence. *British Journal of Hospital Medicine* **51**: 614.

Cox, D., Findley, L. (1994b) Is chronic fatigue syndrome treatable in an NHS environment? *Clinical Rehabilitation* **8**: 76–80.

Cox, B., Blaxter, M., Buckle, A. et al. (1987) *The Health and Lifestyle Survey.* London: Health Promotion Research Trust.

Crofford, L., Pillemer, S., Kalogeras, K. et al. (1994) Hypothalamic-pituitary-adrenal axis perturbations in patients with fibromyalgia. *Arthritis and Rheumatisim* **37**: 1583–1592.

Dana, C. (1904) The partial passing of neurasthenia. *Boston Medical and Surgical Journal* **60**: 339–344.

David, A., Wessely, S., Pelosi, A. (1988) Post-viral fatigue: time for a new approach. *British Medical Journal* **296**: 696–699.

David, A., Pelosi, A., McDonald, E., et al. (1990) Tired, weak or in need of rest: fatigue among general practice attenders. *British Medical Journal* **301**: 1199–1122.

Deale, A., Chalder, T., Marks, I., Wessely, S. (1996) A randomised controlled trial of cognitive behaviour versus relaxation therapy for chronic fatigue syndrome. *American Journal of Psychiatry* in press.

Deluca, J., Johnson, S., Natelson, B. (1993) Information processing efficiency in chronic fatigue syndrome and multiple sclerosis. *Archives of Neurology* **50**: 301–304.

Deluca, J., Johnson, S., Beldowicz, D., Natelson, B. (1995) Neuropsychological impairments in chronic fatigue syndrome, multiple sclerosis, and depression. *Journal of Neurology Neurosurgery and Psychiatry* **58**: 38–43.

Demitrack, M., Greden, J. (1991) Chronic fatigue syndrome; the need for an integrative approach. *Biological Psychiatry* **30**: 747–752.

Demitrack, M., Dale, J., Straus, S. et al (1991) Evidence for impaired activation of the hypothalamic-pituitary-adrenal axis in patients with chronic fatigue syndrome. *Journal of Clinical Endocrinology and Metabolism* **73**: 1224–1234.

Demitrack, M., Zubieta, J., Engleberg, et al. (submitted) Polysomnographic sleep characteristics of patients with chronic fatigue syndrome; comparison to patients with mood disorders and healthy controls.

Denman, A. (1990) The chronic fatigue syndrome; a return to common sense. *Postgraduate Medical Journal* **66**: 499–501.

Dinerman, H., Steere, A.C. (1992) Lyme disease associated with fibromyalgia. *Annals of Internal Medicine* **117**: 281–285.

Djaldetti, R., Ziv, I., Achiron, A., Melamed, E. (1996) Fatigue in multiple sclerosis compared with chronic fatigue syndrome. *Neurology* **46**: 632–635.

Dowson, D. (1993) The treatment of chronic fatigue syndrome by complementary medicine. *Complementary Therapies in Medicine* **1**: 9–13.

Edwards, R., Gibson, H., Clague, J., Helliwell, T. (1993) Muscle physiology and histopathology in chronic fatigue syndrome. In Kleinman, A., Straus, S. (eds) *Chronic Fatigue Syndrome*, pp. 101–131. Chichester: John Wiley.

Escobar, J., Burnam, A., Karno, M., Forsythe, A., Golding, J. (1987) Somatization in the community. *Archives of General Psychiatry* **44**: 713–718.

Euba, R., Chalder, T., Deale, A., Wessely, S. (1996) A comparison of the characteristics of chronic fatigue syndrome in primary and tertiary care. *British Journal of Psychiatry* **168**: 121–126.

Farmer, A., Jones, I., Hillier, J. et al. (1995) Neuraesthenia revisited: ICD-10 and DSM-III-R psyciatric syndromes in chronic fatigue patients and comparison subjects. *British Journal of Psychiatry* **167**: 503–506.

Feder, H., Dworkin, P., Orkin, C. (1994) Outcome of 48 pediatric patients with chronic fatigue; a clinical experience. *Archives of Family Medicine* **3**: 1049–1055.

Feiden, K. (1990) *Hope and Help for Chronic Fatigue Syndrome: The Official Guide of the CFS/CFIDS Network*. New York: Prentice Hall.

Fekety, R. (1994) Infection and chronic fatigue syndrome. In Straus, S. (ed.) *Chronic Fatigue Syndrome*, pp. 101–180. New York: Dekker.

Finlay, S. (1986) Don't listen if your GP says it's 'just nerves'. *Scotsman* 18 August.

Fischler, B., Cluydts, R., De Gucht, V., Kaufman, L., DeMeirleir, K. (1996a) Generalised anxiety disorders in chronic fatigue syndrome. *Acta Psychiatrica Scandinavica* in press.

Fischler, B., D'Haenen, H., Cluydts, R. et al. (1996b) Comparison of 99m HMPAO SPECT scan between chronic fatigue syndrome, major depression and healthy controls: an exploratory study of clinical correlates of regional cerebral blood flow. *Neuropsychologia* in press.

Frank, J. (1946) Emotional reactions of American soldiers to an unfamiliar disease. *American Journal of Psychiatry* **102**: 631–640.

Franklin, A. (1995) *Children with ME: Guidelines for School Doctors and General Practitioners*. Essex: ME Association.

Friedberg, F., Krupp, L. (1994) A comparison of cognitive behavioral treatment for chronic fatigue syndrome and primary depression. *Clinical Infectious Diseases* **18** (Suppl 1), S105–110.

Fuhrer, R., Wessely, S. (1995) Fatigue in French primary care. *Psychological Medicine* **25**: 895–905.

Fukuda, K., Straus, S., Hickie, I. et al. (1994) The chronic fatigue syndrome: a comprehensive approach to its definition and study. *Annals of Internal Medicine* **121**: 953–959.

Fulcher, K., Cleary, K., White, P. (1994) A placebo controlled study of a graded exercise programme in patients with chronic fatigue syndrome. *European Journal of Applied Physiology* **69** (Suppl 3), S35.

Garralda, M. (1992) Severe chronic fatigue syndrome in childhood; a discussion of pyschopathological mechanisms. *European Journal of Child and Adolescent Psychiatry* **1**: 111–118.

Gibson, H., Carroll, N., Clague, J., Edwards, R. (1993) Exercise performance and fatiguability in patients with chronic fatigue syndrome. *Journal of Neurology, Neurosurgery and Psychiatry* **56**: 993–998.

Ginannopoulou, J., Marriott, S. (1994) Chronic fatigue syndrome or affective disorder? Implications of the diagnosis on management. *European Journal of Child and Adolescent Psychiatry* **3**: 97–100.

Goldenberg, D., Felson, D., Dinerman, H. (1986). Randomised, controlled trial of amitriptyline and naproxen in treatment of patients with fibrositis. *Arthritis and Rheumatism* **29**: 1371–1377.

Goldenberg, D., Kaplan, K., Nadeau, M. et al. (1994) A controlled study of a stress-reduction, cognitive behavioral treatment program in fibromyalgia. *Journal of Musculoskeletal Pain* **2**: 53–65.

Goodnick, P., Sandoval, R. (1993) Psychotropic treatment of chronic fatigue syndrome and related disorders. *Journal of Clinical Psychiatry* **54**: 13–20.

Gow, J., Behan, W., Clements, G. et al. (1991) Enteroviral RNA sequences detected by polymerase chain reaction in muscle of patients with postviral fatigue syndrome. *British Medical Journal* **302**: 692–696.

Gow, J., Behan, P., Simpson, K. et al. (1994) Studies of enteroviruses in patients with chronic fatigue syndrome. *Clinical Infectious Diseases* **18** (Suppl 1), S126–129.

Gracious, B., Wisner, K. (1991) Nortriptyline in chronic fatigue syndrome; a double blind, placebo-controlled single case study. *Biological Psychiatry* **30**: 405–408.

Grafman, J., Schwartz, V., Scheffers, M., Houser, C., Straus, S. (1993) Analysis of neuropsychological functioning in patients with chronic fatigue syndrome. *Journal of Neurology, Neurosurgery and Psychiatry* **56**: 684–689.

Graham, H. (1990) Family interventions in general practice: a case of chronic fatigue. *Journal of Family Therapy* **13**: 225–230.

Greenberg, D. (1990) Neurasthenia in the 1980s: chronic mononucleosis, chronic fatigue syndrome, and anxiety and depressive disorders. *Psychosomatics* **31**: 129–137.

Gunn, W., Connell, D., Randall, B. (1993) Epidemiology of chronic fatigue syndrome: the Centers for Disease Control study. In Kleinman, A., Straus, S. (eds) *Chronic Fatigue Syndrome*, pp. 83–101. Chichester: John Wiley.

Hagnell, O., Grasbeck, A., Ojesjo, L., Otterbeck, L. (1993) Mental tiredness in the Lundby study; incidence and course over 25 years. *Acta Psychiatrica Scandanivica* **88**: 316–321.

Halpin, D., Wessely, S. (1989) VP-1 antigen in chronic postviral fatigue syndrome. *Lancet* **ii**: 1028–1029.

Hay, J., Jenkins, F. (1994) Human herpesviruses and chronic fatigue syndrome. In Straus, S. (ed.) *Chronic Fatigue Syndrome*, pp. 181–198. New York: Dekker.

Hickie, I., Lloyd, A., Wakefield, D., Parker, G. (1990) The psychiatric status of patients with chronic fatigue syndrome. *British Journal of Psychiatry* **156**: 534–540.

Hickie, I., Lloyd, A., Hadzi-Pavlovic, D. et al. (1995) Can the chronic fatigue syndrome be defined by distinct clinical features? *Psychological Medicine* **25**: 925–935.

Hinds, G., McCluskey, D. (1993) A retrospective study of chronic fatigue syndrome. *Proceedings of the Royal College of Physicians of Edinburgh* **23**: 10–14.

Hodgkinson, N. (1987) Virus research doctors finally prove shirkers really are sick. *Sunday Times* 25 January.

Holmes, G., Kaplan, J., Gantz, N. et al. (1988) Chronic fatigue syndrome: a working case definition. *Annals of Internal Medicine* **108**, 387–389.

Howard, L., Wessely, S. (1993) The psychology of multiple allergy. *British Medical Journal* **307**: 747–748.

Ho-Yen, D.O. (1988) The epidemiology of post viral fatigue syndrome. *Scottish Medical Journal* **33**: 368–369.

Ho-Yen, D. (1991) General practitioners' experience of the chronic fatigue syndrome. *British Journal of General Practice* **41**: 324–326.

Ichise, M., Salit, S., Abbey, S. et al. (1992) Assessment of regional cerebral perfusion by 99 Tc HMPAO SPECT in chronic fatigue syndrome. *Nuclear Medicine Communications* **13**: 767–772.

Janet, P. (1919) *Les Obsessions et la Psychasthénie,* vol 1. Paris: Alcan.

Johnson, S., Deluca, J., Natelson, B. (1996a) Assessing somatization disorder in the chronic fatigue syndrome. *Psychosomatic Medicine* **58**: 50–57.

Johnson, S., Deluca, J., Nateson, B. (1996b) Depression in fatiguing illness: comparing patients with chronic fatigue syndrome, multiple sclerosis and depression. *Journal of Affective Disorders* in press.

Jones, D., Newham, D., Round, J., Tolfree, S. (1986) Experimental human muscle damage: morphological changes in relation to other indices of damage. *Journal of Physiology* **375**: 435–448.

Joyce, E., Blumenthal, S., Wessely, S. (1996) Memory, attention and executive function in chronic fatigue syndrome. *Journal of Neurology, Neurosurgery and Psychiatry* **60**: 495–503.

Karno, M., Hoffman, R. (1974) The pseudoanergic syndrome. In Kiev, A. (ed.) *Somatic Manifestations of Depressive Disorders,* pp. 55–85. Amsterdam: Excerpta Medica.

Kaslow, J., Rucker, L., Onishi, R. (1989) Liver extract-folic acid-cyanocobalamin vs placebo for chronic fatigue syndrome. *Archives of Internal Medicine* **149**: 2501–2503.

Katon, W., Russo, J. (1992) Chronic fatigue syndrome criteria: a critique of the requirement for multiple physical complaints. *Archives of Internal Medicine* **152**: 1604–1609.

Katon, W., Buchwald, D., Simon, G., Russo, J., & Mease, P. (1991) Psychiatric illness in patients with chronic fatigue and rheumatoid arthritis. *Journal of General Internal Medicine* **6**: 277–285.

Kendell, R. (1991) Chronic fatigue, viruses and depression. *Lancet* **337**: 160–162.

Kent-Braun, J., Sharma, K., Weiner, M., Massie, B., Miller, R. (1993) Central basis of muscle fatigue in chronic fatigue syndrome. *Neurology* **43**: 125–131.

Klug, G., McAuley, E., Clark, S. (1989) Factors influencing the development and maintenance of aerobic fitness: lessons applicable to the fibrositis syndrome. *Journal of Rheumatology* **16** (Suppl 19): 30–39.

Komaroff, A. (1990) 'Minor' illness symptoms; the magnitude of their burden and of our ignorance. *Archives of Internal Medicine* **150**: 1586–1587.

Kroenke, K., Mangelsdorff, D. (1989) Common symptoms in ambulatory care: incidence, evaluation, therapy and outcome. *American Journal of Medicine* **86**: 262–266.

Kroenke, K., Wood, D., Mangelsdorff, D., Meier, N., Powell, J. (1988) Chronic fatigue in primary care: prevalence, patient characteristics and outcome. *Journal of the American Medical Association* **260**: 929–934.

Kroenke, K., Arrington, M., Mangelsdorff, D. (1990). The prevalence of symptoms in medical outpatients and the adequacy of therapy. *Archives of Internal Medicine* **150**: 1685–1689.

Kroenke, K., Spitzer, R., Williams, J. (1994) Physical symptoms in primary care; predictors of psychiatric disorders and functional impairment. *Archives of Family Medicine* **3**: 774–779.

Kyle, D., DeShazo, R. (1992) Chronic fatigue syndrome: a conundrum. *American Journal of Medical Science* **303**: 28–34.

Lane, R. (1994) Aetiology, diagnosis and treatment of chronic fatigue syndrome. *Journal of Serotonin Research* **1**: 47–60.

Lane, T., Matthews D., Manu, P. (1990) The low yield of physical examinations and laboratory investigations of patients with chronic fatigue. *American Journal of Medical Science* **299**: 313–318.

Lane, T., Manu, P., Matthews, D. (1991) Depression and somatization in the chronic fatigue syndrome. *American Journal of Medicine* **91**: 335–344.

Lask, B., Dillon, M. (1990) Postviral fatigue syndrome. *Archives of Disease in Childhood* **65**: 1198.

Lawrie, S., Pelosi, A. (1995) Chronic fatigue syndrome in the community: prevalence and associations. *British Journal of Psychiatry* **166**: 793–797.

Leese, G., Chattington, P., Fraser, W. et al. (1996) Short-term night-shift working mimics the pituitary-adrenocortical dysfunction of chronic fatigue syndrome. *Journal of Clinical Endocrinology and Metabolism* **81**: 1867–1870.

Levine, P., Kreuger, G., Straus, S. (1989) Postviral chronic fatigue syndrome: a round table. *Journal of Infectious Diseases* **160**: 722-724.

Levy, J. (1994) Introduction; viral studies of chronic fatigue syndrome. *Clinical Infectious Diseases* **18** (Suppl 1), S117–120.

Lewis, G., Wessely, S. (1992) The epidemiology of fatigue: more questions than answers. *Journal of Epidemiology and Community Health* **46**: 92–97.

Liebowitz, M., Quitkin, F., Stewart, J. et al. (1988). Antidepressant specificity in atypical depression. *Archives of General Psychiatry* **45**: 129–137.

Lloyd, A., Hales, J., Gandevia, S. (1988) Muscle strength, endurance and recovery in the postinfection fatigue syndrome. *Journal of Neurology, Neurosurgery and Psychiatry* **51**: 1316–1322.

Lloyd, A., Hickie, I., Boughton, R., Spencer, O., Wakefield, D. (1990) Prevalence of chronic fatigue syndrome in an Australian population. *Medical Journal of Australia* **153**: 522–528.

Lloyd, A., Gandevia, S., Hales, J. (1991) Muscle performance, voluntary activation, twitch properties and perceived effort in normal subjects and patients with the chronic fatigue syndrome. *Brain* **114**: 85–98.

Lloyd, A., Hickie, I., Brockman, A. et al. (1993) Immunologic and psychological therapy for patients with chronic fatigue syndrome. *American Journal of Medicine* **94**: 197–203.

Lloyd, A., Hickie, I., Wilson, A., Wakefield, D. (1994) Immune function in chronic fatigue syndrome and depression; implications for understanding these disorders and for therapy. *Clinical Immunotherapy* **2**: 84–88.

Lynch, S., Seth, R. (1989) Postviral fatigue syndrome and the VP-1 antigen. *Lancet* **ii**: 1160–1161.

Lynch, S., Seth, R., Montgomery, S. (1991) Antidepressant therapy in the chronic fatigue syndrome. *British Journal of General Practice* **41**: 339–342.

MacDonald, K., Osterholm, M., LeDell, K. et al. (1996). A case control study to assess possible triggers and cofactors in chronic fatigue syndrome. *American Journal of Medicine* **100**: 548–554.

Maes, M., Jacobs, J., Lambreckhts, J. (1992) Evidence for a systemic immune activation during depression; results of leucocyte enumeration by flow cytometry in conjunction with antibody staining. *Psychological Medicine* **22**: 45–53.

Manu, P., Matthews, D., Lane, T. (1993) Food intolerance in patients with chronic fatigue. *International Journal of Eating Disorders* **13**: 203–209.

Martin, R., Ogston, S., Evans, J. (1994) Effects of vitamin and mineral supplementation on symptoms associated with chronic fatigue syndrome with Coxsackie B antibodies. *Journal of Nutritional Medicine* **4**: 11–23.

Masuda, A., Nozoe, S., Matsuyama, T., Tanaka, H. (1994) Psychobehavioral and immunological characteristics of adult people with chronic fatigue and patients with chronic fatigue syndrome. *Psychosomatic Medicine* **56**: 512–518.

McArdle, A., McArdle, F., Jackson, M. et al. (1996) Investigation by polymerase chain reaction of enteroviral infection in patients with chronic fatigue syndrome. *Clinical Science* **90**: 295–300.

McCain, G., Bell, D., Mai, F., Holliday, P. (1988) A controlled study of the effects of a supervised cardiovascular fitness program on the manifestations of primary fibromyalgia. *Arthritis and Rheumatism* **31**: 1135–1141.

McCluskey, D. (1993) Pharmacological approaches to the therapy of chronic fatigue syndrome. In Kleinman, A., Straus, S. (eds) *Chronic Fatigue Syndrome*, pp. 280–297. Chichester: John Wiley.

McCully, K., Sisto, S., Natelson, B. (1996) Use of exercise for treatment of chronic fatigue syndrome. *Sports Medicine* **21**: 35–48.

McDonald, E., David, A., Pelosi, A., Mann, A. (1993) Chronic fatigue in general practice attenders. *Psychological Medicine* **23**: 987–998.

McEvedy, C., Beard, A. (1970) Royal Free epidemic of 1955; a reconsideration. *British Medical Journal* **i**: 7–11.

Medical Staff of the Royal Free Hospital Group (1955) An outbreak of encephalomyelitis in the Royal Free Hospital Group. *British Medical Journal* **ii**: 895–904.

Merikangas, K., Angst, J. (1994) Neurasthenia in a longitudinal cohort study of young adults. *Psychological Medicine* **24**: 1013–1024.

Mihill, C. (1992) Brainwaves suggest ME is a physical illness, not a psychiatric disorder. *Guardian* 29 August.

Miller, H., Carmichael, H., Calder, B. et al. (1991) Antibody to Coxsackie B virus in diagnosing postviral fatigue syndrome. *British Medical Journal* **302**: 140–143.

Morrell, D., Wale, C. (1976) Symptoms perceived and recorded by patients. *Journal of Royal College of General Practitioners* **26**: 398–403.

Morris, D., Stare, F. (1993) Unproven diet therapies in the treatment of chronic fatigue syndrome. *Archives of Family Medicine* **2**: 181–186.

Morriss, R., Sharpe, M., Sharpley, A. et al. (1993) Abnormalities of sleep in patients with the chronic fatigue syndrome. *British Medical Journal* **306**: 1161–1164.

Moss-Morris, R. (1996) The role of illness cognitions and coping in the aetiology and maintenance of the chronic fatigue syndrome (CFS). In Weinman, J., Patrie, K. (eds) *The Patient's Perception of Illness and Treatment: Current Research and Applications*, Reading: Harwood Academic Publishers.

Moss-Morris, R., Petrie, K., Largem R., Kydd, R. (1996) Neuropsychological deficits in chronic fatigue syndrome: artifact or reality? *Journal of Neurology, Neurosurgery and Psychiatry* **60**: 474–477.

Mountz, J., Bradley, L., Modell, J. et al. (1995) Fibromyalgia in women: abnormalities of regional cerebral blood flow in the thalamus and the caudate nucleus are associated with low pain threshold levels. *Arthritis and Rheumatism* **38**: 926–938.

Natelson, B., Cohen, J., Brassloff, I., Lee, H.-J. (1994) A controlled study of brain magnetic resonance imaging in patients with the chronic fatigue syndrome. *Journal of Neurological Science* **120**: 213–217.

Natelson, B., Cheu, J., Pareja, J. et al. (1996) Randomized, double-blind, controlled placebo-phase in trial of low dose phenelzine in the chronic fatigue syndrome. *Psychopharmacology* **124**: 226–230.

Newham, D. (1988) The consequences of eccentric contractions and their relationship to delayed onset muscle pain. *European Journal of Applied Physiology* **57**: 353–359.

Nielsen, W., Walker, C., McCain, G. (1992) Cognitive behavioral treatment of fibromyalgia syndrome. *Journal of Rheumatology* **19**: 98–103.

Ormel, J., VonKorff, M., Ustun, B. et al. (1994) Common mental disorders and disabilities across cultures: results from the WHO collaborative study on psychological problems in general health care. *Journal of the American Medical Association* **272**: 1741–1748.

Pagani, M., Lucini, D., Mela, G., Langewitz, W., Malliani, A. (1994) Sympathetic overactivity in subjects complaining of unexplained fatigue. *Clinical Science* **87**: 655–661.

Patterson, J., Aitchinson, F., Wyper, D. et al. (1995) SPECT brain imaging in chronic fatigue syndrome. *Revista di Immunologia ed Immunofarmacologia* **15**: 53–58.

Pawlikowska, T., Chalder, T., Hirsch, S. et al. (1994) A population based study of fatigue and psychological distress. *British Medical Journal* **308**: 743–746.

Pelcovitz, D., Septimus, A., Friedman, S. et al. (1995) Psychosocial correlates of chronic fatigue syndrome in adolescent girls. *Journal of Developmental and Behavioral Paediatrics* **16**: 333–338.

Pepper, C., Krupp, L., Friedberg, F., Doscher, C., Coyle, P. (1993) A comparison of neuropsychiatric characteristics in chronic fatigue syndrome, multiple sclerosis and major depression. *Journal of Neuropsychiatry and Clinical Neurosciences* **5**: 200–205.

Petrie, K., Moss-Morris, R., Weinman, J. (1995) The impact of catastrophic beliefs on functioning in chronic fatigue syndrome. *Journal of Psychosomatic Research* **39**: 31–37.

Pipe, R., Wait, M. (1995) Family therapy in the treatment of chronic fatigue syndrome in adolescence. *ACPP Review and Newsletter* **17**: 9–16.

Ramsay, M. (1986) *Postviral Fatigue Syndrome: The Saga of Royal Free Disease*. London: Gower Medical.

Ray, C., Phillips, L., Weir, W. (1993) Quality of attention in chronic fatigue syndrome; subjective reports of everyday attention and cognitive difficulty, and performance on tasks of focused attention. *British Journal of Clinical Psychology* **32**: 357–364.

Ray, C., Jeffries, S., Weir, W. (1995) Coping with chronic fatigue syndrome: illness responses and their relationship with fatigue, functional impairment and emotional status. *Psychological Medicine* **25**: 937–945.

Richman, J., Flaherty, J., Rospenda, K. (1994) Chronic fatigue syndrome: have flawed assumptions been derived from treatment-based studies? *American Journal of Public Health* **84**: 282–284.

Ridsdale, L. (1989) Chronic fatigue in family practice. *Journal of Family Practice* **29**: 486–488.

Ridsdale, L., Evans, A., Jerrett, W. et al. (1993) Patients with fatigue in general practice: a prospective study. *British Medical Journal* **307**: 103–106.

Rikard-Bell, C., Waters, B. (1992) Psychosocial management of chronic fatigue syndrome in adolescence. *Australian and New Zealand Journal of Psychiatry* **26**: 64–72.

Riley, M., O'Brien, C., McCluskey, D., Bell, N., Nicholls, D. (1990) Aerobic work capacity in patients with chronic fatigue syndrome. *British Medical Journal* **301**: 953–956.

Roberts, L., Byrne, E. (1994) Single fibre EMG studies in chronic fatigue syndrome: a reappraisal. *Journal of Neurology, Neurosurgery and Psychiatry* **57**: 375–376.

Rosen, S.D., King, J.C., Wilkinson, J.B., Nixon, P.G.F. (1990) Is chronic fatigue syndrome synonymous with effort syndrome. *Journal of the Royal Society of Medicine* **83**: 761–764.

Rutherford, O., White, P. (1991) Human quadriceps strength and fatigability in patients with post-viral fatigue. *Journal of Neurology, Neurosurgery and Psychiatry* **54**: 961–964.

Saisch, S., Deale, A., Gardner, W., Wessely, S. (1994) Hyperventilation and chronic fatigue syndrome. *Quarterly Journal of Medicine* **87**: 63–67.

Saltin, B., Blomquist, G., Mitchell, J. et al. (1968) Response to exercise after bed rest and training: a longitudinal study of adaptive changes in oxygen transport and body composition. *Circulation* **38** (Suppl 7), 1–55.

Schepank, H. (1987) *Epidemiology of Psychogenic Disorders; The Mannheim Study*. Berlin: Springer-Verlag.

Schluederberg, A., Straus, S., Peterson, P. et al. (1992) Chronic fatigue syndrome research: definition and medical outcome assessment. *Annals of Internal Medicine* **117**: 325–331.

Schmaling, K., DiClementi, J., Cullum, M., Jones, J. (1994) Cognitive functioning in chronic fatigue syndrome and depression: a preliminary comparison. *Psychosomatic Medicine* **56**: 383–388.

Schwartz, R., Komaroff, A., Garada, B. et al. (1994) SPECT imaging of the brain: comparison of findings in patients with chronic fatigue syndrome, AIDS dementia complex, and major unipolar depression. *American Journal of Roentgenology* **162**: 943–951.

Schweitzer, R., Robertson, D., Kelly, B., Whiting, J. (1994) Illness behaviour of patients with chronic fatigue syndrome. *Journal of Psychosomatic Research* **38**: 41–50.

Scott, S., Deary, I., Pelosi, A. (1995) General practitioners' attitudes to patients with a self-diagnosis of myalgic encephalomyelitis. *British Medical Journal* **310**: 508.

Shahar, E., Lederer, J. (1990) Asthenic symptoms in a rural family epidemiologic characteristics and a proposed classification. *Journal of Family Practice* **31**: 257–262.

Sharpe, M. (1996) Cognitive-behavioral therapy for patients with chronic fatigue syndrome: How? In Demitrack, M., Abbey, S. (eds) *Chronic Fatigue Syndrome: An Integrative Approach to Evaluation and Treatment*, pp. 240–262. New York: Guildford Press.

Sharpe, M., Bass, C. (1992) Pathophysiological mechanisms in somatization. *International Review of Psychiatry* **4**: 81–97.

Sharpe, M., Chalder, T. (1994) Management of the chronic fatigue syndrome. In Illis, L. (ed.) *Neurological Rehabilitation*, pp. 282–294. Oxford: Blackwell.

Sharpe, M., Archard, L., Banatvala, J. et al. (1991) Chronic fatigue syndrome: guidelines for research. *Journal of the Royal Society of Medicine* **84**: 118–121.

Sharpe, M., Hawton, K., Seagroatt, V., Pasvol, G. (1992) Follow up of patients with fatigue presenting to an infectious diseases clinic. *British Medical Journal* **302**: 347–352.

Sharpe, M., Hawton, K., Simkin, S. et al. (1996) Cognitive behaviour therapy for chronic fatigue syndrome; a randomized controlled trial. *British Medical Journal* **312**: 22–26.

Shefer, A., Dobbins, J., Fukuda, K. et al. (1994) Investigation of chronic fatigue syndrome among employees in two state office buildings in California, 1993. In *American Association for Chronic Fatigue Syndrome Research Conference*, Fort Lauderdale, Florida.

Shorter, E. (1992) *From Paralysis to Fatigue: A History of Psychosomatic Illness in the Modern Era*. New York: Free Press.

Shorter, E. (1995) Sucker-punched again! Physicians meet the disease-of-the-month syndrome. *Journal of Psychosomatic Research* **39**: 115–188.

Sidebotham, P., Skeldon, I., Chambers, T., Clements, S., Culling, J. (1994) Refractory chronic fatigue syndrome in adolescence. *British Journal of Hospital Medicine* **51**: 110–112.

Simon, G., VonKorff, M. (1991) Somatization and psychiatric disorder in the NIMH epidemiologic catchment area study. *American Journal of Psychiatry* **148**: 1494–1500.

Sisto, S., MaManca, J., Cordero, D. et al. (1996) Metabolic and cardiovascular effects of a progressive exercise test in patients with chronic fatigue syndrome. *American Journal of Medicine* **100**: 634–640.

Smith, M., Mitchell, J., Corey, L. et al. (1991) Chronic fatigue in adolescents. *Pediatrics* **88**: 195–201.

Smith, R., Greenbaum, D., Vancouver, I. et al. (1990) Psychological factors are associated with health care seeking rather than diagnosis in irritable bowel syndrome. *Gastroenterology* **98**: 293–301.

Stokes, M., Cooper, R., Edwards, R. (1988) Normal strength and fatigability in patients with effort syndrome. *British Medical Journal* **297**: 1014–1018.

Stopp, C. ME sufferers forced to battle with insurers. *Independent on Sunday* 27 June.

Straus, S. (1988) The chronic mononucleosis syndrome. *Journal of Infection* **157**: 405–412.

Straus, S. (1990) Intravenous immunoglobulin treatment for the chronic fatigue syndrome. *American Journal of Medicine* **89**: 551–553.

Straus, S., Dale, J., Wright, R., Metcalfe, D. (1988) Allergy and the chronic fatigue syndrome. *Journal of Allergy and Clinical Immunology* **81**: 791–795.

Straus, S., Fritz, S., Dale, J., Gould, B., Strober, W. (1993) Lymphocyte phenotype and function in the chronic fatigue syndrome. *Journal of Clinical Immunology* **13**: 30–40.

Strober, W. (1994) Immunological function in chronic fatigue syndrome. In Straus, S. (ed.) *Chronic Fatigue Syndrome*, pp. 207–240. New York: Dekker.

Surawy, C., Hackmann, A., Hawton, K., Sharpe, M. (1995) Chronic fatigue syndrome: a cognitive approach. *Behaviour Research and Therapy* **33**: 535–544.

Swanink, C., Melchers, W., van der Meer, J. et al. (1994) Enteroviruses and the chronic fatigue syndrome. *Clinical Infectious Diseases* **19**: 860–864.

Swanink, C., Vercoulen, J., Bleijenberg, G. et al. (1995) Chronic fatigue syndrome: a clinical and laboratory study with a well matched control group. *Journal of Internal Medicine* **237**: 499–506.

Swartz, M. (1988) The chronic fatigue syndrome – one entity or many? *New England Journal of Medicine* **319**: 1726–1728.

Valdini, A., Steinhardt, S., Feldman, E. (1989) Usefulness of a standard battery of laboratory tests in investigating chronic fatigue in adults. *Family Practice* **6**: 286–291.

Van Hemert, A., Hengeveld, M., Bolk, J., Rooijmans, H., Vandenbroucke, J. (1993) Psychiatric disorder in relation to medical illness among patients of a general medical out-patient clinic. *Psychological Medicine* **23**: 167–173.

Vercoulen, J., Hommes, O., Swanink, C. et al. (1996a) The measurement of fatigue in patients with multiple sclerosis: a multi-dimensional comparison with patients with chronic fatigue syndrome and healthy subjects. *Archives of Neurology* **46**: 632–635.

Vercoulen, J., Swanink, C., Fennis, J. et al. (1996b) Prognosis in chronic fatigue syndrome: a prospective study on the natural course. *Journal of Neurology, Neurosurgery and Psychiatry* **60**: 489–494.

Vercoulen, J., Swanink, C., Zitman, F. et al. (1996c) Fluoxetine in chronic fatigue syndrome; a randomized, double-blind, placebo-controlled study. *Lancet* **347**: 858–861.

Vereker, M. (1992) Chronic fatigue syndrome: a joint paediatric–psychiatric approach. *Archives of Disease in Childhood* **1992**: 550–555.

Wachsmuth, J., MacMillan, H. (1991) Effective treatment for an adolescent with chronic fatigue syndrome. *Clinical Pediatrics* **30**: 488–490.

Wagenmakers, A., Coakley, J., Edwards, R. (1988) The metabolic consequences of reduced habitual activities in patients with muscle pain and disease. *Ergonomics* **31**: 1519–1527.

Walford, G., McNelson, W., & McCluskey, D. (1993) Fatigue, depression and social adjustment in children with chronic fatigue syndrome. *Archives of Disease in Childhood* **68**: 384–388.

Walker, E., Katon, W., Jemelka, R. (1993) Psychiatric disorders and medical care utilisation among people who report fatigue in the general population. *Journal of General Internal Medicine* **8**: 436–440.

Wearden, A., Appleby, L. (1996) Research on cognitive complaints and cognitive functioning in patients with chronic fatigue syndrome (CFS): what conclusions can we draw? *Journal of Psychosomatic Research* in press.

Wearden, A., Morriss, R., Mullis, R. et al. (submitted) A double-blind, placebo controlled treatment trial of fluoxetine and a graded exercise programme for chronic fatigue syndrome.

Wells, K., Stewart, A., Hays, R. et al. (1989) The functioning and well-being of depressed patients: results from the Medical Outcomes Study. *Journal of the American Medical Association* **262**: 914–919.

Wessely, S. (1991) History of the postviral fatigue syndrome. *British Medical Bulletin* **47**: 919–941.

Wessely, S. (1994) Neurasthenia and chronic fatigue: theory and practice in Britain and America. *Transcultural Psychiatric Research Review* **31**: 173–209.

Wessely, S. (1995) The epidemiology of chronic fatigue syndrome. *Epidemiologic Reviews* **17**: 139–151.

Wessely, S. (1996) Cognitive behavioral therapy for patients with chronic fatigue syndrome: Why? In Demitrack, M., Abbey, S. (eds) *Chronic Fatigue Syndrome: An Integrative Approach to Evaluation and Treatment*, pp. 212–239. New York: Guildford Press.

Wessely, S., Powell, R. (1989) Fatigue syndromes: a comparison of chronic 'postviral' fatigue with neuromuscular and affective disorder. *Journal of Neurology, Neurosurgery and Psychiatry* **52**: 940–948.

Wessely, S., Butler, S., Chalder, T., David, A. (1991) The cognitive behavioural management of the post-viral fatigue syndrome. In Jenkins, R., Mowbraw, J. (eds) *Postviral Fatigue Syndrome*, pp. 305–334. Chichester: John Wiley.

Wessely, S., Chalder, T., Hirsch, S. et al. (1995) Post infectious fatigue: a prospective study in primary care. *Lancet* **345**: 1333–1338.

Wessely, S., Chalder, T., Hirsch, S., Wallace, P., Wright, D. (1996a) Psychological symptoms, somatic symptoms and psychiatric disorder in chronic fatigue and chronic fatigue syndrome: a prospective study in primary care. *American Journal of Psychiatry* **153**: 1050–1059.

Wessely, S., Chalder, T., Hirsch, S., Wallace, P., Wright, D. (1996b) The prevalence and morbidity of chronic fatigue and chronic fatigue syndrome: a prospective primary care study. *American Journal of Public Health* in press.

White, P., Thomas, J., Amess, J. et al. (1995) The existence of a fatigue syndrome after glandular fever. *Psychological Medicine* **25**: 907–916.

White, P., Thomas, J., Amess, J. et al. (submitted) The incidence, prevalence and prognosis of the fatigue syndrome which follows Epstein–Barr virus infection.

Wilson, A., Hickie, I., Lloyd, A. et al. (1994a) Longitudinal study of the outcome of chronic fatigue syndrome. *British Medical Journal* **308**: 756–760.

Wilson, A, Hickie, I., Lloyd, A., Wakefield, D. (1994b) The treatment of chronic fatigue syndrome; science and speculation. *American Journal of Medicine* **96**: 544–549.

Wolfe, F., Cathey, M., Hawley, D. (1994) A double-blind placebo controlled trial of fluoxetine in fibromyalgia. *Scandanavian Journal of Rheumatology* **23**: 255–259.

Wood, G., Bentall, R., Gopfert, M., Edwards, R. (1991) A comparative psychiatric assessment of patients with chronic fatigue syndrome and muscle disease. *Psychological Medicine* **21**: 619–628.

Yousef, G., Bell, E., Mann, G. et al. (1988) Chronic enterovirus infection in patients with postviral fatigue syndrome. *Lancet* **i**: 146–150.

Zola, I. (1966) Culture and symptoms; an analysis of patients presenting complaints. *American Sociological Review* **31**: 398–403.

Zorbas, Y., Matveyev, I. (1986) Man's desirability in performing physical exercises under hypokinesia. *International Journal of Rehabilitation* **9**: 170–174.

3

Clinical Controversies and Biological Models of Obsessive–Compulsive Disorder

James V. Lucey, Jogin H. Thakore and Timothy G. Dinan

INTRODUCTION

The first adequate description of obsessive–compulsive disorder (OCD), a condition characterized by recurrent intrusive thoughts or images and by ritualistic repetitive behaviours, was given by Esquirol in 1838. Sigmund Freud (1924) in his influential paper on 'Character and Anal Erotocism' described the orderly and parsimonious nature of such individuals as a partial sublimation of, or reaction formation to, their anal erotic activities. Such psychoanalytic thinking, which was to remain instrumental in determining the clinical attitude and management of OCD for many years, has proved largely ineffective. Modern techniques in behaviour therapy are effective strategies for OCD (Marks and O'Sullivan, 1988). and these are often used in combination with biological treatments such as serotonin transport inhibitors (Greist et al., 1995). Thus paradigms used to consider OCD have shifted significantly in recent years from psychoanalytic to biological perspectives. Neuroimaging and also clinical studies support the view that OCD is a neuropsychiatric disorder. A distinct neuroendocrine profile is emerging from a large number of published studies, including abnormal prolactin and possibly also growth hormone release mechansims. This review will examine various biological models of OCD and controversies regarding its clinical presentation.

OCD DEFINITION

In the DSM-IV definition (APA, 1994), obsessions are recurrent thoughts, impulses or images, that are experienced at some time as intrusive or inappropriate. They cause marked anxiety or distress. The person attempts to suppress them through some other action or thought, and recognizes that these experiences are the product of his/her own mind. Compulsions are repetitive obsessional acts, which the person feels compelled to perform, often in response to an obsession. There is no realistic connection between the obsessions and compulsions and at some point the patient must recognize these experiences are unreasonable. Crucially, these experiences cause marked distress and/or handicap. Their content must be distinct from another axis I disorder (if another is present) and they must not be the product of substance abuse or general medical disorder (APA, 1994). The operational definition of OCD in ICD-10 (WHO, 1992) is similar. In addition, it also provides helpful subcategories such as: predominantly obsessional (which is closely related to depression), predominantly compulsive (which is not so closely associated with depression and may be more amenable to behavioural therapies), and mixed obsessive–compulsive presentation (WHO, 1992).

CLINICAL PHENOMENOLOGY

OCD was described over a century ago by Westphal (1878), and its classic features have never been in dispute. However, the predictive value of OCD's phenomenology still remains unclear. Swedo et al. (1989b) described a remarkable similarity in the style and content of OCD's symptoms between adults and children, thereby allowing the authors to propose an ethological explanation for this condition. Nonetheless, rigorous evidence for clinical stability is still lacking. In Zurich, Degonda et al. (1993) followed patients with OCD over 11 years and found a certain amount of stability in terms of symptoms but none at a diagnostic level. Despite data suggesting that OCD syndrome as a whole is stable (Swedo et al., 1989b), individual follow-up studies of sufficient duration are rare and inconclusive (Degonda et al., 1993).

Repeated washing, checking, thoughts of the past, embarrassing behaviour and depression emerged as commonly occurring phenomena in a study by Khanna et al. (1990), indicating that symptom clusters do exist. Applying a principal components analysis to the Yale–Brown Obsessive–Compulsive Subscale checklist results of 107 patients with OCD, Baer (1994) found that three symptom clusters existed. The first cluster (symmetry/hoarding) (20.7% of symptom variance) correlated with comorbid obsessive–compulsive personality disorder and tic spectrum disorder (Baer, 1994). No correlates with the other two clusters were found; contamination/checking (16%), and pure obsessions (Religious and/or Sexual) (11.3%). Baer (1994) and McDougle et al. (1990) proposed appropriate therapeutic procedures with these apparently distinct sub-groupings in mind. Those with pure obsessional phenomena might benefit from selective serotonin reuptake inhibitors, those with symmetry/hoarding with comorbid tics might require the addition of a neuroleptic, while those with symptoms of contamination and checking may respond best to behaviour therapy. Similar predictions were made for the clinical subdivisions in ICD-10 (WHO, 1992), but the therapeutic and predictive value of clinical subtypes still needs to be established.

PREVALENCE

With a prevalence rate of 0.05%, OCD was considered to be relatively rare for many years. The original figure was incorrectly attributed to a paper in German by Rudin and Beitrag (1953) with many subsequent European investigators perpetuating the error. Using non-operationally defined ICD-9 criteria, these studies confirmed the low prevalence rate of this condition. For example, in a study of 1495 people in Munich only one case of obsessive–compulsive neurosis was found (Fichter, 1990). With the advent of operationally defined criteria, higher rates of OCD were detected. The Epidemiologic Catchment Area (ECA) study, used the Diagnostic Interview Schedule (DIS), recruited over 18 500 subjects and detected lifetime prevalence rates of between 1.9% and 2.4%; rates over 60 times higher than previously reported (Karno et al., 1988). Furthermore, OCD was most common amongst white, young, divorced and the unemployed. The presence of OCD increased the probability of having another lifetime psychiatric diagnosis; but OCD patients did not differ from other DSM-IIIR diagnoses in the degree of comorbidity (Karno et al., 1988). Though the surveys were conducted over five separate communities across the United States, a major criticism of this study was the use of trained lay observers in gathering information (Rasmussen and Tsuang, 1986).

Clinican-based interviews, using more restrictive criteria have found lower prevalence rates than the ECA study (Karno et al., 1988). Angst et al. (1984) and Degonda et al. (1993) in their longitudinal study of a Swiss population found OCD to be a rarity, with rates of 0.002%. A series of eight studies conducted in the USA, Taiwan, Europe and New Zealand using the DIS found lifetime prevalence rates of between 0.5% and 3.2% (Degonda et al., 1993). Methodological differences between high and low prevalence studies may explain the observed discrepancies, as secondary depression, lifetime depression or axis II (DSM-IIIR) diagnoses were not exclusion criteria in the latter studies. However, Weissman et al. (1994) using DIS noted that the prevalence of OCD, 1.1% to 1.8%, is remarkably similar in diverse societies (ranging from the USA, New Zealand, Korea, Puerto Rico and Germany), indicating that this condition is a common disorder worldwide.

OCD onset age is later in women than in men (mean difference is three years) (Noshirvani et al., 1986). The mean onset age for men is 21 years and for women is 24 years (Noshirvani et al., 1986). Early onset (between five and 15 years) is more common in men and this may reflect a greater proportion of organic factors (Noshirvani et al., 1991). The estimated average delay between symptom onset and first psychiatric presentation is 7.5 years (Pollit, 1957; Rasmussen and Tsuang, 1986).

The sex ratio in OCD is nearly equal, since females account for approximately 50% of most large studies (Black, 1974; Yaryura-Tobias and Neziroglu, 1983; Noshirvani et al., 1986; Karno et al., 1988; Degonda et al., 1993). There are sex differences in OCD symptom subtypes, so that women are more likely to present with compulsive washing, a history of anorexia nervosa or treated depression (Noshirvani et al., 1986). The lifetime prevalence of eating disorders in OCD is between 6% and 12%, and this is accounted for almost entirely by women (Noshirvani et al., 1991). Males are more likely to have coexistent psychotic features (Eisen and Rasmussen, 1993). In general, OCD's equal sex ratio is a feature which distinguishes it from other types of anxiety disorder, such as phobic disorders, where there is a marked female preponderance (Marks, 1987).

COMORBIDITY

OCD is quite a distinctive illness which is characterized by obsessions and compulsions (Rasmussen and Tsuang, 1986). Some would say that its inclusion under the rubric of anxiety disorders is mistaken since these cardinal features are uncommonly found in other illnesses (Montgomery, 1993). Nonetheless, OCD is loosely associated with other conditions, particularly phobic disorders (Angst, 1993). Lifetime prevalence of depression is common, though OCD is most closely associated with agoraphobia and social phobia (Lucey et al., 1994). Primary phobic disorders are differential diagnosis of prime importance to exclude, though depression, dysthymia and generalized anxiety disorders do occur with some frequency (Swedo et al., 1989b; Angst and Wicki, 1992). Personality disorders are commonly associated with OCD, though to no greater extent than with other DSM-IV (1994) axis I disorders (Joffe et al., 1988; Black, 1993). Of 96 patients with OCD who were given the structured DSM-III personality disorder interview, over half (52%) fulfilled the criteria for an axis II disorder; mixed, histrionic and dependent being the most common subcategories (Baer and Minichiello, 1990). Surprisingly, only 6% had compulsive personality disorder. Whatever the reason for comorbidity, the presence of another diagnosis is of prognostic importance as these conditions are more severe, and have an increased risk of suicide (Angst, 1993).

PSYCHOSIS, INSIGHT AND RESISTANCE

Traditionally, two key features which have served to distinguish OCD from psychotic disorders are the absence of delusional intensity and the preservation of insight. However, many believe that OCD may lie along a psychopathological spectrum of insight with patients at the severe end having 'obsessive–compulsive psychosis' (Insel and Akiskal, 1986). Janet (1903) described over 300 patients with OCD, of which 8% had psychotic features (see also Pitman, 1984). Eisen and Rasmussen (1993) studied 475 patients with a DSM-IIIR diagnosis of OCD and found 16% to have psychotic symptoms. Psychotic features in 6% of these patients consisted of a lack of insight and an intense conviction about the reasonableness of their obsessions ('OCD without insight'). The remainder had hallucinations, delusions and/or thought disorder which met criteria for schizophrenia, delusional disorder and schizotypal personality disorder. A poor outcome was determined by the presence of 'frank psychosis' with these patients tending to be young, male and having a more degenerative course. The 'OCD without insight' group had a more benign course.

Maintenance of insight into OCD phenomena is frequently absent (Lewis, 1935) and is not a diagnostic requirement (APA, 1994). True OCD symptoms are subjectively unwelcome but often, only initially resisted. Only 50% of OCD patients had even moderate resistance to their compulsions (Stern and Cobb, 1978). Similarly, in 432 patients with DSM-IIIR OCD (Foa and Kozak, 1995) only 13% of patients were certain their feared consequence would not occur. Treatment-resistance patients must be screened for psychotic features and/or comorbid schizotypy, as symptom heterogeneity appears to be an integral part of OCD (Jenike et al., 1986). Some of these patients may require the addition of a dopamine antagonist to their serotonin (5HT) re-uptake inhibitor (McDougle et al., 1994).

NEUROLOGY AND OCD

Gross neurological abnormality is present in only a minority of OCD cases (Kettl and Marks, 1993). OCD has developed following head injury (Hillbom, 1960; Lishman, 1968; McKeon et al., 1984), birth injury (Capstick and Seldrup, 1977) and temporal lobe epilepsy (Kettl and Marks, 1986). Clinical syndromes involving striatal disease are associated with increased incidence of OCD symptoms; these include post-encephalitic Parkinson's disease (Von Economo, 1931) and Sydenham's chorea (Freeman et al., 1965; Swedo et al., 1989a). Discrete lesions of the basal ganglia are also associated with obsessive–compulsive phenomena (Laplane et al., 1984, 1989; Denckla, 1989; Tonkonogy and Barreira, 1989). However, most OCD patients do not have gross lesions of the basal ganglia (Kettl and Marks, 1986).

Forty medication-free patients with OCD were compared with 20 normal controls by a neurologist who was blind to their diagnostic status, using videotaped interviews (Hollander et al., 1990). Soft neurological signs, consisting of abnormalities of fine motor co-ordination, involuntary movements, sensory dysfunction and visuo-spatial errors appeared to occur with greater frequency in OCD than expected. Similar results were found in a study of 39 OCD patients,

43 healthy controls and 23 non-OCD anxiety disorder patients (Bihari et al., 1991). A preliminary study, awaiting replication, has shown that OCD patients with high scores on a soft-signs neurological investigation have increased ventricular volumes on computerized tomography (Stein et al., 1993). However, the evidence is growing that subtle neurological dysfunction is present in at least some OCD patients (Hollander et al., 1990; Bihari et al., 1991).

MOVEMENT DISORDERS

Symptoms of OCD can also occur in patients with Sydenham's chorea and Gilles de la Tourette's syndrome (Swedo and Leonard, 1994). The presence of chorea implies disease of the basal ganglia and the earliest case report of obsessional symptoms was by Chapman et al. (1953) who described eight children with rituals following an infection. Swedo et al. (1989a) report on 23 children with Sydenham's chorea of which three developed obsessional phenomena. Movement disorders arising from other striatal diseases are also associated with increased incidence of OCD symptoms (Von Economo, 1931; Swedo et al., 1989a; Laplane et al., 1984, 1989; Denckla, 1989; Tonkonogy and Barreira, 1989).

Gilles de la Tourette's syndrome (GTS) is a related chronic neuropsychiatric disorder with clinical and, possible, genetic links to OCD (Pauls et al., 1986). The onset of GTS is in childhood and is characterized by motor and phonic tics which wax and wane in intensity. Nearly 70% of GTS patients have interfering obsessive–compulsive symptoms (Pauls et al., 1986; Pitman et al., 1987). OCD is prevalent in between 7% (Pitman et al., 1987) and 23% (Pauls et al., 1986) of first-degree relatives of GTS probands. In some OCD samples, 6% meet criteria for GTS (Pitman et al., 1987). The association between OCD and tics is also long established (Schilder, 1938; Grimshaw, 1964; Inouye, 1965; Green and Pitman, 1986). Tics are repetitive, involuntary, motor actions. Unlike compulsions, they are not designed to produce or prevent some dreaded situation. Tics are purposeless and prevalent in up to 38% of OCD patients (Pitman et al., 1987). In our study of 50 OCD outpatients, GTS was rare ($N=1$), but tics were common (Lucey et al., 1994). It may be that specific forms of OCD, GTS or tic-spectrum disorder are genetically related (McDougle et al., 1994; Pauls et al., 1995).

GENETICS

Evidence for a genetic influence in the pathogenesis of OCD exists, as monozygotic concordance rates of between 53% and 87% have been reported (Rasmussen and Tsuang, 1986; Carey and Gottesman, 1981). Others have suggested that there is a general genetic predisposition to develop anxiety disorders as opposed to any vulnerability specific for OCD (Torgerson, 1983; Andrews et al., 1990). Interpretation of genetic data best fits a non-specific neurotic syndrome in keeping with Janet's (1903) original observations on the neuroses (Andrews et al., 1990). However, methodological differences between the various studies mentioned make them impossible to compare.

Pauls et al. (1995) have determined the rates of OCD and movement disorders in patients and their first-degree relatives and have provided further evidence that OCD is a heterogeneous condition. On examining 466 relatives of 100 probands with OCD and healthy volunteers, Pauls et al. (1995) found that the rates of index illness were higher in affected (10.3%) versus healthy individuals (2%). Furthermore, the prevalence of tics (Tourette's syndrome and chronic tics) was greater in relatives of OCD patients (4.6%) than comparison subjects (1%). Relatives of female probands were more likely to have OCD and early onset increased the likelihood of OCD and tics (Pauls et al., 1995). Therefore, some cases are familial and associated with tics, others are familial and not associated with tics and a third group has neither a family history of OCD nor movement disorders.

NEUROIMAGING STUDIES

Luxenberg et al. (1988) undertook a computerized tomography (CT) scan study of childhood onset OCD. Ten male patients with a long duration of illness underwent a quantitative volumetric analysis of their CT scans. The patients had significantly smaller caudate nuclei bilaterally than did healthy controls. Such a gross structural abnormality in the basal ganglia of male patients with early onset OCD is intriguing. Baxter and his colleagues at the University of California have conducted a series of positron emission tomography (PET) studies in patients with OCD. In the first of these (Baxter et al., 1987), 14 patients with OCD were shown to have significantly increased metabolic rates in the left orbital gyrus and bilaterally in the caudate nuclei in comparison with a group of 14 normal controls and 14 unipolar depressives. In a related PET scan study, in which earlier criticisms of the heterogeneity of the patient population were addressed, Baxter et al. (1988) found increased metabolic rates in the left orbital gyrus and bilaterally in the caudate nuclei.

Swedo et al. (1992) working at the National Institute of Mental Health (NIMH) undertook a similar PET scan investigation of childhood-onset OCD. Eighteen patients with severe OCD were included. Nine of these had a lifetime history of major depression but none were currently depressed. They found a trend towards increased metabolism in the caudate nuclei with significant increases in metabolic rates in frontal regions. The regions included the prefrontal area bilaterally, the left orbital frontal, the left premotor and right sensorimotor. Increased metabolism in the anterior cingulate gyri bilaterally was also noted.

The French study of Martinot et al. (1990) reported global grey matter hypometabolism and prefrontal lateral cortex hypometabolism. The patients were more chronically disabled than those in the previous studies and the glucose utilization in the controls was higher than in the American studies. There were also methodological differences in relation to the extent of sensory stimulation during the studies. In the NIMH study, patients had their eyes closed and ears plugged. The latter was not carried out in the French study. It may be that glucose utilization is acutely increased but chronically decreased in OCD.

Swedo et al. (1992) observed that pharmacotherapy in patients with OCD resulted in a decrease in right orbitofrontal metabolism which correlated with two measures of improvement as determined by various rating scales. In a similar study, Baxter et al. (1992) found that post-treatment levels of glucose metabolism were significantly reduced in the head of the right caudate nucleus in those who had responded to either behaviour therapy or drug therapy. Percentage changes in obsessive–compulsive disorder symptom scores positively correlated with the decreased local cerebral activity.

Rauch et al. (1994) used oxygen-15-labelled carbon dioxide, a short half-life tracer, to allow for repeated PET determinations of regional blood flow on each of eight subjects with OCD, during a resting or a provoked state. Individually tailored provocative stimuli were used to provoke symptoms. Omnibus subtraction of images demonstrated a statistically significant increase in relative regional cerebral blood flow during the OCD symptomatic state versus the resting state in the right caudate nucleus, left anterior cingulate cortex with a trend towards increase in the left thalamus. McGuire et al. (1994) using PET scanning also demonstrated that there was a graded relationship between the intensity of induced urges to ritualize and regional cerebral blood flow.

Magnetic resonance imaging (MRI) scan abnormalities have been described in the orbital frontal cortex, cingulate gyrus and lenticular nuclei (Garber et al., 1989). Thirty-two patients, 19 of whom were taking clomipramine, were investigated. Although no gross structural abnormalities were detected, the spin lattice relaxation time (T1) was prolonged in the above regions. The authors conclude that their findings are largely in agreement with the PET findings. Kellner et al. (1991) compared various brain regions, including the head of the caudate nucleus and corpus callosum and found no consistent differences between controls and those with OCD. Calabrese et al. (1993) also using MRI found higher signal intensity in the left caudate nucleus compared with the right. No asymmetry was found in the control group. Contrary to the previous research cited, Robinson et al. (1995) found that patients with OCD had significantly smaller caudate nuclei than control subjects. However, there was no correlation between actual volume and the severity/duration of symptoms. Likewise, single photon emission computerized tomography (SPECT) scanning studies using 99mTc-exametazine (99mTc-HMPAO) show reduced perfusion in the basal ganglia of patients with OCD as opposed to controls (Rubin et al., 1992; Lucey et al., 1995; Edmonstone et al., 1994; Adams et al., 1993). Despite varying methodologies, a large number of neuroimaging studies support the view that there are abnormalities in OCD orbital frontal regions and in the basal ganglia.

NEUROENDOCRINE STUDIES

There are now numerous published papers on the neuroendocrinology of OCD (Table 3.1). Overall these studies indicate that 5HT receptor systems are dysfunctional in OCD. The release of prolactin from the anterior pituitary is under serotoninergic control (Preziosi, 1983). D-Fenfluramine, which brings about a release and prevents the uptake of 5HT, stimulates prolactin release in healthy controls. There is blunting of this release mechanism in patients with OCD (Lucey et al., 1992a). Hollander et al. (1992) found that PRL responses to m-CPP were blunted, though the same was not true in response to the racemic mixture of fenfluramine (60 mg); conclusions are difficult to

Table 3.1   Summary of endocrine stimulation tests in obsessive–
compulsive disorder

Hormone	Probe	Result	Investigators
Cortisol	Dexamethasone	Normal	Monteiro et al. (1986)
Cortisol	mCPP	Blunted	Zohar et al. (1987)
Cortisol	mCPP	Normal	Charney et al. (1988)
Prolactin	MK212	Blunted	Bastani et al. (1990)
Prolactin	D-Fenfluramine	Blunted	Lucey et al. (1992a)
Prolactin	Buspirone	Normal	Lucey et al. (1992b)
Prolactin	L-Tryptophan	Blunted	Montgomery et al. (1992)
Prolactin	mCPP	Blunted	Hollander et al. (1992)
Prolactin	D,L-Fenfluramine	Normal	Hollander et al. (1992)
Prolactin	D,L-Fenfluramine	Blunted	Hewlett et al. (1992)
Growth hormone	Clonidine	Blunted	Siever et al. (1983)
Growth hormone	Clonidine	Normal	Lee et al. (1990)
Growth hormone	Desipramine	Normal	Lucey et al. (1992c)
Growth hormone	Pyridostigmine	Enhanced	Lucey et al. (1993b)
ACTH	CRF	Blunted	Bailly et al. (1994)
ACTH/cortisol	Ipsapirone	Normal	Lesch et al. (1991)
ACTH/cortisol	Buspirone	Normal	Norman et al. (1994)

draw from this study as neither of these agents are specific for the serotonergic system. Yet, Hewlett et al. (1992) using the same dose of fenfluramine as Hollander et al. (1992), observed that PRL responses were blunted in comparison with control subjects.

Abnormal cortisol responses following challenge with mCPP and MK212, the 5HT agonists, have also been reported (Zohar et al., 1987; Charney et al., 1988; Bastani et al., 1990). The data support the view that there is 5HT receptor subsensitivity rather than an abnormality at a pituitary level. When Lucey et al. (1993a) stimulated prolactin release with thyroid-releasing hormone (TRH), which acts directly on the pituitary, normal responses were seen. Two separate studies examined the function of 5HT1A receptors in OCD. Buspirone- and ipsapirone-induced corticotropin and cortisol release were no different between controls and those with OCD (Lesch et al., 1991; Lucey et al., 1992b; Norman et al., 1994). Together these studies indicate that serotonergic dysfunction may lie at a receptor other than the 5HT1A binding site.

Adolescents presenting with OCD are shorter and weigh less than their disease-free male counterparts (Hamburger et al., 1989). Lucey et al. (1992c, 1993b) have used a variety of somatotropic probes in order to explore potential growth hormone (GH) pathophysiology in OCD. GH plasma levels reflect a balance between the antagonistic actions of GH-releasing hormone (GHRH) and somatostatin (SS) (Dieguez et al., 1988). In turn these hypothalamic neuropeptides are under the influence of various neurotransmitters. Stimulation of GH secretion in response to noradrenergic probes probably occurs via GHRH (Katakami et al., 1984) while cholinergic-induced release of GH may occur via inhibition of SS secretion (Penalva et al., 1990).

Lucey et al. (1992c) found normal GH release in response to nor-adrenergic challenge. Administration of pyridostigmine, a potent inhibitor of SS secretion, led to augmented GH release in patients with OCD as opposed to controls (Lucey et al., 1993b). This may be due either to enhanced cholinergic receptor sensitivity or enhanced SS tone (Lucey et al., 1993b). The latter might explain the stunted growth patterns and is supported by the fact that OCD patients have increased SS levels in their cerebrospinal fluid. When such enhanced SS tone is reduced with pyridostigmine, robust GH release takes place.

Other neuroendocrine disturbances have also recently been reported, including disturbance of the hypothalamic-pituitary-adrenal axis with altered release of ACTH in response to intravenous injection of the hypothalamic peptide, corticotropin-releasing hormone (CRH) (Bailly et al., 1994). As in the case of depressed patients, subjects with OCD show impaired ACTH release. This abnormality was reported in the absence of elevated cortisol, and suggests an abnormality in central release mechanisms, rather than in feedback control.

An intriguing hypothesis, regarding the role of oxytocin, has been put forward by Leckman et al. (1994) who examined various posterior pituitary hormone levels in the CSF of patients with OCD and of healthy controls. Oxytocin-containing neurones not only project to the posterior pituitary, but also from the paraventricular nucleus of the hypothalamus to limbic structures and to midbrain regions such as the locus coeruleus (possibly the largest condensation of nor-adrenergic cell bodies) (Wagner and Clemens, 1993). The ritualistic handwashing one sees in OCD could be considered to be a behav-ioural correlate of grooming which occurs in response to oxytocin. A total of 29 patients with OCD, 23 patients with Tourette's syndrome and 31 normal controls were included in the study. Oxytocin levels were significantly increased in those patients with OCD but without a personal or family history of tic disorder. A strong correlation was established between oxytocin levels and severity of symptoms and between oxytocin levels and the main 5HT metabolite 5HIAA. The study provides evidence to implicate both oxytocin and 5HT in the aetiology of the disorder.

CONCLUSIONS

The prevalence of OCD is still a controversial issue. Evidence indicates that it occurs more frequently than previously thought, though issues regarding its natural history are still contested. OCD appears to be a common heterogeneous and neuropsychiatric disorder. Future OCD research needs to adhere to operational illness definitions, with well-defined clinical subgroups. Neuroimaging and neuroendocrine investigations lend credibility to the notion that OCD has a biological basis. This change in perspective must rank as one of the most important paradigm shifts to take place in psychiatric practice in recent times.

References

Adams, B.L., Warneke, L.K., McEewan, A.J. et al. (1993) Single photon emission tomography in obsessive compulsive disorder: a preliminary study. *Journal of Psychiatry and Neuroscience* **18**: 109–112.

American Psychiatric Association (1994) *Diagnostic and Statistical Manual of Mental disorders*, 4th edn (DSM-IV). Washington, DC: APA.

Andrews, G, Stewart, G., Allen, R. et al. (1990) Evidence for a general neurotic syndrome. *British Journal of Psychiatry* **157**: 6–12.

Angst, J. (1993) Co-morbidity of anxiety, phobia, compulsion and depression. *International Clinical Psychopharmacology* **8** (Suppl): 21–25.

Angst, J., Wicki, W. (1992) The Zurich study. XIII. Recurrent brief anxiety. *European Archives of Psychiatry and Clinical Neuroscience* **241**: 296–300.

Angst, J., Dobler-Mikola, A., Binder, J. (1984) The Zurich study: a prospective epidemiological study of depressive, neurotic and psychosomatic syndromes. *European Archives of Psychiatry and Neurological Science* **234**: 13–20.

Baer, L. (1994) Factor analysis of symptom subtypes of obsessive compulsive disorder and their relation to personality and tic disorders. *Journal of Clinical Psychiatry* **55** (Suppl): 18–23.

Baer, L., Minichiello, W.E. (1990) Behaviour therapy for obsessive compulsive disorder. In Jenike, M.A., Baer, L., Minichiello, W.E. (eds) *Obsessive Compulsive Disorders: Theory and Management*, pp. 203–232. Chicago, Illinois: Year Book.

Baer, L., Janike, M.A., Ricciardi, J.N. et al. (1990) Standardised assessment of personality disorders in obsessive–compulsive disorder. *Archives of General Psychiatry* **47**: 826–830.

Bailly, D., Servant, D., Dewailly, D. et al. (1994) Corticotropin releasing factor stimulation test in obsessive compulsive disorder. *Biological Psychiatry* **35**: 143–146.

Bastani, B., Nash, J.F., Meltzer, H.Y. (1990) Prolactin and cortisol responses to MK-212, a serotonin agonist in obsessive compulsive disorder. *Archives of General Psychiatry* **47**: 833–839.

Baxter, L.R., Phelps, M.E., Mazziotta, J.C. et al. (1987) Local cerebral glucose metabolic rates in obsessive compulsive disorder. *Archives of General Psychiatry* **44**: 211–218.

Baxter, L.R., Schwartz, J.M., Mazziotta, J.C. et al. (1988) Cerebral glucose metabolic rates in non-depressive-obsessive-compulsive disorder. *American Journal of Psychiatry* **145**: 1560–1563.

Baxter, L.R., Schwartz, J.M., Mazziotta, J.C. et al. (1989) Reduction of prefrontal cortex glucose metabolism common to three types of depression. *Archives of General Psychiatry* **46**: 243–250.

Baxter, L.R., Schwartz, J.M., Bergman, K.S. et al. (1992) Caudate nucleus metabolic rate changes with both drug and behaviour therapy in obsessive compulsive disorder. *Archives of General Psychiatry* **49**: 681–689.

Bihari, K., Pato, M.T., Hill, J.L. et al. (1991) Neurological soft-signs in obsessive compulsive disorder. *Archives of General Psychiatry* **48**: 278–279.

Black, A. (1974) The natural history of obsessional neurosis. In Beech, H.R. (ed.) *Obsessional States*, pp. 19–54. London: Methuen.

Black, D.W., Noyes, R., Bfohl, B. et al. (1993) Personality disorders amongst obsessive compulsive volunteers, well comparison subjects, and their first degree relatives. *American Journal of Psychiatry* **150**: 1226–1232.

Calabrese, G., Colombo, C., Bonfanti, A. et al. (1993) Caudate nucleus abnormalities in obsessive-compulsive disorder: measurements of MRI signal intensity. *Psychiatry Research* **50**: 89–92.

Capstick, N., Seldrup, J. (1977) Obsessional states: a study of the relationship between abnormalities occurring at birth and the subsequent development of obsessional symptoms. *Acta Psychiatrica Scandinavia* **56**: 427–431.

Carey, G., Gottesman, I. (1981) Twin and familial aspects of anxiety, phobic and obsessive disorders. In Klein, D.F., Rabkin, J. (eds) *Anxiety: New Research and Changing Concepts*. New York: Raven Press.

Chapman, A.H., Pilkey, L., Gibbons, M.J. (1953) A psychosomatic study of eight children with Sydenham's chorea. *Paediatrics* **21**: 582–595.

Charney, D.S., Goodman, W.K., Price, L.H. et al. (1988) Obsessive compulsive disorder: a comparison of the effects of tryptophan and *m*-chlorophenyl-piperazine in patients and healthy subjects. *Archives of General Psychiatry* **45**: 177–185.

Degonda, M., Wyss, M., Angst, J. (1993) The Zurich study: XVIII. Obsessive compulsive disorders and syndromes in the general population. *European Archives of Psychiatry and Clinical Neuroscience* **243**: 16–22.

Denckla, M.B. (1989) The neurological examination. In Rappoport, J.L. (ed.) *Obsessive-Compulsive Disorder in Children and Adolescents*, pp. 107–118. Washington DC: American Psychiatric Press.

Dieguez, C., Page M.D., Scanlon, M.F. (1988) Growth hormone neuroregulation and its alterations in disease states. *Clinical Endocrinology* **28**: 109–143.

Edmonstone, Y., Austin, M.P., Prentice, N. et al. (1994) Uptake of 99mTc-exametazime shown by single photon emission computerized tomography in obsessive compulsive disorder compared with major depression and normal controls. *Acta Psychiatrica Scandinavia* **90**: 298–303.

Eisen, J.L., Rasmussen, S.A. (1993) Obsessive compulsive disorder with psychotic features. *Journal of Clinical Psychiatry* **54**: 373–379.

Esquirol, J.E.D. (1838) *Des Maladies Mentals Considérées sous les Rapports Médicals, Hygiéneques et Médico-legals*, Vol 1. Paris: Baillière.

Fichter, M.M. (1990) *Verlauf psychischer Erkränkungen in der Bevölkerung.* Berlin: Springer.

Foa, E.B., Kozak, M.J. (1995) DSM-IV field trial: obsessive-compulsive disorder. *American Journal of Psychiatry* **152**: 90–96.

Freeman, J., Aron, A., Collard, J. et al. (1965) The emotional correlates of Sydenham's chorea. *Paediatrics* **35**: 42–49.

Freud, S. (1924) Obsessions and phobias: their psychological mechanisms and their aetiology. In *Collected Papers* 1. pp. 153–154. London: Hogarth Press.

Garber, H.J., Ananth, J.V., Chiu, L.C. et al. (1989) Nuclear magnetic resonance study of obsessive compulsive disorder. *American Journal of Psychiatry* **146**: 1001–1005.

Green, R.C., Pitman, P.K. (1986) Tourette syndrome and obsessive compulsive disorder. In Jenike, M.A., Baer, L., Minichello, W.E. (eds) *Obsessive Compulsive Disorders: Theory and Management*. Littleton Massachusetts: PSG.

Griest, J.H., Jefferson, J.W., Kobak, K. et al. (1995) Efficacy and tolerability of serotonin transport inhibitors in obsessive-compulsive disorder. *Archives of General Psychiatry* **52**: 53–60.

Grimshaw, L. (1964) Obsessional disorders and neurological illness. *Journal of Neurology, Neurosurgery and Psychiatry* **27**: 229–231.

Hamburger, S.D., Suedo, S., Whitaker, A. et al. (1989) Growth rate in adolescents with obsessive–compulsive disorder. *American Journal of Psychiatry* **146**: 652–655.

Hewlett, W.A., Vinogradov, S., Martin, K. et al. (1992) Fenfluramine stimulation of prolactin in obsessive compulsive disorder. *Psychiatry Research* **42**: 81–92.

Hillbom, E. (1960) After effects of brain injuries. *Acta Psychiatrica et Neurologica Scandinavia* **35** (Suppl 142): 125.

Hollander, E., Schiffman, E., Cohen, B. et al. (1990) Signs of central nervous system dysfunction in obsessive compulsive disorder. *Archives of General Psychiatry* **47**: 37–42.

Hollander, E., DeCaria, C.M., Nitescu, A. et al. (1992) Serotonergic function in obsessive compulsive disorder. Behavioural and neuroendocrine responses to oral *m*-chlorophenylpiperazine and fenfluramine in patients and healthy volunteers. *Archives of General Psychiatry* **49**: 21–28.

Inouye, E. (1965) Similar and dissimilar manifestations of obsessive compulsive neurosis in monozygotic twins. *American Journal of Psychiatry* **121**: 1171–1175.

Insel, T.R., Akiskal, H.S. (1986) Obsessive-compulsive disorder with psychotic features: a phenomenological analysis. *American Journal of Psychiatry* **143**: 1527–1533.

Janet, P. (1903) *Les Obsessions et la Psychasthenie*, Vol 1. Paris: Alcan. (Reprinted New York 1976.)

Jenike, M.A., Baer, L., Minichiello, W.E. et al. (1986) Co-existent obsessive-compulsive disorder and schizotypal personality disorder: a poor prognostic indicator. *Archives of General Psychiatry* **43**: 296.

Joffe, R.T., Swinson, R.P., Regan, J.J. (1988) Personality features of obsessive compulsive disorder. *American Journal of Psychiatry* **145**: 1127–1129.

Karno, M., Golding, J.M., Sorenson, S.B. et al. (1988) The epidemiology of obsessive compulsive disorder in five US communities. *Archives of General Psychiatry* **45**: 1094–1099.

Katakami, H., Kato, Y., Matsushita, N. et al. (1984) Effects of neonatal treatment with monosodium glutamate on growth hormone release induced by clonidine and prostaglandin E in conscious male rats. *Neuroendocrinology* **38**: 1–5.

Kellner, C.H., Jolley, R.R., Holgate, R.C. et al. (1991) Brain MRI in obsessive compulsive disorder. *Psychiatry Research* **36**: 45–49.

Kettl, P.A., Marks, I.M. (1986) Neurological factors in obsessive compulsive disorder; two case reports and a review of the disorder. *British Journal of Psychiatry* **149**: 315–319.

Khanna, S., Kaliaperumal, V.G., Channabasavanna, S.M. (1990) Clusters of obsessive compulsive phenomena in obsessive compulsive disorder. *British Journal of Psychiatry* **156**: 51–54.

Laplane, D., Baulac, M., Widlocher, D. et al. (1984) Pure psychic akinesia with bilateral lesions of the basal ganglia. *Journal of Neurology, Neurosurgery and Psychiatry* **47**: 377–385.

Laplane, D., Levasseur, M., Pilloni, B. et al. (1989) Obsessive compulsive and behavioural changes with bilateral basal ganglia lesions. *Brain* **112**: 649–725.

Leckman, J.F., Goodman, W.K., North, W.G. et al. (1994) The role of central oxytocin in obsessive compulsive disorder and related normal behaviour. *Psychoneuroendocrinology* **19**: 723–749.

Lee, M.A., Cameron, O.G., Guirguis, G.N.M. et al. (1990) Alpha-2 adrenoceptor status in obsessive-compulsive disorder. *Biological Psychiatry* **27**: 1083–1093.

Lesch, K-P., Hoh, A., Disselkamp-Tietze, J. et al. (1991) 5-Hydroxytryptamine1A receptor sensitivity in obsessive compulsive disorder: a comparison of patients and controls. *Archives of General Psychiatry* **48**: 540–547.

Lewis, A. (1935) Problems of obsessional illness. *Proceedings of The Royal Society of Medicine* **29**: 325–326.

Lishman, W.A. (1968) Brain damage in relation to psychiatric disability after head injury. *British Journal of Psychiatry* **114**: 373–410.

Lucey, J.V., O'Keane, V., Butcher, G. et al. (1992a) Cortisol and prolactin responses to d-fenfluramine in non-depressed patients with obsessive compulsive disorder. A comparison with depressed and healthy controls. *British Journal of Psychiatry* **161**: 517–522.

Lucey, J.V., Butcher, G., Clare, A.W. et al. (1992b) Buspirone/prolactin responses in obsessive compulsive disorder: is OCD a $5HT_2$ receptor disorder? *International Clinical Pharmacology* **7**: 45–51.

Lucey, J.V., Barry, S., Webb, M.G. et al. (1992c) Normal alpha-2 nor-adrenergically mediated growth hormone response to desipramine in obsessive-compulsive disorder: further support for the serotonergic theory of OCD? *Acta Psychiatrica Scandinavia* **86**: 367–371.

Lucey, J.V., Butcher, G., Clare, A.W. et al. (1993a) The anterior pituitary responds normally to protirelin in obsessive-compulsive disorder: evidence to support a neuroendocrine serotonergic deficit. *Acta Psychiatrica Scandinavia* **87**: 384–388.

Lucey, J.V., Clare, A.W., Dinan, T.G. (1993b) Elevated growth hormone responses to pyridostigmine in obsessive compulsive disorder: evidence for cholinergic dysfunction. *American Journal of Psychiatry* **150**: 961–963.

Lucey, J.V., Butcher, G., Clare, A.W. et al. (1994) The clinical characteristics of a patient with obsessive compulsive disorder: a descriptive study of an Irish sample. *Irish Journal of Psychological Medicine* **11**: 11–14.

Lucey, J.V., Costa, D.C., Blanes, T. et al. (1995) Regional cerebral blood flow in obsessive–compulsive disordered patients at rest: different correlates with obsessive–compulsive and anxious avoidant dimensions. *British Journal of Psychiatry* **167**: 629–634.

Luxenberg, J.S., Swedo, S.E., Flament, F. et al. (1988) Neuroanatomical abnormalities in obsessive compulsive disorder detected with quantitative x-ray computed tomography. *American Journal of Psychiatry* **145**: 1089–1093.

Marks I.M. (ed.) (1987) *Fears, Phobias and Rituals: Panic Anxiety and Their Disorders*, pp. 423–453. Oxford: Oxford University Press.

Marks, I.M., O'Sullivan, G. (1988) Drugs and psychological treatments for agoraphobia/panic and obsessive compulsive disorders: a review. *British Journal of Psychiatry* **153**: 650–658.

Martinot, J.L., Allilaire, J.F., Huret, J.D. et al. (1990) Obsessive compulsive disorder: a clinical, neuropsychological and PET study. *Journal of Cerebral Blood Flow and Metabolism* **9** (Suppl 1): S588.

McDougle, C.J., Goodman, W.K., Price, L.H. et al. (1990) Neuroleptic addition in fluvoxamine-refractory obsessive-compulsive disorder. *American Journal of Psychiatry* **147**: 652–654.

McDougle, C.J., Goodman, W.K., Price, L.H. (1994) Dopamine antagonists in tic-related and psychotic spectrum obsessive compulsive disorder. *Journal of Clinical Psychiatry* **55** (Suppl 3): 24–31.

McGuire, P.K., Bench, C.J., Frith, C.D. et al. (1994) Functional anatomy of obsessive compulsive disorder. *British Journal of Psychiatry* **164**: 459–468.

McKeon, J., McGuffin, P., Robinson, P. (1984) Obsessive compulsive neurosis following head injury – a report of four cases. *British Journal of Psychiatry* **144**: 190–192.

Monteiro, W., Marks, I.M., Noshirvani, H. et al. (1986) Normal dexamethasone suppression test in obsessive compulsive disorder. *British Journal of Psychiatry* **148**: 326–329.

Montgomery, S.A. (1993) Obsessive compulsive disorder is not an anxiety disorder. *International Clinical Psychopharmacology* **8**: 57–62.

Montgomery, S.A., Fineberg, N., Montgomery, D. et al. (1992) L-Tryptophan in obsessive compulsive disorder: a placebo controlled study. *European Neuropsychopharmacology* **2**: 384–385.

Norman, T.R., Apostolopoulos, A., Burrows, G.D. et al. (1994) Neuroendocrine responses to single doses of buspirone in obsessive compulsive disorder. *International Clinical Psychopharmacology* **9**: 89–94.

Noshirvani, H.F., Kasvikis, Y.G., Tsakiris, F. et al. (1986) Demographic characteristics of 280 cases of obsessive-compulsive disorder. In Marks, I.M. (ed.) *Fears, Phobias and Rituals: Panic Anxiety and their disorders*, pp. 423–453. Oxford: University Press.

Noshirvani, H.F., Kasvikis, Y., Marks, I.M. et al. (1991) Gender divergent aetiological factors in obsessive compulsive disorder. *British Journal of Psychiatry* **158**: 260–263.

Pauls, D.L., Towbin, K.E., Leckman, J.F. et al. (1986) Gilles de la Tourette's syndrome and obsessive compulsive disorder. *Archives of General Psychiatry* **43**: 1180–1182.

Pauls, D.L., Alsobrook, J.P., Goodman, W. et al. (1995) A family study of obsessive–compulsive disorder. *American Journal of Psychiatry* **152**: 76–84.

Penalva, A., Muruais, C., Casanueva F.F. et al. (1990) Effect of enhancement of endogenous cholinergic tone with pyridostigmine on the dose–response relationships of growth hormone (GH) releasing hormone-induced GH secretion in normal subjects. *Journal of Clinical Endocrinology and Metabolism* **70**: 324–327.

Pitman, R.K. (1984) Janet's obsessions and psychaesthenia: a synopsis. *Psychiatric Quarterly* **56**: 291–315.

Pitman, R.K., Green, R.C., Jenike, M.A. et al. (1987) Clinical comparison of Tourette's disorder with obsessive–compulsive disorder. *American Journal of Psychiatry* **144**: 1166–1171.

Pollit, J. (1957) Natural history of obsessional states. *British Medical Journal* **1**: 194–198.

Preziosi, P. (1983) Serotonin control of prolactin release: an intriguing puzzle. *Trends in Pharmacological Sciences* **4**: 171–174.

Rasmussen, S.A., Tsuang, M.T. (1986) Epidemiology and clinical features of obsessive compulsive disorder. In Jenike, M.A., Baer, L., Minichiello, W.E. (eds) *Obsessive Compulsive Disorders*, pp. 23–44. Littleton, Massachusetts: PSG Publishing Company.

Rauch, S.L., Jenike, M.A., Alpert, N.M. et al. (1994) Regional cerebral blood flow measured during symptom provocation in obsessive compulsive disorder using oxygen 15-labelled carbon dioxide and positron emission tomography. *Archives of General Psychiatry* **51**: 62–70.

Robinson, D., Wu, H., Munne, R.A. et al. (1995) Reduced caudate nucleus volume in obsessive compulsive disorder. *Archives of General Psychiatry* **52**: 393–398.

Rubin, R.T., Villanvera-Meyer, J., Ananth, J. et al. (1992) Regional xenon 133 cerebral blood flow and cerebral technetium 99m HMPAO uptake in unmedicated patients with obsessive–compulsive disorder and matched normal control subjects. *Archives of General Psychiatry* **49**: 695–702.

Rudin, E., Beitrag, Z.U. (1953) Frage der Zwangskrankheit insbesondere inheritaren Beiziechunger. *Archiv für Psychiatrie und Nervenkrankheiten* **191**: 14–54.

Schilder, P. (1938) The organic background of obsessions and compulsions. *American Journal of Psychiatry* **94**: 1397–1416.

Siever, L.J., Insel, T.R., Jimerson, D.C. et al. (1983) Growth hormone response to clonidine in obsessive–compulsive disorder. *British Journal of Psychiatry* **142**: 184–187.

Stein, D.J., Hollander, E., Chan, S. (1993) Computed tomography and neurological soft signs in obsessive compulsive disorder. *Psychiatry Research Neuroimaging* **50**: 143–150.

Stern, R.S., Cobb, J.P. (1978) Phenomenology of obsessive compulsive neurosis. *British Journal of Psychiatry* **132**: 233–239.

Swedo, S.E., Rappoport, J.L., Cheslow, D.L. et al. (1989a) High prevalence of obsessive compulsive symptoms in patients with Sydenham's chorea. *American Journal of Psychiatry* **146**: 246–249.

Swedo, S.E., Rappoport, J.L., Leonard, H. et al. (1989b) Obsessive compulsive disorder in children and adolescents: clinical phenomenology of 70 cases. *Archives of General Psychiatry* **46**: 335–341.

Swedo, S.E., Pietrini, P., Leonard, H.L. et al. (1992) Cerebral glucose metabolism in childhood-onset obsessive compulsive disorder: revisualisation during pharmacotherapy. *Archives of General Psychiatry* **49**: 690–694.

Swedo, S.E., Leonard, H.L. (1994) Childhood movement disorders and obsessive compulsive disorder. *Journal of Clinical Psychiatry* **55** (Suppl): 32–37.

Tonkonogy, J., Barreira, P. (1989) Obsessive-compulsive disorder and caudate-frontal lesion. *Neuropsychiatry, Neuropsychology and Behavioural Neurology* **2**: 203–209.

Torgerson, S. (1983) Genetic factors in anxiety disorder. *Archives of General Psychiatry* **40**: 1085–1089.

Von Economo, C. (1931) *Encephalitis Lethargic: Its Sequelae and Treatment*. Oxford: Oxford University Press.

Wagner, C.K., Clemens, L.G. (1993) Neurophysin-containing pathway from the paraventricular nucleus of the hypothalamus to a sexually dimorphic nucleus in the lumbar spinal cord. *Journal of Comparative Neurology* **336**: 106–116.

Weissman, M.M., Bland, R., Canino, G.J. et al. (1994) The cross national epidemiology of obsessive compulsive disorder. *Journal of Clinical Psychiatry* **55** (Suppl): 5–10.

Westphal, C. (1878) Dwangforstellungen. *Archiv Psychiatrie und Nervenkrankheiten* **8**: 734–750.

World Health Organisation (1992) The ICD-10 Classification of Mental and Behavioural Disorders: clinical description and diagnostic guidelines, pp. 132–173. Geneva: World Health Organisation.

Yaryura-Tobias, J.A., Neziroglu, F.A. (1983) *Obsessive Compulsive Disorders: Pathogenesis – Diagnosis – Treatment*. Basel: Marcel Dekker.

Zohar, J., Mueller, E.A., Insel, T.R. et al. (1987) Serotonergic responsivity in obsessive–compulsive disorder. Comparison with healthy controls. *Archives of General Psychiatry* **44**: 948–951.

4

Psychiatric Disorders in Women

Uriel Halbreich

THE PREVALENCE OF SPECIFIC MENTAL DISORDERS IN WOMEN

Several dysphoric disorders have been found to be more prevalent among women compared to men (Robins and Regier, 1992; Regier et al., 1988; Robins et al., 1992). This gender difference is apparent worldwide and mostly so during reproductive age (Weissman and Olfson, 1995; Wolk and Weissman, 1995). Most prominently, gender differences occur in major depressive disorder (MDD), the prevalence of which was quite consistently found to show a 2:1 female-to-male ratio (Weissman et al., 1987, 1993; Kessler et al., 1993). However, several other dysphoric disorders are more prevalent in women as well (Hamilton and Halbreich, 1993), including 'atypical depression' (with increased sleep and appetite, decreased energy, hostility and sensitivity to rejection), anxious depression (Van Valkenburg et al., 1984), seasonal affective disorder (SAD) (Parry, 1989), rapid cycling mood in response to treatment with tricyclic antidepressants and probably other depressive spectrum disorders, as well as panic disorders and other anxiety disorders.

The predominance of some depressions in women is associated with a higher ratio of prescriptions of antidepressants to women (Baum et al., 1988) which introduces an array of other factors to the equation. Women differ from men in pharmacokinetics of many drugs, treatment outcome, time-to-response, and side-effects (reviews: Hamilton and Halbreich, 1993; Jensvold et al., 1996). This aspect, which will be addressed later, underscores the utmost necessity to consider gender differences in research trials, as well as in a day-to-day clinical practice. The processes that might contribute to the high prevalence of dysphoric disorders in women will be discussed in a later section. However, it should be emphasized that gender differences are not limited to depression, they have been demonstrated in schizophrenia and response to antipsychotic medications as well as their side-effects (Jensvold et al., 1996). Gender differences in neurostructural autoimmune disorders (e.g. multiple sclerosis, systemic lupus erythematosus) and their mood and behaviour manifestations (Halbreich, 1994), sensitivity to alcohol couples with lower rates of alcohol abuse (Robins and Regier, 1992) as well as some other disorders were also demonstrated.

In addition to the higher prevalence of several mental disorders in women compared to men, there is a group of female-specific disorders which include menstrually related disorders (mostly premenstrual dysphoric disorder), peripartum disorders, motherhood stress, menopause and peri-menopause related dysphorias, side-effects of contraceptive pills and gonadal hormones, and stress-related amenorrhoea, just to mention a few. The pathobiology of these situations might suggest several common biological processes that might contribute to the higher vulnerability to, and higher prevalence of, affective disorders in women.

PSYCHOSOCIAL AND IDEOLOGICAL ASPECTS

Even though the emphasis in the current chapter is on a biomedical model, the psychosocial aspects of dysphoric states in women cannot be ignored. Regretfully, the weight of psychosocial factors as contributing to the higher prevalence of diagnosis of depression in women is more aggressively promoted by people with well-defined political agendas, which sometimes obscures the issues.

The social contribution to depression as well as the different emphases given by different professionals can be demonstrated by the conclusion drawn by some (e.g. Brown and Harris, 1978) that 'the major factors leading to the provocation and generalization of hypertension' are: (a) the loss of the mother to a child under 11 years old; (b) lack of an intimate confiding marital relationship; (c) lack of paid employment outside the home; and (d) three or more children under 14 (cited by Subotsky, 1991), or women's general low status (Weissman and Klerman, 1977). Indeed, one can go as far as suggesting that the lives of women will be perpetually affected by decisions in which they do not take part for as long as they are over-represented among mental patients and family care-givers while being under-represented in medicine, psychiatry, and politics (Brooks-Bertam and Halbreich, 1996). Despite the attempts of professionals with social constructionist perspectives to question the validity of the finding of gender differences, claiming that they are artifactual and based on the psychiatrist's sexist approach (which this author views very critically), this literature is of utmost importance because it provides sometimes an extreme social causative approach, examining the features of women's lives that enhance or undermine mental disorders and well-being, and therefore provides some balance and a more rounded picture in the sometimes equally extreme exclusively-biological approach.

Therefore, the current communication is based on the assumption that gender differences in well-being and some mental disorders are real, but biological explanations are only part of the picture (even though some, like Nolen-Hoeksema (1990) probably would not fully agree even to this limited approach); social and environmental factors and processes contribute to vulnerability as well as to the expression of symptoms. The social constructionists are very constructive in this framework; their critique and doubts might not only complement the social approach but introduce doubt and scepticism which are needed in the process of any serious scientific discourse. Needless to say, we believe that there is no need for two or three opposing camps here when a well-rounded conceptualization is necessary for an efficient and efficacious remedy (or treatment, depending on the semantics used). In this context, it is also important to note that the change in women's role in society and their self-perception cause changes in the quality and quantity of mental disorders and distress, and eventually would mask some of the non-biological factors contributing to gender differences, leading sex ratios in some disorders to be more equal (e.g. Klerman and Weissman, 1989), and allow for a more focused evaluation of the actual biological processes that lead to the 'pure core' of situations in which real gender differences exist.

SEX DIFFERENCES IN PSYCHOPHARMACOLOGY

Women consume more psychotropic medications than men (Skegg et al., 1977; Rawson and D'Arcy, 1991), with a ratio of greater than

2:1. This is mostly true for anxiolytics and antidepressants (Baum et al., 1988). Women also report more side-effects to medications (Bottiger et al., 1979), and have different treatment outcomes (Halbreich et al., 1995). From these survey data, it is quite safe to deduce that not only do women show sex-specific features that are manifested in mental symptoms, but they also have some features that influence treatment response.

Pharmacokinetics of Psychotropic Medications

Pharmacokinetics are the processes involved in the delivery of a drug to its site of action and its removal. They include absorption, distribution, bioavailability, metabolism, clearances and excretion. Women have slower gastric emptying than men, affecting the absorption and causing lower and slower peak blood levels (Hamilton and Yonkers, 1996; Yonkers and Hamilton, 1995). The distribution and bioavailability is different because on average women weigh less than men, have lower blood volume, and higher percentage of body fat. Therefore, despite initial lower serum levels, they eventually increase. Lipophilic drugs are stored in higher levels and for longer periods, increasing the half-life time, and further contributing to higher serum levels (Yonkers et al., 1992). Cerebral blood flow (CBF) in women of reproductive age is higher than in men (Shaw et al., 1979). In post-menopausal women in whom it is decreased, the CBF is increased with oestrogen replacement therapy (Ohkura et al., 1995a), improving site delivery of psychotropic medications. Especially in younger women, liver metabolic pathways are slower, and further contribute to higher psychotropic blood levels. This effect is even more notable by the higher renal clearance in males, which is another mechanism contributing to higher blood levels of psychotropic medications for longer periods in women.

Pharmacodynamics

Pharmacodynamics are the processes of drug action once it is delivered to its target site. They include receptor sites, sensitivity and binding, signal transduction, and genomic effects. Genomic-organization effects are involved in the tendency or proneness of women to respond differently to various drugs. However, there is an accumulation of data showing that non-genomic-activational effects of steroid hormones, including gonadal hormones, have a direct effect on symptom formation and treatment response. Oestrogen has been shown to selectively influence several serotonergic receptor subtypes, binding sensitivity, and responsivity. It decreases activity of the enzyme monoamine oxidase (MAO) and thus decreases the metabolism of monoamine transmitters. It also influences binding and sensitivity of norepinephrine (adrenaline)-related receptors (Halbreich, 1997, in press). The overall influence of oestrogen is such that it increases activity of several serotonergic systems and might be responsible for the observed better response of women to specific serotonergic re-uptake inhibitors (SSRIs) (Yonkers et al., 1995). In many cases, progesterone counteracts oestrogen activity. The picture here is more complicated because some progesterone metabolites and other progestins are anxiolytics, while others are anxiogenic. In both cases, the main neurotransmitter system studied in this context is the γ aminobutyric acid$_A$ (GABA$_A$) receptors (e.g. Finn and Gee, 1994) but indeed the monoamine systems are involved as well, especially in the same areas that are sites of action of oestrogen: e.g. the hypothalamus, hypocampus and the preoptic area.

The biological determinants of pharmacokinetics and pharmacodynamics cannot be studied and interpreted without the context of psychosocial factors. There are gender differences in the attitudes of men and women about initiation, continuation, and termination of the use of tranquillizers, even if the gender difference in drug use in the certain population studied is small (Ettorre et al., 1994; Ettorre, 1992). For instance, women seek treatment with tranquillizers through 'not coping' or sleeplessness, while men cite work-related reasons. Physicians also encourage men more than women to stop medications. The psychosocial aspects are of further importance because they are different in various cultures and are influenced by traditions, the role of women in society, the social change and its rate, as well as by the structure and availability of health services.

PREMENSTRUAL SYNDROMES

Premenstrual syndromes (PMS) are quite prevalent. Up to 80% of women of reproductive age report some physical, mood and behaviour change during their late-luteal-premenstrual phase of the menstrual cycle. Up to 8% of women report dysphoric PMS that are severe and associated with impairment of day-to-day activity, or induce distress, and therefore warrant treatment (Woods et al., 1982a and 1982b; Andersch et al., 1986; Haskett et al., unpublished data 1987). Regretfully, there is no agreed-upon definition of PMS. Most researchers and clinicians agree that symptoms or syndromes are to be considered as PMS if they exist cyclically during the late-luteal phase, disappear shortly after the beginning of the menstrual flow and do not exist during the mid-follicular phase of the menstrual cycle. In most cases, the definitions of the nature, duration, and severity of symptoms are debatable. Probably the most elaborate definition of a specific PMS is that of the American Psychiatric Association task force for the DSM IV (*Diagnostic and Statistical Manual*, 4th Edition (APA, 1994)) which sets criteria for a premenstrual dysphoric disorder (PMDD) based on a list of symptoms, their timing, impairment of function, and prospective confirmation. The International Classification of Disease (ICD) (WHO, 1992) include PMS (or premenstrual tension syndrome – PMTS) under 'Diseases of the Genito-Urinary System' and its details are less formulated. For clinical purposes, however, any symptom or cluster of symptoms that are severe enough to cause distress and treatment-seeking, should be treated as PMS if they are menstrually related, do not exist for a period including the mid-follicular phase of the menstrual cycle and their cyclicity and phase-selectivity can be confirmed by prospective daily monitoring of symptoms (Halbreich, 1993a).

The diagnostic process relies mostly on the woman-patient's reports. For efficiency some of the information can be gathered and self-reported prior to the first office visit. This includes medical, obstetric/gynaecological and psychiatric history and monitoring of symptoms on a daily basis with daily rating forms (DRF) for two menstrual cycles. The DRF and other forms can be brought in for the first office visit that should be scheduled for the expected late-luteal-symptomatic phase. During that visit, the DRF are examined in detail, history is taken, and the PMS or PMDD are differentiated from other disorders. If there are doubts concerning the existence of the symptom-free period, the patient should be seen again during the mid-follicular phase. At present, there are no biological tests or other objective measurements for the diagnosis of PMS.

Dysphoric PMS has been shown to be associated with major depressive disorder (MDD) (Halbreich and Endicott, 1985) and women with PMS are at a high risk of developing MDD in the future (Graze et al., 1990). Dysphoric PMS has also been shown to be statistically associated with other hormonally related and biological disorders in women's lives, such as postpartum depression, dysphoric adverse effects to contraceptive hormones and hormonal replacement therapy, panic disorder, and seasonal affective disorder, just to mention a few (Halbreich et al., 1988). Many women who seek treatment for PMS actually have chronic disorders or the exacerbation of chronic MDD, dysthymic disorder, panic disorders, and other dysphoric disorders. These situations have to be distinguished from PMS to allow for an adequate treatment decision.

The Aetiology of PMS

The pathobiology of PMS is still obscure. It has been extensively reviewed by many (e.g. Halbreich et al., 1988; Smith and Schiff, 1993; Gold and Severing, 1994; Halbreich, 1995). Gonadal steroids (oestrogen and progesterone) have been postulated to be the main culprit of PMS since Frank (1931). Hypotheses included lack of oestrogen, lack of progesterone and differences in their ratios. Special attention was given to the lack of progesterone which led to progesterone suppository treatment – one of the most publicized treatment modalities for PMS (Dalton, 1964). However, that treatment modality has not been confirmed in any well-controlled studies. Others, including this author, believe that even though there are probably no group differences in absolute levels of gonadal hormones in women with PMS, they might show differences in cyclicity or rate of fluctuations as well as increased sensitivity to 'normal' fluctuations (Halbreich et al., 1986, 1988). If any, most women with PMS might have increased and not decreased levels of progesterone. Changes occurring during the early luteal phase might be no less important than those occurring during the symptomatic period itself. The reports that women do not have PMS in anovulatory cycles and that suppression of ovulation is a very effective treatment modality (e.g. Halbreich et al., 1991) support the notion that fluctuations in gonadal hormones and other ovulation-related processes are important factors in the pathobiology of PMS. Gonadal hormones probably interact with neurotransmitters and other processes that are putatively involved in regulation of mood and behaviour. Vulnerability also plays a major role in expression of symptoms and their individual nature. It has been shown (review: Halbreich, 1995) that women with PMS are different from women with no PMS in a variety of variables, including personality, cognition, serotonergic processes, thyroid functions and NE related receptors even when they do not have any symptoms – emphasizing the interaction and accumulated impact of vulnerability, hormonal changes and brain processes. To that equation, environmental and psychosocial aspects should be added.

Treatment of PMS

Currently several effective treatment modalities are available. For women with mild PMS, changes in lifestyle, exercise, general healthy nutrition, relaxation, and social support are sometimes sufficient for improvement. Women with severe dysphoric PMS respond well to antidepressant medications, mostly to SSRIs (Steiner et al., 1995; Yonkers et al., 1995), but also to benzodiazepines like alprezolam (Harrison, et al., 1990). Alprezolam may be administered in a cyclic regimen limited to the late-luteal phase. It is still unclear if SSRIs can be limited to the luteal phase or should be given continuously. In any case, up to 60–70% success rate has been reported.

The most effective treatment for a wide range of PMS is suppression of ovulation, mostly with GnRH analogues, but also with danazole or high dosages of oestrogen. This treatment modality was demonstrated to be effective for physical as well as dysphoric PMS. Its disadvantage is the inducement of 'pharmacological menopause' with its array of undesirable effects. The addition of cyclic oestrogen–progesterone replacement is not so effective because it simulates the physiological hormonal fluctuation. Treatment with oestrogen also might prove to be effective if given in dosages high enough to suppress ovulation and in a cyclic fashion in order to allow for a withdrawal and endometrial shedding.

With an adequate diagnosis and proper treatment, almost all women with PMS can be successfully treated.

PSYCHIATRIC DISORDERS DURING PREGNANCY AND POSTPARTUM

About 10% of pregnant women might meet criteria for some mood disorder (Gotlieb et al., 1989). This rate is markedly lower if symptoms that are usually associated with both depression and pregnancy, such as changes in appetite, sleep, and energy, are taken into account (Klein and Essex, 1995). Nonetheless chronic and de-novo dysphoric states during pregnancy pose a treatment problem due to the possible impact on the fetus and the unique hormonal milieu, which is characterized by increasing levels of oestrogen and progesterone. Immediately following delivery, levels of gonadal hormones abruptly plunge, and between days 4 and 10 postpartum up to 85% of women experience the postpartum or maternity 'blues' (Stein, 1982).

Symptoms are usually short-lived. The woman feels that dysphoria, crying, irritability, and mood lability are 'imposed' on her despite her expectation to be happy. In most women, these endogenously imposed states last for less than a day. This should be considered normal and it calls for no treatment beyond the assurance that it is normal.

A dysphoria is beyond normal if it persists for a long period of time and becomes more severe (Kendell et al., 1981; Kelly and Deakin, 1992). The prevalence of the more-severe postpartum depression (PPD) is 10–15% of women (Carothers and Murray, 1990). In most cases, the depression improves spontaneously within a few months. Symptoms are those of MDD. In addition to the timing, risk factors to develop PPD include: previous history of PPD or MDD; family history of affective disorders; psychosocial stress or adverse life events; marital discord; and having twins (Stowe and Nemeroff, 1995). If depression appears beyond six months following delivery, this author does not consider it as a postpartum depression, even though some others might diagnose the MDD as such. In very few women (about 1:1000) a postpartum psychosis might occur very shortly following delivery. These women might present with dysphoric mood, confusion, delirium-like state, cognitive impairment, perplexity, and other symptoms of acute-transient organic brain syndrome. This state might be unique to the postpartum period (Brockington et al., 1982); it has a very good prognosis, and might be the result of the abrupt disordered homeostasis immediately following parturition.

Despite the suggestion that the abrupt and substantial hormonal withdrawal is the culprit of postpartum pathology, this assumption has not yet been proven. The changes in gonadal hormones are also associated with dysfunction of the thyroid system (Pedersen et al., 1993), 'positive' or 'negative' changes in the hypothalamo-pituitary-adrenal (HPA) system (Nomura and Okano, 1992; Fleming et al., 1995), rapid postpartum withdrawal of endorphins (Smith et al., 1990) and a gonadal-hormone-associated decrease in serotonergic activity (Dean et al., 1989), and probably also in some other neurotransmitter systems. It is quite plausible that, as is the case with some other mental disorders, the pathobiology of postpartum disorders involves vulnerability to affective disorders and to disrupted homeostasis, the actual disruption of homeostasis, which is probably triggered by the abrupt withdrawal of gonadal hormones, and the influence of that withdrawal on a wide range of other biological systems that are involved in the regulation of mood and behaviour. An important factor in that mechanism is the restoration of homeostasis. Almost all women have 'blues' shortly following delivery; but there is probably a strong stabilizing mechanism that restores the euthymic state. In some women, that mechanism is deficient; they continue to be dysphoric with increased severity for longer periods. In these cases, treatment is warranted.

Treatment of PPD is mostly symptomatic, with antidepressants or electroconvulsive therapy (ECT) (NIH, 1995). Because of the higher risk of PPD in women with previous PPD, past history of other affective disorders and bipolar disorders (Cooper and Murray, 1995; Leibenluft, 1996), there are some recommendations for prophylactic or preventive treatment with SSRIs or a tricyclic antidepressant, with or without lithium. An interesting approach for a pharmacological treatment of PPD or its prevention stems from the notion that the main trigger of psychopathology is the abrupt decrease in oestrogen and/or progesterone levels (e.g. Wieck et al., 1991); therefore, oestrogen or progesterone administration might soften this withdrawal (e.g. Sichel et al., 1995). These hormonal treatment modalities are intriguing and promising but have not been confirmed yet.

In every treatment decision of PPD, the transfer of medication to the baby through breast-feeding should be taken into account. Breast-feeding by itself has been proposed to worsen the possibility of depression because of high levels of prolactin; and its discontinuation should be seriously considered in cases of PPD. Both tricylic anti-depressants (TCA) (Wisner and Perel, 1996; Wisner et al., 1995) and SSRIs (Isenberg, 1990; Ratan and Friedman, 1995) are excreted in the mother's breast milk. Their safety for the baby is not clear and, because of high levels of lithium in breast milk, it is not advisable to prescribe it to nursing mothers (Pons et al., 1994). Such is also the case with valproic acid, because of hepatotoxicity (Goldberg and Nissim, 1994). In both cases, if the mother absolutely needs the medication she should discontinue breast-feeding. Otherwise carbamazapine might be safer for the baby (Mortola, 1989). Benzodiazepines and antipsychotics are not recommended either.

In all cases of psychopharmacologic treatment, the psychosocial aspects should be taken into account, especially the mother–child interactions and the impact of a depressed or psychotic mother on her child. Psychotherapy should be an integral component of the therapeutic effort.

Pharmacotherapy during Pregnancy

Virtually all psychotropic medications pass through the placenta from the pregnant mother to her fetus. Therefore, they might induce teratogenic as well as behavioural and developmental short- and long-term effects on the fetus and later the child. Nonetheless, in many cases, the actual effects are unknown and knowledge in humans is accumulated on a trial-and-error basis. Because mental illnesses are quite prevalent among pregnant women and do not improve due to pregnancy, the risk/benefit evaluations in these cases are very complicated and carry a heavy ethical load. As concluded by Steiner (1996), it appears that 'although no controlled studies have been done on pregnant women, the overall emerging picture is less alarming than was previously thought (Altshuler and Szube, 1994; Goldberg and Nissim, 1994; Shader, 1994). It appears that some, but not all, current psychotropic drugs are fairly safe for use in pregnancy'.

This generalized opinion is not pertinent to carbamazepine and valproate, both of which show high teratogeneity (e.g. Lindhout and Schmidty, 1986). Even though there are recent reports that lithium is not as teratogenic as has been previously believed, it is still safer to discontinue lithium maintenance immediately when pregnancy is suspected and reinstate it only in the third trimester or immediately postpartum with discontinuation of breast feeding (Stewart et al., 1991; Cohen et al., 1995).

The safety of benzodiazepines is still unclear despite early reports of cleft palate and lip. Most TCAs are safe, but high dosages are needed during the third trimester due to increased hepatic metabolism (Nau et al., 1984) which might cause withdrawal effects in the baby. Data on SSRIs are still not sufficient, even though no teratogeneity has yet been demonstrated. Most antipsychotics are probably not teratogenic and should be given in acute or chronic psychosis during pregnancy (Sitland-Marken et al., 1989) but antiparkinsonian drugs should be avoided.

In many individual cases, the obvious risk of not treating a pregnant woman when treatment is definitely warranted should be individually compared to the probable risk to the fetus, which is in many cases unknown.

PSYCHIATRIC PROBLEMS DURING THE PERIMENOPAUSE AND MENOPAUSE

The perimenopause is the period of transition from women's reproductive life, when ova are produced associated with menstrual cycles, and oestrogen and progesterone secretion, to the post-menopausal period when follicules no longer mature, ovulation is absent, there are no menstrual cycles and their associated oestradiol and progesterone secretion, and LH and FSH levels are continuously high due to the lack of gonadal feedback mechanism. The perimenopause occurs in most women in their late 40s to early 50s and is characterized by irregular menstrual cycles and the appearance of menopausal symptoms.

The menopause, and especially the perimenopause, were observed to be associated with severe depression for at least two centuries. Kraepelin (1907) coined 'involutional melancholia' as a very severe depression, despondency and hypochondrial delusions with no prior history of depression, which was later classified as a form of manic-depressive illness. The first appearances of depression during the perimenopause and menopause were later doubted (Weissman, 1979) and dismissed. We, as well as others (Schmidt and Rubinow, 1991) believe that this notion still deserves a better elucidation. The studies of prevalence of affective disorders during the perimenopause and menopause focus on criteria for MDD, subsyndromal and 'atypical' depression were not adequately studied (Winokur, 1973), even though they are prevalent during periods of hormonal change in women's life (e.g. the premenstrual period). The report of an increased female-to-male ratio of affective disorders during mid-life (from 2:1 to 3–4:1) (Kessler et al., 1993; Weissman et al., 1988a and 1988b) suggests that a broader spectrum of affective symptoms should be studied. Further support for this suggestion is provided by Angst (1978) who reported a second peak of onset of bipolar affective disorder in women aged 45–55 but not in men of the same age. It is plausible that the hormonal instability or substantial hormonal changes during that period of life might be associated with that destabilized mood disorder.

Even though no increase in MDD during menopause and the perimenopause has been definitely found, it is now well established that oestrogen replacement therapy (ORT) improves well-being and selective cognitive performance. Oestrogen does not act as an antidepressant in its own right but acts as a potent adjunct to antidepressants in cases of non-response. Due to its accumulated action on several neurotransmitter systems, it might also act as a preventative measure in women who are vulnerable to affective disorders (Ottowitz and Halbreich, 1995), even though this possibility has not been fully confirmed yet. The almost total lack of oestrogen during menopause might decrease the threshold for depressions of women who are vulnerable to developing them. This is an area that is still in need of clarification. The situation might be rectified by hormonal replacement therapy (HRT).

The regimen of HRT might be important from the standpoint of mood and well-being. Most HRT regimens employ sequential administration of oestrogen and progesterone (in order to induce endometrial shedding and bleeding) and thus simulate the normal menstrual cycle. However, it has been reported (Hammerbäck and Bäckström, 1985) that this regimen produces PMS-like symptoms, especially in women who had them during their reproductive lives. Some progestins might induce depression, anxiety, and other dysphoric symptoms even when not given in a sequential cyclic fashion. Therefore, the clinical recommendation of the type of HRT should take these issues into account, especially when the mood side-effects might decrease compliance.

The administration of oestrogen with no progesterone is not very prevalent even though cyclic administration with short withdrawal periods every 30–60 days induces endometrial bleeding in almost all cases. An interesting HRT is the combination of oestrogen and androgen, with no progesterone. Androgens were shown to have a positive cognitive effect; they also increase libido, assertiveness and energy. On the other hand, they might induce masculinization and increase aggression and irritability. In an adequate dosage of an adequate androgen, the combination of oestrogen and androgen approximates the normal hormonal secretion of the ovary. Its cyclic administration with no progesterone shows a promising potential. The main indications for the above HRTs are the prevention of osteoporosis and cardiovascular disorders. The improvement of mood and cognition are at present only secondary and are not yet approved. However, it has been reported that women who received HRT for a long time tended to be less prone to Alzheimer's disease than their age-matched peers, and that patients who have Alzheimer's and who received HRT have less cognitive impairment. If this is indeed the case, then the central nervous system (CNS) effect of oestrogen might be an additional major indication for HRT.

An interesting practical issue is when to start HRT. In the opinion of this author, due to the effects of oestrogen on hot flushes and other early menopause symptoms and due to the possibility that perimenopausal women are more vulnerable to a varity of dysphoric disorders, an early initiation of ORT might be recommended.

CONCLUSION

Gender difference in the prevalence of affective disorders is well documented. The higher and selective prevalance of some disorders but not of others, in many women suggests that gender differences are not only due to psycho-socio-cultural factors, which obviously do play an important role in the dynamics and manifestation of disorders as well as in treatment-seeking, delivery, and availability of health services to women in various countries and communities.

A major role is played by biological sex-related differences. First among them are the gonadal hormones: oestrogen and progesterone. Genomic-organizational and non-genomic-activation effects of these hormones are well documented in animals. The knowledge of their effects on humans is rapidly accumulating and is pointing in the direction of an important role for gonadal hormones in the regulation of mood and behaviour, and therefore also as potential remedies.

In this chapter, we focused on women's specific states and events such as the menstrual cycle, pregnancy, postpartum period, the perimenopause and menopause, as well as specific considerations in women who have affective disorders and receive psychotropic medications. It should be pointed out that the association between mood, psychotropic medications and gonadal hormones is bidirectional. Psychotropic medications by themselves influence the reproduction system and might cause a myriad of side-effects in women as well as in men. Their side-effects range from impairment of libido and sexual performance (e.g. SSRIs) to amenorrhoea (e.g. neuroleptics), and transient infertility. These aspects, however, are beyond the scope of the current discussions and are discussed in further detail elsewhere (Halbreich, 1996).

Acknowledgements

The preparation of this chapter was partially supported by NIMH Grant R01-MH 45901. Some of the sections are based on chapters in the book *Psychiatric Issues in Women* (Halbreich, 1996).

References

Altshuler, L.L., Szuba, M.P. (1994) Course of psychiatric disorders in pregnancy: dilemmas in pharmacologic management. *Neurologic Clinics of North America* **12**: 613–635.

Andersch, B., Wendestam, C., Hahn, L., Ohman, R. (1986) Premenstrual complaints. I. Prevalence of premenstrual symptoms in a Swedish urban population. *Journal of Psychosomatic Obstetrics and Gynaecology* **5**: 39–49.

Angst, J. (1978) The course of affective disorders. II: Typology of bipolar manic-depressive illness. *Archiv für Psychiatrie und Nervenkrankheiten* **226**: 65–73.

APA (American Psychiatric Association) (1994) Premenstrual dysphoric disorder. In *Diagnostic and Statistical Manual of Mental Disorders* 4th edn, pp. 714–718. Washington DC: American Psychiatric Association.

Baum, C., Kennedy, D., Knapp, D.E. et al. (1988) Prescription drug use in 1984 and changes over time. *Medical Care* **26**: 105–114.

Berg, G., Hammar, M. (eds) (1994) *The Modern Management of the Menopause: A Perspective for the 21st Century*. New York: Parthenon Publishing Group.

Bottiger, L.E., Furhoff, A.K., Holmberg, L. (1979) Fatal reactions to drugs. *Acta Medica Scandinavica* **102**: 451–456.

Brockington, I.F., Winokur, G., Dean, C. (1982) Puerperal psychosis. In Brockington, I.F., Kumar, R. (eds) *Motherhood and Mental Illness*, pp. 37–69. London: Academic Press.

Brooks-Bertram, P., Halbreich, U. (1996) Social and psychological aspects of women's well-being: a diversified perspective. In Halbreich, U. (ed.) *Psychiatric Issues in Women: Bailliere's Clinical Psychiatry,* vol. 4, pp. 619–648. London: Bailliere Tindall.

Brown, G.W., Harris, T.O. (1978) *Social Origins of Depression*. New York: Free Press.

Carothers, A.D., Murray, L. (1990) Estimating psychiatric morbidity by logistic regression: applications to post-natal depression in a community sample. *Psychological Medicine* **20**: 695–702.

Cohen, L.S., Sichel, D.A., Robertson, L.M. et al. (1995) Postpartum prophylaxis for women with bipolar disorder. *American Journal of Psychiatry* **152**: 1641–1645.

Cooper, P.J., Murray, L. (1995) Course and recurrence of postnatal depression: evidence for the specificity of the diagnostic concept. *British Journal of Psychiatry* **166**: 191–195.

Dalton, K. (1964) *The Premenstrual Syndrome*. Springfield, IL: Charles C. Thomas.

Dean, C., Williams, R.J., Brockington, I.F. (1989) Is puerperal psychosis the same as bipolar manic-depressive disorder? A family study. *Psychological Medicine* **19**: 637–647.

Ettore, E. (1992) *Women and Substance Use*. New Jersey: Rutgers University Press.

Ettore, E., Klaukka, T., Riska, E. (1994) Psychotropic drugs: long-term care use dependency and the gender factor. *Social Science and Medicine* **39**: 1667–1673.

Finn, D.A., Gee, K.W. (1994) The significance of steroid action on the GABA-A receptor complex. In Berg, G., Hammar, M. (eds) *The Modern*

Management of the Menopause, pp. 301–313. Lancs: The Parthenon Publishing Group.

Fleming, A.S., Corter, C., Steiner, M. (1995) Sensory and hormonal control of maternal behaviour in rat and human mothers. In Pryce, C.R., Martin, R.D., Skuse, D. (eds) *Motherhood in Human and Nonhuman Primates*, pp. 106–114. Basel: S. Karger.

Frank, R.T. (1931) The hormonal causes of premenstrual tension. *Archives of Neurological Psychiatry* **26**: 1053.

Gold, J., Severino, S. (1994) *Premenstrual Dysphorias, Myths and Realities*. Washington, DC: American Psychiatric Association Press.

Goldberg, H.L., Nissim, R. (1994) Psychotropic drugs in pregnancy and lactation. *International Journal of Psychiatry in Medicine* **24**: 129–149.

Gotlieb, I.H., Whiffen, V.E., Mount, J.H. et al. (1989) Prevalence rates and demographic characteristics associated with depression in pregnancy and postpartum. *Journal of Consulting and Clinical Psychology* **57**: 269–274.

Graze, K.K., Nee, J., Endicott, J. (1990) Premenstrual depression predicts future major depressive disorder. *American Journal of Psychiatry* **81**: 201.

Halbreich, U. (1993a) Menstrually-related changes and disorders; conceptualization and diagnostic considerations. *Neuropsychopharmacology*, **9**: 25.

Halbreich, U. (1993b) Multiple sclerosis: a neurostructural model of affective and cognitive disorders. In: Halbreich, U. (ed.) *Multiple Sclerosis: A Neuropsychiatric Structural Disorder*, pp 171–184. Washington, DC: American Psychiatric Association Press.

Halbreich, U. (1994) Gender-related biological research: methodological and ethical considerations. In *XIX CINP Congress*. Washington, DC, June.

Halbreich, U. (1995) Menstrually related disorders: what we do know, what we only believe we know, and what we know that we do not know. *Critical Reviews in Neurobiology* **9**: 163–175.

Halbreich, U. (ed.) (1996) *Psychiatric Issues in Women*. Bailliére's International Practice and Research: Clinical Psychiatry. London: Bailliére-Tindall.

Halbreich, U. (ed.) (1997) *Hormonal Modulation of Brain and Behavior*. Washington DC: American Psychiatric Press. (In press).

Halbreich, U., Endicott, J. (1985) The relationship of dysphoric premenstrual changes to depressive disorders. *Acta Psychiatrica Scandinavica* **71**: 331.

Halbreich, U., Endicott, J., Goldstein, S. et al. (1986) Premenstrual changes and changes in gonadal hormones. *Acta Psychiatrica Scandinavica* **74**: 576.

Halbreich, U., Holtz, A.I., Paul, L. (1988) Premenstrual changes, impaired hormonal endocrinology. *Metabolic Clinics of North America* **17**: 173.

Halbreich, U., Rojansky, N., Wang, K. (1991) Psychological, hormonal and neurotransmitter aspects of menstrually related symptoms. In Nappi, G., Bono, G., Sandrini, G. et al. (eds) *Headache and Depression: Serotonin Pathways as a Common Clue*, pp. 191–203. New York: Raven Press.

Halbreich, U., Piletz, J.E., Carson, S., Halaris, A., Rojansky, N. (1993) Increased imidazoline and alpha-2 adrenergic binding in platelets of women with dysphoric premenstrual syndrome. *Biological Psychiatry* **34**: 676.

Hamilton, J.A., Halbreich, U. (1993) Special aspects of neuropsychiatric illness in women: focus on depression. *Annual Review of Medicine* **44**: 355–364.

Hamilton, J.A., Yonkers, K.A. (1996) Sex differences in pharmacokinetics of psychotropic medications. Parts I and II. In Jensvold, M.F., Halbreich, U., Hamilton, J.A. (eds). *Psychopharmacology and Women*, pp. 11–72. Washington DC: American Psychiatric Press.

Hammarbäck, S., Bäckström, T. (1988) Induced ovulation as treatment for premenstrual syndrome: a double-blind crossover study with GnRH-agonist versus placebo. *Acta Obstetrics and Gynecology Scandinavica* **67**: 159–166.

Hammarbäck, S., Bäckström, T., Holst, J. et al. (1985) Cyclical mood changes as in the premenstrual tension syndrome during sequential estrogen-progestagen postmenopausal replacement therapy. *Acta Obstetrics and Gynecology Scandinavica* **64**: 393–397.

Harrison, W.M., Endicott, J., Nee, J. (1990) Treatment of premenstrual dysphoria with alprazolam: a controlled study. *Archives of General Psychiatry* **47**: 270–275.

Isenberg, K.E. (1990) Excretion of fluoxetine in human breast milk. *Journal of Clinical Psychiatry* **51**: 169.

Jensvold, M.F., Halbreich, U., Hamilton, J.A. (eds) (1996) *Psychopharmacology and Women: Sex, Gender and Hormones*. Washington DC: American Psychiatric Press.

Kraepelin, E. (1907) *Lehrbuch der Psychiatrie*. New York: Macmillan.

Kelly, A., Deakin, B. (1992) Postnatal depression and antenatal morbidity. *British Journal of Psychiatry* **161**: 577–578.

Kendell, R.E., McGuire, R.J., Connor, Y., Cox, J.L. (1981) Mood changes in the first three weeks after childbirth. *Journal of Affective Disorders* **3**: 317–326.

Kessler, R., McGonagle, K., Swartz, M. et al. (1993) Sex and depression in the National Comorbidity Survey. I: lifetime prevalence, chronicity, and recurrence. *Journal of Affective Disorders* **29**: 85–96.

Klein, M.H., Essex, M.J. (1995) Pregnant or depressed? The effect of overlap between symptoms of depression and somatic complaints of pregnancy on rates of major depression in the second trimester. *Depression* **2**: 308–314.

Klerman, G.L., Weissman, M.M. (1989) Increasing rates of depression. *Journal of the American Medical Association* **261**: 2229–2235.

Leibenluft, E. (1996) Women with bipolar illness: clinical and research issues. *American Journal of Psychiatry* **153**: 163–173.

Lindhout, D., Schmidty, D. (1986) In utero exposure to valproate and neural defects. *The Lancet* **1**: 392–393.

Mortola, J.F. (1989) The use of psychotropic agents in pregnancy and lactation. *Psychiatric Clinics of North America* **12**: 69–87.

Nau, H., Loock, W., Schmidt-Gollwitzer, M., Kuhnz, W. (1984) Pregnancy-specific changes in hepatic drug metabolism in man. *Drugs and Pregnancy* **50**: 45–62.

NIH (1995) National Institutes of Health Consensus Conference: electro-convulsive therapy. *Journal of the American Medical Association* **254**: 2103–2108.

Nolen-Hoeksma, S. (1990) *Sex Differences in Depression.* Palo Alto, CA: Stanford University Press.

Nomura, J., Okano, T. (1992) Endocrine function and hormonal treatment of postpartum psychosis. In Hamilton, J.A., Harberger, P.N. (eds) *Postpartum Psychiatric Illness – A Picture Puzzle*, pp. 176–190. Philadelphia, PA: University of Pennsylvania Press.

Ohkura, T., Isse, K., Alazawa, K., Hamamoto, M., Yaoi, Y., Hagino, N. (1995a) Long-term estrogen replacement therapy in female patients with dementia of the Alzheimers type: 7 case reports. *Dementia* **6**: 99–107.

Ohkura, T., Teshima, Y., Isse, K. et al. (1995b) Estrogen increases cerebral and cerebellar blood flows in postmenopausal women. *Menopause* **2**: 13–18.

Ottowitz, W.E., Halbreich, U. (1995) Mood and cognitive changes following estrogen replacement therapy to postmenopausal women. *CNS Drugs* **4**: 161–167.

Parry, B.I. (1989) Reproductive factors affecting the course of affective illness in women. *Women's Diseases* **12**: 207–220.

Pedersen, C.A., Stern, R.A., Pate, J. et al. (1993) Thyroid and adrenal measures during late pregnancy and the puerperium in women who have been major depressed or who become dysphoric postpartum. *Journal of Affective Disorders* **29**: 201–211.

Pons, G., Rey, E., Matheson, I. (1994) Excretion of psychoactive drugs into breast milk. *Clinical Pharmacokinetics* **27**: 270–289.

Ratan, D.A., Friedman, T. (1995) Antidepressants in pregnancy and breast-feeding. *British Journal of Psychiatry* **167**: 824.

Rawson, N.S.B., D'Arcy, C. (1991) Sedative hypnotic drug use in Canada. *Health Reports* **3**: 33–57.

Regier, D.A., Boyd, J.H., Burk, J.D. et al. (1988) One month prevalence of mental disorders in the United States. Based on five epidemiologic catch-ment area sites. *Archives of General Psychiatry* **45**: 977–986.

Robins, L.N., Regier, D.A. (eds) (1992) *Psychiatric Disorders in America.* New York: Free Press.

Robins, L.N., Locke, B.Z., Regier, D.A. (1992) An overview of psychiatric disorders in America. In Robins, L.N., Reigier, D.A. (eds) *Psychiatric Disorders in America*, pp. 328–366. New York: Free Press.

Schmidt, P.J., Rubinow, D.R. (1991) Menopause-related affective disorders: a justification for further study. *American Journal of Psychiatry* **148**: 844–852.

Shader, R.I. (1994) Is there anything new on the use of psychotropic drugs during pregnancy? *Journal of Clinical Psychopharmacology* **14**: 438.

Shaw, T., Meyer, J.S., Mortel, K. et al. (1979) Effects of normal aging, sex and risk factors for stroke on regional cerebral blood flow (rCBF) in normal volunteers. *Acta Neurologica Scandinavica* **72** (Suppl): 462–463.

Sichel, D.A., Cohen, L.S., Robertson, L.M. et al. (1995) Prophylactic estrogen in recurrent postpartum affective disorder. *Biological Psychiatry* **38**: 814–818.

Sitland-Marken, P.A., Rickman, L.A., Wells, B.G., Mabie, W.C. (1989) Pharmacologic management of acute mania in pregnancy. *Journal of Clinical Psychopharmacology* **9**: 78–87.

Skegg, D.C.G., Doll, R., Perry, J. (1977) Use of medicines in general practice. *British Medical Journal* **1**: 1561–1563.

Smith, S., Schiff, I. (eds) (1993) *Modern Management of Premenstrual Syndrome*. New York: WW Norton.

Smith, R., Cubis, J., Brinsmead, M. et al. (1990) Mood changes, obstetric experience and alterations in plasma cortisol, beta-endorphin and corticotrophin releasing hormone during pregnancy and the puerperium. *Journal of Psychosomatic Research* **34**: 53–69.

Stein, G. (1982) The maternity blues. In Brockington, I.F., Kumar, R. (eds) *Motherhood and Mental Illness*, pp. 119–154. London: Academic Press.

Steiner, M. (1996) Psychiatric disorders during the menopause and perimenopause. In Halbreich, U. (ed.) *Psychiatric Issues in Women*. Baillière's International Practice and Research: Clinical Psychiatry. London: Baillière-Tindall.

Steiner, M., Steinberg, S., Stewart D. et al. (1995) Fluoxetine in the treatment of premenstrual dysphoria. *New England Journal of Medicine* **332**: 1529–1533.

Stewart, D.E., Klompenhouwer, J.L., Kendell, R.E., Van Hulst, A.M. (1991) Prophylactic lithium in puerperal psychosis: the experience of three centres. *British Journal of Psychiatry* **158**: 393–397.

Stowe, Z.N., Nemeroff, C.B. (1995) Women at risk for postpartum-onset major depression. *American Journal of Obstetrics and Gynecology* **173**: 639–645.

Subotsky, F. (1991) Issues for women in the development of mental health services. *British Journal of Psychiatry* **10**: 17–21.

Van Valkenburg, C., Akiskal, H.S., Puzantian, V., Rosenthal, T. (1984) Anxious depression: clinical, family history, and naturalistic outcome – comparisons with panic and major depressive disorders. *Journal of Affective Disorders* **6**: 67–82.

Weissman, M.M. (1979) The myth of involutional melancholia. *Journal of the American Medical Association* **242**: 742–744.

Weissman, M.M., Klerman, G.L. (1977) Sex differences and the epidemiology of depression. *Archives of General Psychiatry* **34**: 98–111.

Weissman, M.M., Klerman, G. (1987) Gender and depression. In Formanek, R., Gurian, A. (eds) *Women and Depression: A Lifespan Perspective*, pp. 3–15. New York: Springer Publishing Company.

Weissman, M.M., Olfson, M. (1995) Depression in women: implications for health care research. *Science* **269**: 799–801.

Weissman, M.M., Leaf, P.J., Bruce, M.L., Florio, L. (1988a) The epidemiology of dysthymia in five communities: rates, risks, comorbidity, and treatment. *American Journal of Psychiatry* **145**: 815–819.

Weissman, M.M., Leaf, P.J., Tischler, G.L. et al. (1988b) Affective disorders in five United States communities. *Psychological Medicine* **18**: 141–153.

Weissman, M.M., Leaf, P.J., Bruce, M.L. (1987) Single parent women. *Social Psychiatry* **22**: 29–36.

Wieck, A., Kumar, R., Hirst, A.D. et al. (1991) Increased sensitivity of dopamine receptors and recurrence of affective psychosis after childbirth. *British Medical Journal* **303**: 613–616.

Winokur, G. (1973) Depression in the menopause. *American Journal of Psychiatry* **30**: 92–93.

Wisner, K.L., Perel, J.M., Foglia, J.P. (1995) Serum clomipramine and metabolite levels in four nursing mother–infant pairs. *Journal of Clinical Psychiatry* **56**: 17–20.

Wisner, K.L., Perel, J.M. (1996) Psychopharmacologic treatment during pregnancy and lactation. In Jensvold, M.F., Halbreich, U., Hamilton, J.A. (eds) *Psychopharmacology and Women: Sex, Gender and Hormones*. Washington DC: American Psychiatric Press.

Wolk, S.I., Weissman, M.M. (1995) Women and depression: an update. In Oldham, J.M., Riba, M.B. (eds) *Review of Psychiatry*, Vol. 14, pp. 227–259. Washington, DC: American Psychiatric Press.

Woods, N.F., Dery, G.K. and Most, A. (1982a) Stressful live events and perimenstrual symptoms. *Journal of Human Stress* **8**, 23–31.

Woods, N.F., Most, A., Dery, G.K. (1982b) Estimating perimenstrual distress: comparison of two methods. *Research Nursing and Health* **5**: 123–136.

Woods, N.F., Lentz, M., Mitchell, E., Oakley, L.D. (1994) Depressed mood and self-esteem in young Asian, black and white women in America. *Health Care for Women International* **15**: 243–262.

World Health Organization (1992) *International Classification of Diseases*, 10th edn. Geneva: World Health Organization.

Yonkers, K.A., Hamilton, J.A. (1995) Psychotropic medications. In Oldham, J.M., Riba, M.B. (eds) *Review of Psychiatry*, Vol. 14, pp. 307–332. Washington, DC: American Psychiatric Press.

Yonkers, K.A., Kando, J.L., Cole, J.O. et al. (1992) Gender differences in pharmacokinetics and pharmacodynamics of psychotropic medication. *American Journal of Psychiatry* **149**: 587–595.

Yonkers, K., Halbreich, U., Freeman, E., Brown, C., Pearlstein, T. (1995) Sertraline treatment for premenstrual dysphoric disorder (abstract). Orlando, FL: NCDEU.

5

Borderline Personality Disorder – History and Current Dilemmas

Anthony W. Bateman

Over the last decade dynamic and descriptive psychiatry have had a fertile marriage, producing integrated and accurate descriptions of personality disorder which are clinically relevant to ordinary practitioners. Although dynamic psychiatrists are primarily interested in the development and internal structure of the personality and its dynamic function within relationships, and descriptive psychiatrists are concerned more with reliable descriptions of behaviour and social functioning, together they have produced a successful progeny in borderline personality disorder. Nevertheless the term may still be accused of imprecision and meaning all things to all men or 'Humpty Dumptyism' –

> *"When I choose a word," Humpty Dumpty said in a rather scornful tone, "it means just what I choose it to mean, – neither more nor less."*
> *"The question is," said Alice, "whether you can make words mean so many different things."*
>
> *(Lewis Carrol, Through the Looking Glass)*

The inherently ambiguous term 'borderline' evokes an ambivalent response in both the psychoanalytic and psychiatric community. Higgit and Fonagy (1992) have predicted its eventual replacement by some more satisfactory formulation. However, the term, like hysteria, may outlive its obituarists, having survived already for nearly a century; Kraepelin (1909), in reviving interest in Prichard's 'moral insanity', described 'morbid personalities' as 'borderline states between insanity and day-to-day eccentricities of normal individuals'.

HISTORICAL BACKGROUND

The term 'borderline' emerged from a confluence of psychiatric and psychoanalytic research. At the turn of the century, European psychiatrists identified a group of patients characterized by cyclical emotions. Jules Falret (1890) elucidated 'folie hysterique' consisting of emotional volatility, impulsivity, contradictoriness, and proneness to controversy. Kraepelin (1909–1915) described subaffective personalities and Kretschmer (1921) defined patients with a 'mixed cycloid-schizoid' temperament. However the first use of the term is usually attributed to Stern (1938), a psychoanalyst, who used it to describe a heterogeneous group of patients who, for all intents and purposes, appeared neurotic but in treatment or under stress were prone to brief psychotic episodes. Further papers appeared describing similar observations. Deutsch (1942) wrote of the 'as if' personality, and Zetzel (1968) of the 'so-called good hysteric' (who turns out in treatment to be highly disturbed and difficult), Winnicott (1965) and Laing (1960) of the 'false self'. All were trying to capture the essence of people who, while not diagnostically psychotic, evince psychotic mechanisms, often regress dangerously within psychoanalytic treatment, and yet prove challenging and sometimes rewarding patients. They exist, as Rey (1994) summarizes it, on the borderline between oedipal and pre-oedipal, between psychosis and neurosis, between male and female, between paranoid–schizoid and depressive positions, between fear of the object and need for the object, between inner and outer, between body and mind.

In parallel with these developments, similar observations were emerging from genetic and descriptive studies, although the conclusions were very different. Zilboorg (1941) described individuals who appeared normal but showed shallow emotions, dereistic thinking, incapacity for true friendships, and inability to settle in life. He regarded this condition as a variant of schizophrenia. Hoch and Polatin (1949) described a different condition, coining the term 'pseudoneurotic schizophrenia' on the basis that individuals showed underlying core features of schizophrenia. The patients suffered from pananxiety, panneurosis, and pansexuality. Their whole life was riddled with conflict, their sexual life characterized by promiscuity and perversion, and they displayed multiple neurotic symptoms. The link with schizophrenia continued in the adoption studies of Rosenthal et al. (1968).

The two developmental lines, psychodynamic psychiatry and genetic/descriptive psychiatry, laid the foundation for attempts at a clearer definition of the concept. Although the conclusions of the two approaches differed, they both highlight a process that is germaine to the present concept of 'borderline', namely that an apparent normality or neurotic facade can hide a much 'sicker' inner core. Grinker et al. (1968) were the first to attempt to establish objective criteria for borderline disorder. In a study of hospitalized patients they arrived at four characteristics of borderline patients, namely persistent anger, volatile interpersonal relationships, identity disturbance, and depression and loneliness. These criteria have continued to form a central part of the borderline concept ever since.

Nonetheless, over the next decade, the relationship of the disorder to schizophrenia gained further credence through the adoption studies of Wender et al. (1974) and Kety et al. (1975). A further complication was added by the finding that many borderline patients were depressed. An association with depressive disorders was suggested (Klein 1975, 1977). The impulsive behaviour, drug abuse, and desperate relationships of borderlines were conceptualized as an attempt to stabilize an underlying affective disorder – an idea not far removed from psychoanalytic views of symptom formation in which an individual's attempt to maintain psychic equilibrium leads to compromises in the form of symptoms. Nor is it far away from some cognitive–behavioural formulations of borderline as emotional dysregulation. However, the link between borderline disorder and affective disorder has been clarified further. Gunderson and Eliot (1985) noted the association of affective illness with borderline disorder and proposed four possible explanations. Two of the possibilities imply that one disorder is a consequence of the other. Firstly drug abuse, promiscuity etc. are used to relieve unbearable feelings of depression, or, secondly that depression results from poor impulse control and constant failure in relationships. In other words borderline personality either predisposes to affective disorder or is itself a subaffective disorder. A third possibility is that the two disorders coexist but are unrelated, and a fourth that both disorders arise from an interaction of symptoms particular to each individual. Six years later, Gunderson and Phillips (1991) concluded that the third possibility was the most tenable.

Examination of the family histories of borderline patients showed that the occurrence of affective disorder in relatives was related to whether or not the borderline patient had a comorbid affective disorder. Family studies showed a high frequency of impulse disorders such as drug and alcohol abuse as well as a five-fold increase of borderline personality disorder itself in relatives of an index patient. Furthermore, clinicians recognized that the depression found in borderline disorders was qualitatively different from that found in patients without a personality disorder. Affective changes in borderline patients are more rapid and less episodic than those in unipolar depressed patients and characterized by anhedonia, boredom, loneliness, and emptiness rather than guilt and feelings of worthlessness (Bateman, 1989).

DIAGNOSTIC CRITERIA

Some of the muddle between the two developmental lines of borderline disorder was clarified by the pioneering work of Gunderson and Kolb (1978) and Spitzer et al. (1979). In 1980 borderline disorder received official status in the DSM-III. The DSM-III and its successors, the DSM-III-R (American Psychiatric Association, 1987) and DSM-IV (American Psychiatric Association, 1994), act as a recipe book for defining psychiatric disorders – appropriate ingredients are mixed in relevant ratios to form a diagnosis. Since the inception of DSM-III, changes in the recipe for borderline personality disorder have been largely semantic but the DSM-IV has partially rectified a severe weakness in earlier versions. Despite increasing evidence that borderline patients experience short-lived psychotic episodes and show an impetuousness in decision making, reference to such symptoms was omitted from both the DSM-III and DSM-III-R. In the DSM-IV, a ninth criterion has been added referring to transient, stress-related paranoid ideation or severe dissociative symptoms.

From a psychodynamic perspective this addition is important as it addresses, from a symptomatic point of view, the disturbance in the sense of self that is central to the borderline. Paranoid ideas arise through inappropriate use of splitting and projective mechanisms, both of which are pivotal in psychodynamic formulations. Derealization and depersonalization also disrupt the sense of self, leaving the borderline patient at the mercy of impulses that are then experienced as discontinuous with the self. Impulse turns immediately into action, such as self-mutilation, which is in turn experienced as inexplicable or alien to the non-dissociated self. The other eight criteria are:

1. Frantic efforts to avoid real or imagined abandonment.
2. A pattern of unstable and intense interpersonal relationships characterized by alternating between extremes of idealization and devaluation.
3. Identity disturbance: markedly and persistently unstable self-image or sense of self.
4. Impulsivity in at least two areas that are potentially self-damaging.
5. Recurrent suicidal behaviour, gestures, or threats, or self-mutilating behaviour.
6. Affective instability due to marked reactivity of mood.
7. Chronic feelings of emptiness.
8. Inappropriate, intense anger or difficulty controlling anger.

Five or more of the criteria have to be present in a variety of contexts.

Although this approach is satisfactory to the descriptive psychiatrist, it leaves a number of problems for the psychotherapeutically orientated practitioner. As only five criteria are needed and none is given more weight than the others, it is possible theoretically to make a diagnosis of borderline personality disorder without identity disturbance being present and without pathological splitting and projective processes (see p.129) resulting in paranoid ideation and cognitive distortions. Both elements are essential to the psychodynamic formulation. Akhtar (1992) has offered a synthesis of descriptive and psychodynamic views by using overt and covert characteristics of the borderline according to self-concept, interpersonal relations, social adaptation, love and sexuality, ethics, standards and ideas, and finally cognitive style. Overtly the borderline views his/herself as a victim who is self-righteously enraged, who relishes intense relationships which oscillate between idealization and devaluation, who compulsively socializes looking for romance and sexual adventures, who is fleetingly enthusiastic about new ideas becoming involved in cults, who impetuously takes decisions believing in the law of the talion, seeing things as black and white, and feeling quietly superior to others. Covertly the borderline feels empty, is uncertain about gender and attractiveness, is mistrustful of others often perceiving them as hostile, is socially unpredictable and yet unable to be alone, idealizes lovers and yet denigrates them when threatened by perceived abandonment, tends to become involved in perverse sexuality some-times as a pawn to an unscrupulous partner, is unable to experience true concern for others, lacks recognition of others as independent agents, and suffers from ideas of reference and excessive self-referential perceptions of reality.

The advent of DSM criteria has allowed the development of a number of diagnostic instruments. These include the Diagnostic Interview for Borderlines (DIB; Gunderson et al., 1981), Structured Clinical Interview for DSM personality disorders (SCID II), Personality Interview Question (PIQ-II; Widiger et al., 1986) and Diagnostic Interview for Personality Disorders (DIPD; Zanarini et al., 1987). However, the problem of comorbidity has not gone away.

COMORBIDITY

Early in the development of the concept of borderline, a great deal of energy was expended in differentiating it from affective disorders and schizophrenia. The overlap of borderline personality disorder and affective disorders has already been discussed (see p. 129). The phenomenological difference between inpatients diagnosed either as schizophrenic or borderline has become clearer. Their distinction is now beyond reasonable doubt (Berelowitz and Tarnopolsky, 1993) although outpatient populations have been less well studied. In contrast to early concerns about the overlap of borderline personality disorder with major psychiatric disorders, the focus has now moved to the differentiation of borderline from other personality disorders. This is more problematic.

The independent overlap between several disorders is called comor-bidity. Comorbidity as an explanation may mitigate against intellec-tual rigour – once it is found that categories of personality overlap, comorbidity can be used as an explanation and further attempts to tease apart differing disorders abandoned. Fortunately this has not yet happened, although some authors (Widiger and Frances, 1987) have suggested developing a dimensional system rather than using categorical diagnoses. Nevertheless categorical attempts at differenti-ating personality disorders continue. In the DSM-IV, personality disorders are grouped into clusters. Borderline, a Cluster B disorder, shares its home with antisocial, histrionic, and narcissistic personal-ities from which it must be distinguished if such a classification is to be useful. Furthermore, partly because of their common develop-mental history, schizotypal personality (Cluster A) needs to be differentiated. This is especially the case as all these disorders show similar phenomenological characteristics and, from a psychodynamic point of view, evince comparable use of primitive mental mechanisms and intrapsychic structure. Nurnberg et al. (1991) studied a group of outpatients and found that 82% of patients meeting criteria for borderline personality disorder had at least one additional personality disorder diagnosis. A similar result has been found with an inpatient population (Dolan et al., 1995). In Nurnberg's study, factor analysis revealed a group of borderline patients who overlapped with paranoid, histrionic, narcissistic, antisocial and passive–aggressive personality and another group who overlapped with schizoid, schizotypal, avoidant, obsessive–compulsive, and self-defeating personalities. Some of these categories have been dropped from the DSM-IV. However, one conclusion to be drawn is that borderline personality represents a heterogeneous category which encompasses a general concept of personality disorder.

Dissocial Personality

Dissocial individuals demonstrate impulsive behaviour, show irritability and aggressiveness, disregard their own and others' safety, use primitive mental mechanisms (see discussion on projective identification p. 129), and are consistently irresponsible. However, they may be differentiated from borderline patients by their capacity to leave relationships, moving to another with almost callous ease, their conscious manipulation which is unencumbered by guilt, and their often sustained delinquent behaviour. Their psychic structure and use of primitive mechanisms tends to be more stable than those found in borderline individuals, leading to a fixed paranoid view of the world. In contrast, borderline patients tend to cling desperately to relationships, feel intense attachments which are alternately idealized and denigrated, feel ashamed about their behaviour, and show fluctuating use of primitive mental mechanisms.

Histrionic Personality

Patients with histrionic personality disorder may be the most difficult to differentiate from borderline individuals. Not only do they show the same impulsive behaviour but also they develop clinging relationships and demand excessive attention from partners and the helping professions alike. However, they do not demonstrate the chronic rage of borderline patients and their investment in self-destructive acts is less. Although these features are itemized in more detail in the DSM-IV, the clinical picture is often very similar to borderline patients.

Narcissistic Personality

The concept of narcissistic personality has developed out of psychodynamic psychiatry and psychoanalysis just like that of borderline personality. It may be considered as another disorder of the self. The narcissistic personality is consistently self-assured, self-important, and grandiose on the surface. He is full of his achievements, believes he is special and he should only associate with others of equal or higher status. Beneath he is wracked with nagging fears of inferiority. He is insecure and craves admiration. His self is well defended, cohesive, and in little danger of dissolution. In contrast, the self of the borderline is chronically threatened by identity diffusion (Erikson, 1968) and undermined by regression leading to a persistent tendency to revert to earlier maladaptive coping strategies. The resulting instability leads to self-mutilation, overdosing and other self-destructive acts. Such events are rare in narcissistic disorders in which the body is more likely to be invested with special importance and form part of a grandiose self. Self-destructive acts only occur if the covert feelings of inferiority and insecurity break through.

In contrast to this differentiation, Kernberg (1984) views narcissistic personality disorder as a more mature, but no less therapeutically problematic variant of borderline personality organization, in which there is a fusion between an ideal self and an actual self. Real intersubjectivity is obliterated in an attempt to avoid feelings of rage, disappointment, envy, contempt and despair. Two types of narcissism may be distinguished. Rosenfeld (1987) writes of the 'thick skinned' oblivious insensitive type of narcissist, obsessed with himself and his achievements, whose relationships reflect the need to be admired and lack depth or substance. By contrast, the hypervigilant, 'thin skinned', oversensitive, often hypochondriachal type of narcissist, whose emotional life is the subject of intense and constant scrutiny is perhaps best seen as vulnerable to 'impingement', due to a deficit of maternal attunement (Stern, 1985).

Schizotypal Personality

The word 'schizotype' (Rado, 1953) is an elision of schizophrenia and genotype and arose from the observation that non-psychotic relatives of patients with schizophrenia showed peculiarities suggestive of autistic thinking, shallow interpersonal relationships, hypochondriasis, inability to maintain a steady life pattern, and an inner life suffused with hatred (Zilboorg 1941, 1952). Development of this idea in the work of Meehl (1962), who suggested an inherited neural deficit as the underlying cause, Kety et al. (1968, 1975), Rosenthal et al. (1968, 1971), and Wender et al. (1974), culminated in the survey of Spitzer et al. (1979) which differentiated borderline from schizotypal disorders. Schizotypal personalities show ideas of reference, magical thinking or odd beliefs, unusual perceptual experiences including bodily illusions, social isolation, odd speech and thinking, inadequate rapport, suspiciousness, lack of close friends or confidants, and undue social anxiety. Whilst the perceptual–cognitive distortions are often used on clinical grounds to differentiate schizotypal from borderline patients, this is not fully supported by research. McGlashan (1987) reported that the most discriminating features are odd communications, suspiciousness and social isolation, whilst the least discriminating criteria involved illusions, depersonalization and derealization. Markar et al. (1991) found that the presence of schizotypal features predicted some borderline features but not vice versa. This rather surprising finding suggests that a hierarchical model may be useful in the relationship between schizotypal and borderline disorder. Schizotypal individuals may be linked with the 'tail-end of schizophrenia' (Kernberg, 1984) and therefore superordinate to borderline disorder and perhaps should be classified with the parent disorder rather than within personality disorders.

PSYCHODYNAMIC FORMULATIONS OF BORDERLINE PERSONALITY

Borderline personality disorder has evoked intense theorizing among psychoanalysts, and, perhaps because of its clinical difficulty and variability, represents a battlefield upon which many of the controversies and schizms of contemporary psychoanalyis have been played out. The main difference is between authors who emphasize conflict and those who stress deficit as the central psychopathological theme, each group advocating apparently very different treatment approaches. The 'conflict' group includes both the classical Freudians and neo-classical Lacanians, and the Kleinians and their followers, . while the 'deficit' group comprises, in Britain the Independents, and in the USA the Interpersonalists and Self-psychologists. In practice this divide is somewhat artificial: as we shall see, the evidence suggests that both conflict *and* deficit are important in the aetiology of borderline personality, that both intrapsychic and environmental factors play an important part, and that different authors are probably describing and treating different patient populations with different clinical needs.

Conflict Models of Borderline

Kernberg (1984) addresses comorbidity head-on. He combines classical instinct theory with object relations, to define an underlying *borderline personality organization* found in many psychopathological situations, including borderline, narcissistic, histrionic personality disorders, psychotic disorders, some eating disorders, and in normal individuals who are exposed to extreme stress. Borderline personality organization becomes a supra-ordinate diagnosis.

Kernberg's borderline personality organization has the following features:

1. *Ego weakness.* This leads to poor impulse control, a deficient capacity to cope with anxiety, and therefore difficulty in sublimating instinctual demands into socially acceptable channels.
2. *A shift from secondary to primary process thinking.* This is particularly manifest in the dream-like quasi-psychotic states common in borderline personality disorder, in which the capacity for reality-testing disappears. Thus they may feel that those who care for or love them actually detest and hate them, which, indeed, by projective identification they may be induced to do.
3. *The use of 'primitive' defence mechanisms.* These include splitting and projective identification, idealization, denial, omnipotence and devaluation (see p. 129). Such people swing between feeling all-powerful (often all-powerfully destructive) or helplessly inadequate; rushing from one idealized 'answer' to another, only to be bitterly disappointed as each god turns out to have feet of clay. Perceptions of the world are powerfully coloured by projection and a characteristic feature of analytic work with these patients is projective identification in which feelings are communicated not by symbolism or words but by direct transfer into the therapist's inner world.
4. *Pathological internal object relations.* The inner world in borderline personality organization mirrors these external manifestations of splitting and projection. Instead of stable and smoothly integrated

internal representations of people and their relationships, the self and others are experienced in chiaroscuro, or as part-objects – breasts, penises, and objects for evacuation or exploitation. At different times the subject is in the grip, in Fairbairn's (1952) terms, of a split-off libidinal or antilibidinal self, choosing perversity or self-destruction as a defence against inner emptiness or complete fragmentation –

things fall apart; the centre cannot hold;
mere anarchy is loosed upon the world,
the blood-dimmed tide is loosed, and everywhere
the ceremony of innocence is drowned.

(*Yates, The Second Coming*).

Kernberg relates borderline personality organization to Mahler's 'rapprochement subphase' in which the child begins to separate and to explore the world for him/herself, but needs to rush back to his/her mother for comfort and reassurance and 'narcissistic supplies'. If the mother is physically or psychologically unavailable the child may not be able to integrate good and bad maternal images. The child then reacts to abandonment with an excess of aggression which is projected outwards onto his/her objects and reintrojected into a split self in a way that often resists therapeutic efforts.

This position of an identified-with internal 'bad parent' object, who is clung to, who punishes and persecutes in the way that the original 'bad object' did in reality, combined with elements of revenge and triumph over the object, is a common constellation in borderline personality disorder. One patient described this split-off identificate as 'him', an evil male who took over her personality and made her do destructive things, reminiscent of multiple personality.

Masterson (1976) also focuses on the rapprochement subphase of separation–individuation, although emphasizing the mother's response rather than the innate aggression of the child. In essence, Masterson and Rinsley found that the mothers of borderline patients seemed to have been conflicted about their child growing up. Attempts on the part of the child to become independent are met by threats of loss of love. As a result the child becomes stuck between attempts at independence and terrors of abandonment resulting in the claustrophobic–agoraphobic dilemma so commonly found in borderline patients (Bateman, 1995).

Steiner (1993) describes the inner world of the borderline in spatial terms. Between the splitting of the paranoid–schizoid position and the pain of the depressive position lies the 'borderline position'. The sufferer seeks out 'psychic retreats', safe havens, free from pain, but also sequestered from real emotional contact with people and the flux of life. Steiner suggests that silent, aloof, overtalkative or pseudo-co-operative patients may be operating from such retreats, which are often symbolized in dreams as caves, fortresses, houses, or parts of the body. Fanatical affiliation to political or religious groups may have a similar defensive function as a way of containing disturbance, but also potentially impeding psychic growth.

Deficit Models

Deficit models identify similar features of borderline personality organization but tend to put a different emphasis on the clinical phenomena:

1. *Aggression*. For Kernberg, excess aggression is the primary abnormality in borderline personality organization. For Kohut and Fairbairn the aggression is secondary to environmental failure, a protest against an unresponsive mother, or a way of holding onto an object through hatred in the absence of the capacity to love. The fragmentation and inner loneliness of the borderline are not seen as defences, but as 'breakdown products' of an individual deprived of vital supplies of love (Adler, 1985).
2. *The ego*. Conflict theorists see the ego as 'weak', and unable to contain aggressive impulses. Deficit theorists emphasize the failure of self-soothing function often found in borderline personality organization. Unable to calm themselves psychologically, patients with borderline personality disorder turn to dependent relationships with others, to drugs, compulsive sex, binge-eating, or self-harm. Many 'cutters' describe escalating agitation which, at the moment of self-injury, turns into an almost post-orgasmic sense of calm.
3. *The role of the environment*. Kohut and Winnicott have a rather idealized view of early mother–infant relationship, in which the mother's responsiveness and attunement, that is her capacity to reciprocate meaningfully her child's moods and needs, her capacity to foster transitional space or to modulate her presence and absence, and to supply 'self-object' needs, leads to a secure, stable sense of self. Where the basic 'good enough' maternal functions were missing, the child is vulnerable to borderline personality disorder in later life.
4. *The necessity of narcissism*. For Kernberg, the narcissist is in a

state of conflict between his need for an object and the rage he feels towards his objects – hence he obliterates the gap and self-absorbedly 'becomes' his ideal self. For Kohut and Winnicott the narcissist is faced by an insensitive, absent, or abusive primary object, and so retreats into himself, trying vainly to 'be' the missing mother he so desperately needed, in order to preserve some sense of inner coherence.

The divergence between Kernberg's conflict theory and Kohut's deficit formulation may partly be explained by the different patient populations studied. Kohut's theory was founded on work with relatively well-functioning outpatients who were vulnerable to setbacks because of fragile self-esteem. Kernberg's work was done with inpatients as well as outpatients, many of whom demonstrated severe acting out and showed persistent antisocial features.

Numerous compromise theories have been put forward. One, based on a developmentally based contemporary Freudian theory and 'theory of mind', links intrapsychic conflict with cognitive deficit (Fonagy, 1989, 1991). Essentially, the child is viewed as vulnerable to excessive conflict because of a developmental failure in perceiving the state of mind of others. This deficit arises out of the (usually correct) perception of the child that the primary care-giver harbours hostile and dangerous thoughts about him. In order to protect himself from attack the child inhibits his capacity to recognize what is in the mind of others. This results in an inevitable failure to experience others as human and may leave the child vulnerable to further external trauma, such as sexual abuse, as the child mis-reads the motivation of others. Unfulfilled need creates resentment, distrust, and excessive destructiveness. An incapacity to think about the mental state of others, a deficit, leaves the individual profoundly vulnerable to psychic conflict, which in turn renders the person open to pathological adaptation through the use of defence mechanisms. The severity of the conflict and the developmental level at which the deficit originally occurs results in the mobilization of primitive mental mechanisms, especially splitting and projective identification.

Primitive Mechanisms of Borderline Personality Disorder

Splitting

Following Klein, contemporary psychoanalysts use the term 'splitting' to refer to a division of an object into 'good' and 'bad'. A child, in his mind, will split his mother into two separate persons, the bad, frustrating mother whom he hates and the good, idealized mother whom he loves. By mentally keeping the good and bad mother strictly separate, the ambivalent conflict between loving and hating a mother who is, in reality one and the same person, and a mixture of good and bad, can be avoided.

Klein also recognized that, since internal and external objects are intrinsically related to the ego, a split in the ego may also occur. This was in keeping with Freud's original use of the term splitting. He referred to a splitting of the ego in fetishism, allowing a quasi-psychotic simultaneous holding of contradictory ideas (Freud, 1927). The split coincided with the contradiction between a wishful fantasy and a reality, rather than between object representations – 'the instinct is allowed to retain its satisfaction *and* proper respect is shown to reality' (Freud, 1940). This descriptive use of the term is compatible with Bleuler's (1924) account of the loosening of associations in schizophrenia. However, splitting is now viewed, especially by Kleinian analysts, as a primary phenomenon of mental life in infancy potentially leading to the development of borderline and psychotic disorders later in life (Kernberg, 1975). In these cases splitting is extreme and leads to a distortion of perception, a diminution in the capacity for coherent thought, and fragmentation of objects.

Projection, identification and projective identification

Projective identification is undoubtedly an important but also a complex subject, partly because of its inherent difficulty, partly perhaps because its name is misleading, and partly because, as one of the fundamentals of Kleinian psychoanalysis, it provokes political controversy disproportionate to its clinical role and relevance.

The notion of *projection* is relatively straightforward, and has entered the vernacular of 'folk psychology' (Bruner, 1990). The depressed young man lying on a beach who stated 'everyone on this beach looks utterly miserable' was clearly attributing to others his own affective state. We commonly attribute our more difficult and unacceptable feelings to others, for example blaming those that are close to us for our own shortcomings. Externalization, the outward limb of projection allows us to disown responsibility, and to feel an illusory sense of mastery over our impulses. If our unwanted impulses and feelings boomerang back and result in a feeling of being under constant attack, the projection has gone full circle and leads to anxiety or, if extreme, paranoid delusions.

Identification similarly is relatively straightforward, referring to the process by which self-representations are built up and modified during development, as distinct from the conscious copying of imitation. The little boy who shuffles around in his father's shoes is simply imitating, but as his internal image of himself is influenced and later transformed into a personality characteristic, identification has occurred, especially if he eventually 'steps into his father's shoes' and takes over the family business. Piaget's (1954) concepts of 'assimilation' and 'accommodation' are similar although referring to the development of cognitive ability rather than self-representation. Piaget suggests the young infant has internal 'schemas' of only actions and perceptions, but later the child represents one thing by another through the use of words and symbols. New experiences are 'assimilated' into existing schemas, and may be distorted by them, much as the external world is introjected and modified by unconscious phantasy within a psychoanalytic model. Schemas are modified, extended, and combined to meet new situations through 'accommodation'. Similarly self-representations are modified and built-on through new identifications.

As Klein (1946) originally conceived it, *projective identification* combines these two notions in a highly specific way. She described projective identification as a phantasy in which bad parts of the infantile self are split off from the rest of the self and projected into the mother or her breast. As a result, the infant feels that his mother has 'become' the bad parts of himself. Of particular importance is, firstly, that the projection is 'into' rather than 'onto' the object – prototypically the mother or the analyst, and secondly, that what is projected is not so much a feeling or an attitude, but the self, or part of it. Klein imagined that in the paranoid–schizoid position the infant might project 'bad' sadistic parts of himself into the mother's body in order to control and injure her from within. If these are then reintrojected – 'introjective identification' – the individual contains a 'bad' identificate, a potential source of low self-esteem or self-hatred. In contrast 'good' parts of the self may also be projected and reintrojected, increasing self-esteem and enhancing good object relations if not carried to excess.

In this original formulation projective identification was defensive, intrapsychic, and solipsistic, a mental transaction involving the self and a perception, but not the participation, of the other. How then does projective identification differ, if at all, from projection? Klein, herself, was clear about this. Projection is the mental mechanism under-pinning the process and projective identification is the specific phantasy expressing it. Spillius (1988) suggests that projective identi-fication adds depth to Freud's original concept of projection by empha-sizing the fact that a phantasy of projection is only possible if accompanied by a projection of parts of the self. She comments that British authors rarely consider the distinction between projection and projective identification to be of particular importance. In contrast, many American writers have devoted a great deal of discussion to the topic (Malin and Grotstein, 1966; Langs, 1978; Ogden, 1979), often distinguishing projection and projective identification by whether or not the recipient of the projections is emotionally affected or not by the phantasy. In projection the target of the projections may be bliss-fully unaware of his role – as no doubt were the holidaymakers on the beach in the example above. The paranoid person projects malevolent intentions onto politicians, pop stars, Freemasons etc. with whom he never comes in contact, or indeed onto inanimate objects. This distinction has arisen from developments of Klein's original idea of projective identification emphasizing its *communicative* aspect.

The communicative aspect of projective identification, as opposed to its defensive nature, means that it can be used to describe three distinct processes. First, if projective identification is seen as an inter-active phenomenon, then the recipient of the projection may be induced to feel or act in ways that originate with the projector. This accounts for Heimann (1950), Grinberg (1962) and Racker's (1968) realization that countertransferential feelings evoked in the analyst can reflect aspects of the patient's inner world. Ogden (1979) argues that identification occurs within both projector *and* recipient, while Grotstein (1981) and Kernberg (1987) both feel that the term should be confined to identification within the projector. These ideas, often in a watered-down form, have become widely accepted in psychody-namic circles: if the analyst is feeling bored or irritable or sad, these feelings may well, via projective identification, originate with the patient. Here the 'identification' is occurring within the target of the projective identification, rather than, as Klein first saw it, within the projector.

Second, by extension, projective identification becomes a mutual process in which projector and recipient interact with one another at an unconscious level. The analyst who is unaware of the feelings induced in him by projective identification may *enact* them by, for example, being rejecting or sluggish in the session, feelings which may in turn be identified with by the patient. Spillius (1994) suggests the term 'evocatory projective identification' to describe this pressure put onto the analyst to conform to the patient's phantasy. Sandler (1976a, b) and Sandler and Sandler (1978) see this aspect of projective identification in terms of 'actualization' and 'role responsiveness' in which the analyst has on the one hand to be flexible enough to respond slightly to the role in which he is cast by the patient's projective identification, while remaining sufficiently centred in himself to observe and interpret this process as it happens.

The ramifications of the communicative aspects of projective identification are so great that it can come to cover almost all that happens in the analytic situation. However, it is clinically mistaken to assume that everything that the analyst experiences is a result of what the patient is 'putting into' him. It is important to distinguish between 'patient-derived countertransference' and 'analyst-derived countertransference', however difficult this may be in practice (Money-Kyrle, 1956). The former is based on projective identification, while the latter most definitely is not.

The third extension of projective identification derives from Bion (1962, 1963). Klein saw projective identification primarily in negative terms: the projection of sadistic feelings as part of the paranoid–schizoid position. Bion realized that there was also a 'positive' form of projective identification underlying empathy, and the processes by which the mother contains projected painful and hostile feelings, 'detoxifies' them, and returns them to the infant in a more benign form at a phase-appropriate moment. However, some of Bion's clinical use of the idea of projective identification have been controversial. He advocated speaking to psychotic patients in concrete ways; thus he might say 'you are pushing your fear of murdering me into my insides'. While this kind of interpretation may occasionally be successful, in inexperienced hands it can be at best incomprehensible, at worst dangerous, and as a standard technique has been much criticized (Sandler, 1987). It is rarely used nowadays.

Many authors, including Bion (1955) have stressed the importance of projective identification as a method of control of the object and of unmanageable feelings. In this aspect of projective identification, whole aspects of the ego are split off and projected into another person, animal or inanimate object, who then represents and becomes identified with the split-off parts; attempts are then made to control these split-off parts of the self by asserting control over the other person (Sandler, 1987).

Good aspects of the self can also be projected into others. Projective identification can thus leave an individual feeling deprived of essential aspects of this own personality. A central task of analysis is to help the patient recover these lost aspects of the self.

Projective identification then is important because it tackles the lifeblood of psychoanalysis, the interplay of phantasy in intimate relationships. It is both defensive and communicative and the response of the analyst may be the primary factor in determining which aspect is uppermost (Joseph, 1987). It is 'difficult' because the concept originates in a rather casual definition given by Klein (1952) and retains a title that does not really capture post-Kleinian extensions. Although 'communicative projection' or 'projective interaction' may be preferable expressions, Spillius (1988) suggests that projective identification should be retained as a general term within which various subtypes can be differentiated. The many motives behind the process – to control the object, to acquire its attributes, to evacuate a bad quality, to protect a good quality, to avoid separation, to communicate – may be useful starting points to identify subtypes.

THE SELF

Whatever the divergences of the conflict and deficit models or the compromises of alternative formulations, one factor remains common to all – borderline personality disorder is essentially a disorder in the development and functioning of the 'self'. This agreement is reflected in the changing definition in the DSM-IV which attaches more specificity to distorted self-image and problems with impulse control than hitherto. Unfortunately psychoanalysts and dynamic psychiatrists refer to several different phenomena when using the term 'self' (Westen, 1992), allowing further schisms to take place.

Psychodynamic and Cognitive Self

The focus of Kohut's (1971, 1977) deficit theory became the 'self', and the effect that denial, frustration and fulfilment of wishes has on its development. He depicted the self as a supra-ordinate structure with its own developmental line which subsumed instinctual wishes and defences. Just as Hartmann had postulated a 'conflict-free' zone of the ego, Kohut built on Freud's notion of 'primary narcissism', to suggest that self-love was necessary for psychological health, seeing narcissistic and borderline disorders as resulting from defects in the self brought about by parental empathic failures.

He postulated first a 'bipolar' self and later a 'tripolar' self in which self-assertive ambitions crystallize at one pole, attained ideals and values at the other, and talents and skills at the third. Pathology may arise from a disturbance at each pole and may be compensated for by strength in one of the others.

The idea of the self following a separate developmental pathway, can be seen as an expansion of Freud's view of psychosexual development, and of Anna Freud's (1965) notion of separate development lines along drive-, ego- and object-related pathways. However, X the view that the self has a supra-ordinate or unifying, overarching perspective on personality development is more controversial.

In self-psychology the focus is on the need for empathic and affirming responses from others throughout life, with a move from reliance on archaic objects towards mature dependency. Kohut's view of the self contrasts markedly with that of other writers who commonly use the term when referring to self-representations (Sandler, 1987; Sandler and Rosenblatt, 1962). Most authors then ascribe all sorts of properties to the self-representation including motivation, self-esteem regulation, planning abilities and so on (Markus and Cross, 1990) thereby elevating the concept to virtually all of the personality. But, by definition a self-representation cannot be anything other than a representation of something defined as the 'self'. Thus the self and self-representation cannot be the same thing. A more sensible and theoretically coherent view is given by Westen and Cohen (1993) who define the self as 'the person – body, mental contents, attributes, and the like'. Self-representation becomes but one aspect of the self, namely the view an individual forms of him or herself just like another person might have formed of him or her. Self-representations may be conscious or unconscious. The borderline consciously experiences him/herself as an injured, especially important figure, victimized by the present and past, self-righteously enraged; unconsciously the borderline feels inferior, empty, and defective. Self-representations are a mix of conscious and unconscious psychological processes formed from competing affective and motivational elements from both past and present. They are compromises governed by the pleasure–displeasure principle, maintaining psychic equilibrium to greatest advantage, seeing oneself as one would wish to be seen and how one feels one really is.

Other aspects of the self include:

- self-with-other representations;
- wished for, feared, and ideal self-representations;

- self-esteem;
- self-presentation,
- sense of self;
- identity.

None of these aspects of the self is motivating in itself but may become so if affectively charged. For example, if a patient's conscious self-with-other representation is as a dominant victor, he will continually try to show his prowess over whoever challenges him. In treatment, unconscious feelings of shame and humiliation brought about by seeking and being offered help from a therapist will lead to increasing contempt for the therapist as the patient tries to defend his 'victor' self-with-other representation. Not to take into account such an unconscious affective charge will lead to therapeutic failure.

Each aspect of the self is organized within the mind in many spatial and temporal ways along networks of memories, and experiences, both past and present. These are known as 'relationship schemas'. They have a great deal in common with 'objects' of object relations theory but are clearly more than the 'cognitive schemas' of cognitive–behavioural theory in that there is a greater emphasis on the strength of affective charge and its motivating force. The deification of cognition misses the power of emotion which is so central to borderline pathology and loses the importance of unconscious or underlying forces. The borderline whose manifest cognitive self is angry, victimized and down-trodden is often latently victimizing, bullying and attacking. The grandiose self covers a shrivelled, worthless self.

Self-representations. All aspects of the self are distorted or unstable in the borderline patient. Self-representations are split. Contradictory representations cannot sit side-by-side simultaneously to form a multidimensional whole. Only one memory at a time is evoked and there is a loss of contiguity as memories are described. Contradictory statements separated in time are not questioned, each opposing aspect being true for its specific moment. Thus, one patient described her mother as her best friend but in the next sentence talked about how they never really said anything of importance to each other.

Self-with-other representations are weak and malevolent in borderline personality. The borderline fails to monitor herself as she talks and cannot take into account the 'other'. In Fonagy's terms this represents a failure to develop a theory of mind. Confirming Kernberg's emphasis on the importance of aggression and the ubiquity of projective identification, Nigg et al. (1992) found a preponderance of spiteful, vitriolic relationship schemas in borderline patients. Thus, when the borderline can think about the mind of the other, she feels threatened and endangered.

Wished-for and ideal self-representations are often unrealistic, fleeting and yet yearned for. As soon as frustration arises the ideal is changed leading to inconsistency, a lack of long-term goals, living for the moment, and an inability to sustain relationships. Desperation and a general low level of self-esteem may, however, give rise to a florid, often outrageous performance in an attempt to retrieve a crumbling ideal – more self-presentation than self-expression. In an attempt to prop up an aspect of the self, the self becomes lost and irrelevant leading to an unconscious sense of emptiness. *The* self has become *a* self that is needed, chameleon like, at a given time. No true self exists, leading to identity diffusion and narrative inconsistency. Life, in the experience of the borderline, is a series of dis-crete events, unlinked episodes, each without a history or precursors.

Heard and Linehan (1993) emphasize two aspects of the self in borderline patients, namely the sense of self and *the relational self*. They characterize them from a behavioural point of view rather than from an experiential position and prefer to focus on processes and activities of the individual, and self-referrant behaviours. Nevertheless they recognize the importance of the interaction between the individual and the environment focusing on how the two act as mutually influencing fields. The individual has a powerful effect on his environment and vice versa. This relational definition of the self is less divorced from psychodynamic theory than its authors may wish. In Sullivan's (1953) interpersonal theory, anxiety has an organizing role. It is seen as being stimulated from without, a response to the state of mind of the other. The environment and the self affecting each other. The child forms specific mental representations according to the anxiety that is engendered and imagines that 'bad me' elicited anxiety in the (m)other. In the same way a 'good me', which alleviates anxiety, is also set up along with a 'not me'. The 'not me' is a response to severe panic and confusion which, in the borderline, becomes a nucleus for subsequent psychotic fragmentation. More recent psychoanalytic theory emphasizes the ways in which the individual influences his environment through projective identification, role responsiveness, and actualization. The borderline, like us all, creates responses from others, and others create and mould ours in return – you reap what you sow. Linehan (1993) suggests that the borderline is predisposed to dysfunctions of the self which lead to an interaction with the environment which highlights the full systemic dysfunction.

The focus from both a behavioural and psychodynamic perspective on the influence of the environment in borderline disorders leads to some agreement over aetiology but, perhaps not suprisingly, disagreement over treatment.

AETIOLOGY AND TREATMENT

Psychoanalytic theories offer the most comprehensive understanding of the development of borderline disorders, relating its formation to non-specific developmental factors which lead to pathological development of the self-structure. All psychoanalytic theories stress the interaction between the individual and environment, although their emphasis varies. Kernberg, and Masterson and Rinsley, relate the development of borderline personality to Mahler's rapprochement subphase. Kohut, on the other hand, sees the disorder as an inevitable outcome of a failure of the environmental response to the child. However, all are agreed that problematic, often disrupted, attachments in childhood, chaotic family experiences, lack of attunement between mother and child, and sexual abuse are important. There is now empirical evidence for such views, although it remains unclear which of these factors, under what circumstances, contribute to different elements that make up borderline personality. For example, sexual abuse seems to link to the dissociative experiences of the borderline (Ogata et al., 1990) and also gives rise to identity diffusion and poor self–other differentiation.

Child Sexual Abuse

Over the past few years a great deal of attention has been given to the level of physical and sexual abuse in the childhood and adolescence of borderline patients. Nigg et al. (1991), Brown and Anderson (1991), Byrne et al. (1990) and others have all found raised levels of sexual and physical abuse in the histories of borderline patients when compared with other psychiatric patients and normal populations. Zanarini et al. (1989) tried to tease out which factors, for example, abuse, neglect, separation, or disturbed parenting are most important, as each factor rarely exists alone. Abuse seems to be most discriminating. Neglect and separation, whilst common, are less discriminating.

The evidence for family dysfunction, neglect, instability, and childhood sexual and physical abuse, as important factors in borderline personality disorder is now overwhelming. However, not all children brought up in such circumstances develop such a florid disorder, suggesting that it is the context in which the traumas occur or their admixture, rather than the individual traumas themselves, that may be most important. Parker et al. (1987), Zweig-Frank and Paris (1991), and Patrick et al. (1994) all found low care and high overprotection in families of borderlines. This apparent contradiction may be explained by a mother who is emotionally inaccessible and unable to offer comfort to her distressed child, yet is intrusive and demanding. This view concurs with that founded on biosocial concepts.

Linehan (1987) sees the development of borderline personality as the outcome of the interaction between an emotionally invalidating rearing environment and an emotionally vulnerable child. The primary invalidating phenomenon is a discrediting of the child's emotional and cognitive experiences. In other words the family responds to a child's experience of events and his feelings about them by reinterpreting them to show him he is wrong. The child inevitably feels dysfunctional, cannot rely on his own experience, and fails to develop methods of regulating emotions. Such an environment can exist in either perfect families or chaotic ones. However a constitutionally affectively vulnerable child is also important. Affective vulnerability means an inability to regulate emotions to ensure they return to a baseline relatively quickly, and a biologically determined propensity to over-react emotionally when provoked. This combination results in escalating attempts to obtain a response from the environment to relieve the emotion. As the environment fails to respond, so the individual increases his efforts to provoke care and soothing. Thus for the cognitive-behaviourist the offender is the environment, for the psychoanalyst it is the unattuned mother. However, both assume a constitutional vulnerability and both share the view that the core of the problem is an inability to control intense affects and to test appropriately or to rectify cognitive distortions.

Inevitably the different theoretical viewpoints lead to different treatment modalities. The psychodynamic psychiatrist recommends psychotherapy whilst the cognitive-behaviourist suggests a specific, time-limited, focused, strategic programme. There are now few adherents of a singular pharmacological approach.

TREATMENT APPROACHES

In keeping with the variability of the symptomatology of borderline patients and their rapidly fluctuating mental state, a diverse array of treatment approaches and treatment settings have been used. These range from classical psychoanalysis, inpatient and day hospital psychotherapy, and outpatient psychotherapy to cognitive-behavioural therapy and drug regimens.

Drug regimens have been used extensively in the treatment of borderline disorders but there remains no single drug treatment of choice. There is justification only for short-term use of medication in the treatment of acute symptoms. No drug treatment is going to be effective against the dynamic personality functioning of the borderline, but equally no psychotherapeutic treatment is likely to be effective unless a patient is available for therapeutic work. The question is not so much whether drug treatment is effective but how should it be used to enhance the efficacy of other treatments? Soloff (1994), in reviewing the literature on the use of medication in borderline disorders, recommends pharmacotherapy only as an adjunct to long-term psychotherapy treatment of borderline patients especially to aid control of affective dysregulation, impulsive and aggressive behaviour, and paranoid symptoms and other cognitive distortions. To these ends, tricyclic, MAOI and SSRI anti-depressants, carbamazepine and lithium, and low-dose neuroleptics respectively have all been tried with varying degrees of success.

All psychological treatment methods, whether psychodynamically or behaviourally orientated, have common issues with which to grapple in the treatment of borderline disorders. Once the borderline patient enters any treatment, he feels cared for, understood, and listened to, but gradually feelings of emptiness, depression, and loneliness become evident. Feelings of sympathy are evoked in the clinician who may escalate his attempts to help, only to find that they are rebuffed at a time of a perceived abandonment such as a holiday, ending a session, or weekend. The prospect of loss or rejection by the caring environment arouses rage and coercive attempts to control the environment through destructive acts, either directed against the self or against the abandoning clinician and his property, for example by refusing to leave the building, breaking windows and furniture. When this fails the borderline desperately looks to be cared for through such avenues as promiscuity, substance abuse, and clinging to others. The reactions of the clinician to such provocation may be pivotal to the success of further treatment.

Abend et al. (1983) consider the control in a clinical team of counter-aggressive responses as being an essential part of the treatment of borderline patients. Failure of control leads to a breakdown in treatment. The therapist has constantly to monitor his own emotional reactions to avoid being drawn into constant battles, enticed into endless justifications of an action or interpretation, induced to act outside the therapeutic relationship, and driven to take on an heroic or seducer's role. The capacity of the therapist to survive and to continue thinking under such circumstances is vital to the success of any treatment. The destructive attitude must be addressed if interventions are to be effective. The patient who doesn't do his 'homework' within cognitive analytic therapy (Ryle, 1990) needs to understand why he did not do it before further tasks are undertaken. Otherwise, sabotage, albeit unconsciously driven and influenced by primitive states of mind, will continue to infuse the therapeutic process. As we shall see, the therapeutic approach to distortions, primitive impulses, hostility, denigration and contempt depends on the treatment modality.

Whatever the treatment modality, mood and behavioural fluctuations are dealt with by structure and containment along with a non-anxious attitude on the part of the therapist to crises, acute acting out, and persistent provocation. Structure is maintained through rigid adherence to a treatment contract; containment through interpretation, the treatment setting and milieu, the teaching of cognitive techniques, or even offering 24 hour contact at times of crisis. A calm and thoughtful demeanour on the part of the therapist is established by supervision, working within a specialist team, or understanding one's own reactions better through personal therapy.

Dilemmas of Psychotherapeutic Approaches

The most significant divergence in psychotherapeutic treatment strategies lies between those who emphasize conflict and those who stress deficit. Kernberg and the Kleinian school, emphasizing conflict, stress the importance of verbal interventions and need for early interpretation of negative transference, while the deficit group, following Kohut and to some extent Winnicott, see the creation of a holding environment through empathic responsiveness and validation as the prime necessity. Conflict theorists accuse the deficit group of creating a collusive relationship in which real aggression is denied, mirroring the maternal deprivation in childhood which led to the development of false self and inhibition of autonomy and exploration. Deficit theorists believe that too much emphasis on negative transference reinforces the already fragile self-esteem of the borderline, and even creates the very aggression it attempts to interpret (Ryle, 1994).

Each approach, if rigorously applied, can lead the psychotherapist into serious difficulties. A 'Kohutian' (or 'Winnicottian') strategy can lead to regressive dependency, escalating demands, and erotic transference, with the therapist shifting abruptly from overinvolvement to rejection. An impure culture seems better. Focus on conflict at one moment may be appropriate, recognition of deficit essential at another. Similarly technical interventions may vary according to the stage of therapy. Appropriate shifting to a deficit model in clinical work links with a model put forward by Adler and Buie (1979) who suggest the central deficit in borderline patients is their incapacity to develop and activate soothing introjects. This necessitates a validation by the therapist of past traumas and replacing the emphasis of transference interpretation with techniques aimed at encouraging a trusting and secure relationship. Of course many argue that this is best done through accurate interpretation.

The dangers of excessive confrontation have been outlined by Kernberg (1984) who states 'it is easier to move from expressive to supportive therapy than in the other direction'. If used insensitively, confrontation causes many dropouts in therapies which might otherwise have progressed, since most patients with borderline personality find silence and negative interpretations confusing and unbearable. This may account for the fact that nearly half of borderline patients leave therapy within six months irrespective of the treatment setting. In a study of therapy dropouts in borderline personality disorder, Gunderson and Sabo (1993) found that the majority had left feeling unbearably angry following a confrontation with the analyst.

All practitioners agree that establishing a sound therapeutic alliance is both essential – and extremely difficult. The interpretation of negative transference *and* a high degree of acceptance and holding may, in varying circumstances, be appropriate. Containment and acceptance are needed. The patient, lacking the capacity for self-soothing, needs gentleness; equally needed is some confrontation with a constantly projected inner world, held in the grip of bad objects. Fosshage (1994) relates treatment in borderlines to Gedo and Goldberg's (1973) developmental sequence of empathy, moving from physiological regulation in the newborn, through attunement in infancy, to 'consensual [i.e. verbal] validation' in the toddler. He argues that in order to mobilize analysable transference in borderline patients some non-interpretive work is required. For those patients who move towards a collaborative relationship, permanent internal change becomes possible. For others, the major benefit of treatment may be the prevention at time of crisis of a spiral of self-destructiveness ending in suicide, and ensuring a safe place to which to return at the next crisis. A detailed account of a mixed approach in a day hospital setting has been described by Bateman (1995).

Evidence for the efficacy of psychodynamic treatments is plentiful, although often anecdotal (see Higgit and Fonagy, 1992, for a review). Recent work (Stevenson and Meares, 1992) has suggested that shorter-term interventions of around one year may be helpful in reducing borderline patients' propensity to self-harm, to utilize psychiatric services, and to underfunction. Of particular interest is that 30% of treated subjects no longer fulfilled DSM-III criteria for borderline personality, suggesting that personality functioning had changed markedly. Improvement persisted one year after cessation of therapy.

Overall it is now possible to outline some of the more important ingredients of successful psychodynamic psychotherapy for borderline patients. A stable framework, safeguarding the integrity of the patient, the therapist and the therapy itself, is needed. Limit setting is essential. Any divergence from previously agreed limits may fuel the borderline's wish for immediate gratification of needs and desires. Demands will escalate. Some practitioners set contracts which include forfeits. A focus on interpretation of the here-and-now rather than an emphasis on past traumas and their reconstruction is better. Concentrating on feelings of abandonment in a session as they arise carries more affective meaning to the borderline than an event of the past. The therapist needs to monitor and control his counter-transference reactions whilst using them as a key therapeutic tool. To do so requires vigilant self-scrutiny, supervision, team support, and an internal capacity for personal analysis. Outbursts of self-destructive behaviour, anger, and abject denigration need firm but sensitive handling. Co-operation between agencies is essential and allows therapy to be protected. Pre-arranged social and psychiatric intervention ensure co-ordinated treatment in crises and the patient may be greatly reassured by the example of a collaborative 'parental couple' (Bateman, 1995) who constructively respond in a unified manner.

Cognitive-Behavioural Therapy

Perhaps as a result of the severe difficulties encountered in psycho-analytic psychotherapy, recommendation of long-term treatment

over a period of years, and the inadequacy of pharmacological interventions, attempts have been made to develop short-term, focused
strategies in the treatment of borderline patients. Of particular
importance is the method developed by Linehan (1987) and co-
workers known as dialectical behaviour therapy (DBT). What is also
of interest is how short-term treatments have tended to become
longer once the extent of the pathology of borderline patients is recognized.

DBT consists of weekly individual psychotherapy, skills training,
consultation/supervision meetings for therapists, and telephone
conversations as needed between patient and individual therapist.
Individual sessions are problem-orientated and directive but combine
supportive techniques such as empathy, reflection, acceptance, and
a judicious use of techniques drawn from Zen. Furthermore, paradox
and metaphor, balancing acceptance of problems with change, and
validation of perceptions are also used. Skills training involves model-
ling, didactic instruction, behavioural rehearsal, feedback, coaching
and homework assignments.

Recognition of difficulties in fully implementing a DBT programme
paved the way for increased supervision and support. In supervision
the case is analysed according to behavioural strategies. The
discourse of the meetings is prescribed and agreed to by therapists
before joining the team. Telephone contact is seen as a way of
teaching patients to ask for help before becoming overwhelmed by
their problems. It is also a conduit to teach coping skills in the imme-
diacy of a threatening environment.

Treatment with DBT for one year (see Shearin and Linehan, 1994,
for review) reduces parasuicidal behaviour, inpatient psychiatric
days, and drop-out when compared with treatment as usual.
Although there was improvement on measures of adjustment, both
controls and patients treated with DBT remained in the impaired
range at the end of treatment. Furthermore at 12 months post-
treatment the differences between the two groups levelled out.

Integration

There are some elements of psychodynamic therapy within the DBT
programme as well as some areas of major difference. Both treatments require a collaborative relationship to be built before effective
treatment can begin. In psychodynamic work this is conceptualized
as developing a therapeutic alliance; in cognitive work this is an
orientation phase. The question is, how should it be done? Kernberg

and others set a contract, enforce limits, use interpretive work, presumably including metaphor, maintain a position of neutrality, and show accurate empathy. Dialectical behaviour therapists use an orientation programme, skills training, educational techniques and metaphor. Both use supervision, but have very different aims of the process. In DBT the agenda is problem-orientated, but in psychodynamic therapy careful exploration of counter-transference and its meaning for the patient–therapist dyad is often uppermost. Supervision acts as a 'third object' (Bateman, 1995) allowing the therapist to function creatively rather than a practical, guiding, beacon of knowledge.

Both modes of therapy aim to develop a secure base (Bowlby, 1988) for treatment but the more extensive and ambitious aims of psychodynamic therapy entail longer treatment. DBT focuses on the modification of specific abnormal behaviours, whereas psychodynamic therapy has a more comprehensive aim of restructuring the personality to bring about permanent internal change. A major function of a secure base within both modalities is to foster exploration and to promote affective control of impulses either through coping strategies or the development of internal soothing capacities. However, DBT emphasizes acceptance and validation of experience as well as facilitating adaptive change, seeing changes in the environment and the individual's response to those changes as pivotal. In this way unconscious motivation and distortion of perception through the use of primitive mental mechanisms are not taken into account. From a psychodynamic point of view the validation of a patient's experience may reinforce distortions and maintain maladaptive patterns. The validation of the borderline's experience and the location of the problem within the environment leaves the cognitive-behavioural therapist vulnerable. If the rage and anger are valid, what becomes of the accusations, denigration, and contempt of the therapist? They too must be valid and yet clearly they commonly result from distortion. The ending of a session by a therapist is not really a destructive abandonment any more than is the sending to bed of children by parents. In psychodynamic treatment good technique involves empathizing with the patient's experience whilst challenging those parts that are inappropriate and distorted through splitting and projective identification. Borderline patients do not enter crises solely because the environment fails to match expectation, but primarily because they recreate chaotic and unsatisfactory relationships time and time again. Their internal cognitive, affective, and motivational processes compel them to do so. The unconscious seeking of aggressively charged, chaotic relationships and repetition of negative affects preserves a maladaptive sense of security, a cohesion to a fragile self, and an optimal level of familiar feeling. Any treatment of borderline disorder must take account both of affective dysregulation and of the compulsion to recreate pathological object relationships.

CONCLUSIONS

There is no doubt that some borderline patients are treatable in psychotherapy but it remains unclear whether certain subgroups are either more treatable than others or more responsive to particular treatments. Further outcome studies are necessary but likely to be difficult. Dropout rates are high and Stone et al. (1987) point out that borderline patients are the least likely group of patients to agree to randomization. Furthermore, their fluctuating moods and aggression mitigate against accurate completion of self-assessment questionnaires and compliance with standardized assessment interviews. It is also unclear how outcome needs to be assessed. The overall aim may be to prevent suicide in a group of patients whose long-term prognosis is relatively good. Stone's (1990, 1993) 20-year follow-up suggests that two-thirds of patients end up functioning normally or with minimal symptoms, although those with more severe dysfunction do poorly, ending their lives by suicide.

Problems inherent in the study of borderline patients should not prevent further research. Meanwhile, both patients and therapists must tolerate the limitations of treatment and accept an uncertain outcome.

References

Abend, S.M., Porder, M.S., Willick, M.S. (1983) *Borderline Patients: Psychoanalytic Perspectives*. New York: IUP.

Adler, G. (1985) *Borderline Psychopathology and its Treatment*. New York: Jason Aronson.

Adler, G., Buie, D.H. (1979) Aloneness and borderline psychopathology: the possible relevance of child developmental issues. *International Journal of Psycho-analysis* **60**: 83–96.

Akhtar, S. (1992) *Broken Structures: Severe Personality Disorders and their Treatment*. New York: Jason Aronson.

American Psychiatric Association (1987) *Diagnostic and Statistical Manual of Mental Disorders*, 3rd edn, revised (DSM-III-R). Washington DC: APA.

American Psychiatric Association (1994) *Diagnostic and Statistical Manual of Mental Disorders*, 4th edn (DSM-IV). Washington DC: APA.

Bateman, A.W. (1989) Borderline personality in Britain: a preliminary study. *Comprehensive Psychiatry* **30**: 385–390.

Bateman, A.W. (1995) The treatment of borderline patients in a day hospital setting *Psychoanalytic Psychotherapy*. **9**: 3–16.

Berelowitz, M., Tarnopolsky, A. (1993) The validity of borderline personality: an updated review of recent research. In Tyrer, P., Stein, G. (eds) *Personality Disorder Reviewed*. Royal College of Psychiatrists: Gaskell.

Bion, W.R. (1955) Language and the schizophrenic. In Klein, M., Heimann, P., Money, R. (eds) *Directions of Psychoanalysis*, pp. 220–239. London: Tavistock Publications.

Bion, W. (1962) *Learning from Experience*. London: Heinemann.

Bion, W.R. (1963) *Elements of Psychoanalysis*. London: Heinemann.

Bleuler, E. (1924) *Textbook of Psychiatry*. New York: Macmillan.

Bowlby, J. (1988) *A Secure Base: Clinical Applications of Attachment Theory*. London: Routledge.

Brown, G.R., Anderson, B. (1991) Psychiatric morbidity in psychiatric inpatients with childhood histories of sexual and physical abuse. *American Journal of Psychiatry* **148**: 55–61.

Bruner, J. (1990) *Acts of Meaning*. Cambridge, MA: Harvard University Press.

Byrne, C.P., Velamoor, V.R., Cernovsky, Z.Z. et al. (1990) A comparison of borderline and schizophrenic patients for childhood life events and parent-child relationships. *Canadian Journal of Psychiatry* **35**: 590–595.

Deutsch, H. (1942) Some forms of emotional disturbance and their relationship to schizophrenia. *Psychoanalytic Quarterly* **11**: 301–321.

Dolan, B., Evans, C., Norton, K. (1995) Multiple Axis II diagnoses of personality disorder. *British Journal of Psychiatry* **166**: 107–112.

Erikson, E. (1968) *Identity, Youth and Crisis*. New York: Norton.

Fairbairn, W.R.D. (1952) *Psychoanalysis Studies of the Personality*. London: Routledge.

Falret, J. (1890) *Etudes Cliniques sur les Maladies Mentales*. Paris: Baillière.

Fonagy, P. (1989) On the integration of cognitive behaviour theory with psychoanalysis. *British Journal of Psychotherapy* **5**: 557–563.

Fonagy, P. (1991) Thinking about thinking: some clinical and theoretical considerations in the treatment of a borderline patient. *International Journal of Psychoanalysis* **72**: 639–656.

Fosshage, J. (1994) Towards reconceptualising transference: theoretical and clinical considerations. *International Journal of Psychoanalysis* **75**: 265–280.

Freud, A. (1965) *Normality and Pathology in Childhood*. New York: International Universities Press.

Freud, S. (1927) *Fetishism, S.E. 21*. London: Hogarth.

Freud S. (1940) *An Outline of Psychoanalysis, S.E. 23*. London: Hogarth.

Gedo, J., Goldberg, A. (1973) *Models of the Mind*. Chicago: University of Chicago Press.

Grinberg, L. (1962) On a specific aspect of countertransference due to the patient's projective identification. *International Journal of Psychoanalysis* **43**: 436–440.

Grinker, R.R., Werble, B., Drye, R.C. (1968) *The Borderline Syndrome*. New York: Basic Books.

Grotstein, J.S. (1981) *Splitting and Projective Identification*. New York: Jason Aronson.

Gunderson, J.G., Eliot, G.R. (1985) The interface between borderline personality disorder and affective disorder. *American Journal of Psychiatry* **142**: 277–288.

Gunderson, J.G., Kolb, J.E. (1978) Discriminating features of borderline patients. *American Journal of Psychiatry* **135**: 792–796.

Gunderson, J.G., Phillips, K.A. (1991) A current view of the interface between borderline personality disorder and depression. *American Journal of Psychiatry* **148**: 967–975.

Gunderson, J., Sabo, A. (1993) The phenomenal and conceptual interface between borderline personality disorder and PTSD. *American Journal of Psychiatry* **150**, 19–27.

Gunderson, J.G., Kolb, J.E., Austin, V. (1981) The diagnostic interview for borderline patients *American Journal of Psychiatry* **138**: 896–903.

Heard, H.L., Linehan, M.M. (1993) Problems of self and borderline personality disorder: a dialectical behavioural analysis. In Segal, Z.V., Blatt, S.J. (eds) *The Self in Emotional Distress. Cognitive and Psychodynamic Perspectives*. London: Guilford Press.

Heimann, P. (1950) On countertransference. *International Journal of Psychoanalysis* **31**: 81–84.

Higgitt, A., Fonagy, P. (1992) Psychotherapy in borderline and narcissistic personality disorder. *British Journal of Psychiatry* **161**: 23–43.

Hoch, P., Polatin, P. (1949) Pseudoneurotic forms of schizophrenia. *Psychoanalytic Quarterly* **23**: 248–276.

Kernberg, O. (1975) *Borderline Conditions and Pathological Narcissism*. New York: Jason Aronson.

Kernberg, O. (1984) *Severe Personality Disorders: Psychotherapeutic Strategies*. New Haven, Conn: Yale University Press.

Kernberg, O.F. (1987) Projection and projective identification; developmental and clinical aspects. In Sandler, J. (ed.) *Projection, Indentification, Projective Identification*. pp. 93–115. London: Karnac Books.

Kety, S.S., Rosenthal, D., Wender, P.H., Schulsinger, F. (1968) The types and prevalence of mental illness in the biological and adoptive families of adopted schizophrenics. In Rosenthal, D., Kety, S.S. (eds) *The Transmission of Schizophrenia*. pp. 147–165. Oxford: Pergamon Press.

Kety, S.S., Rosenthal, D., Wender, P.H., Schulsinger, F. (1975) Mental illness and biological and adoptive families of adopted individuals who have become schizophrenic: a preliminary report based on psychiatric

148   Anthony W. Bateman

interviews. In Fieve, R.R., Rosenthal, D., Brill, H. (eds) *Genetic Research in Psychiatry*, pp. 199–208. Baltimore: Johns Hopkins.

Klein, D. (1975) Psychopharmacology and the borderline patient. In Mack, J. (ed.) *Borderline states in Psychiatry*, pp. 75–92. New York: Grune and Stratton.

Klein, D. (1977) Psychopharmacological treatment and delineation of borderline disorders. In Hartocollis, P. (ed.) *Borderline Personality Disorders: The Concept, the Syndrome, the Patient*. New York: IUP.

Klein, M. (1946) Notes on some schizoid mechanisms. In Klein, M., Heimann, P., Isaacs, S., Riviere, J. (eds) *Developments in Psychoanalysis*. London: Hogarth (reprinted London: Karnac Books 1989).

Klein, M. (1952) Some theoretical conclusions regarding the emotional life of the infant. In Riviere, J. (ed.) *Developments in Psychoanalysis*. Reprinted in *The writing of Melanie Klein*, Vol. 3, London: Hogarth.

Kohut, H. (1971) *The Analysis of the Self*. New York: International Universities Press.

Kraepelin, E. (1909–1915) *Psychiatrie: Ein Lehrbuch*, 5th edn. Leipzig: Barth.

Kretschmer, E. (1921) *Physique and Character*. London: Kegan Paul.

Laing, R. (1960) *The Divided Self*. London: Penguin.

Langs, R. (1978) Some communicative properties of the bipersonal field. *International Journal of Psychoanalytic Psychotherapy* 7: 87–135.

Linehan, M.M., (1987) Dialectical behaviour therapy for borderline personality disorder: theory and method. *Bulletin of the Menninger Clinic* 51: 261–276.

Linehan, M.M. (1993) *Cognitive Behavioural Treatment of Borderline Personality Disorder*. New York: Guilford.

Malin, A., Grotstein, J.S. (1966) Projective identification in the therapeutic process. *International Journal of Psychoanalysis* 47: 26–31.

Markar, H.R., Williams, J.M.G., Wells, J., Gordon, L. (1991) Occurrence of schizotypal and borderline symptoms in parasuicidal patients: comparison between subjective and objective indices. *Psychological Medicine* 21: 385–392.

Markus, H., Cross, S. (1990) The interpersonal self. In Pervin, L. (ed.), *Handbook of Personality: Theory and Research*. pp. 576–608. New York: Guilford.

Masterson, J. (1976) *Psychotherapy of the Borderline Adult: A Developmental Approach*. New York: Brunner.

Masterson, J., Rinsley, D. (1975) The borderline syndrome: the role of the mother in the genesis and psychic structure of the borderline personality. *International Journal of Psychoanalysis* 56: 163–177.

McGlashan, T.H. (1987) Testing DSM-III symptom criteria for schizotypal and borderline personality disorders. *Archives of General Psychiatry* 44: 143–148.

Meehl, P.E. (1962) Schizotaxia, schizotypy, schizophrenia. *American Psychologist* 17: 827–838.

Money-Kyrle, R.E. (1956) Normal countertransference and some of its deviations. *International Journal of Psychoanalysis* 37: 360–366.

Nigg, J., Lohr, N.E., Westen, D., Gold, L., Silk, K.R. (1991) Malevolent object representations in borderline personality disorder and major depression. *Journal of Abnormal Psychology* **101**: 61–67.

Nurnberg, H.G., Raskin, M., Levene, P.E. et al (1991) The comorbidity of borderline personality disorder and other DSM-III-R Axis II personality disorders. *American Journal of Psychiatry* **148**: 1371–1377.

Ogata, S., Silk, K.R., Goodrich, S., Lohr, N.E. et al (1990) Childhood abuse and clinical symptoms in borderline personality disorder. *American Journal of Psychiatry* **147**: 1008–1013.

Ogden, T.H. (1979) On projective identification. *International Journal of Psychoanalysis* **60**: 357–373.

Parker, G., Kiloh, L., Hayward, L. (1987) Parental representations of neurotic and endogenous depressives. *Journal of Affective Disorders* **13**: 75–82.

Patrick, M., Hobson, P., Castle, D. et al. (1994) Personality disorder and the mental representation of early social experience. *Development and Psychopathology* **6**: 375–388.

Piaget, J. (1954) *The Construction of Reality in the Child*. New York: Basic Books.

Racker, H. (1968) *Transference and Countertransference*. Reprinted 1985, London: Karnac.

Rado, S. (1953) Dynamics and Classification of disordered behaviour. *American Journal of Psychiatry* **110**: 406–416.

Rey, H. (1994) *Schizoid Modes of Being*. London: Free Association Books.

Rosenfeld, H. (1987) *Impasse and Interpretation: Therapeutic and Anti-Therapeutic Factors in Psychoanalytic Treatment of Psychotic, Borderline and Neurotic Patients*. London: Routledge.

Rosenthal, D., Wender, P.H., Kety, S.S. et al. (1968) Schizophrenics' offspring reared in adoptive homes. Rosenthal, D., Kety, S.S. (eds) *The Transmission of Schizophrenia*. pp. 377–391. Oxford: Pergamon Press.

Rosenthal, D., Wender, P.H., Kety, S.S. et al. (1971) The adopted-away offspring of schizophrenics. *American Journal of Psychiatry* **128**: 307–399.

Ryle, A. (1990) *Cognitive-analytic Therapy: Active Participation in Change*. London: Wiley.

Ryle, A. (1994) Psychoanalysis and cognitive analytic therapy. *British Journal of Psychotherapy* **10**: 404–405.

Sandler, J. (1976a) Dreams, unconscious fantasies and identity of perception. *International Review of Psychoanalysis* **3**: 33–42.

Sandler, J. (1976b) Countertransference and role-responsiveness. *International Review of Psychoanalysis* **3**: 43–47.

Sandler, J. (1987) The concept of projective identification. In Sandler, J. (ed.) *Projection, Identification, Projective Identification*. London: Karnac Books.

Sandler, J., Rosenblatt, B. (1962) The concept of the representational world. *Psychoanalytic Study of the Child* **17**: 128–145.

Sandler, J., Sandler, A.M. (1978) On the development of object relationships and affects. *International Journal of Psychoanalysis* **59**: 285–296.

Shearin, E.N., Linehan, M. (1994) Dialectical behaviour therapy for border-line personality disorder: theoretical and empirical foundations. *Acta Psychiatrica Scandinavica* **89** (suppl. 379): 61–68.

Soloff, P.H. (1994) Is there any drug treatment of choice for the borderline patient? *Acta Psychiatrica Scandinavica* **89** (suppl. 379): 50–55.

Spillius, E. (1988) (ed.) *Melanie Klein Today*. London: Routledge.

Spillius, E. (1994) Developments on Kleinian thought: overview and personal view. *Contemporary Kleinian Psychoanalysis, Psychoanalytic Inquiry* Vol. 14, 324–364.

Spitzer, R.L., Endicott, J., Gibbon, M. (1979) Crossing the border into border-line personality and borderline schizophrenia. *Archives of General Psychiatry*, **36**: 17–24.

Steiner, J. (1993) *Psychic Retreats*. London: Routledge.

Stern, A. (1938) Psychoanalytic investigation of and therapy in the border-line group of neuroses. *Psychoanalytic Quarterly* **7**: 467–489.

Stern, D. (1985) *The Interpersonal World of the Infant*. New York: Basic Books.

Stevenson, J., Meares, R. (1992) An outcome study of psychotherapy for patients with borderline personality disorder. *American Journal of Psychiatry* **149**: 358–362.

Stone, M.H. (1990) Treatment of borderline patients: a pragmatic approach. *Psychiatric Clinics of North America* **13**: 265–286.

Stone, M. (1993) Long-term outcome in personality disorders. *British Journal of Psychiatry* **162**: 299–313.

Stone, M.H., Stone, D.K., Hurt, S. (1987) The natural history of borderline patients treated by intensive hospitalisation. *Psychiatric Clinics of North America* **10**: 185–206.

Sullivan, H. (1953) *The Interpersonal Theory of Psychiatry*. New York: Norton.

Wender, P.H., Rosenthal, D., Kety, S.S. et al. (1974) Crossfostering: a research strategy for clarifying the role of genetic amd experiential factors in the etiology of schizophrenia. *Archives of General Psychiatry* **30**: 121–128.

Westen, D. (1992) The cognitive self and the psychoanalytic self: can we put ourselves together? *Psychological Inquiry* **3**: 1–13.

Westen, D., Cohen, R.P. (1993) The self in borderline personality disorder: a psychodynamic perspective. In Segal, Z.V., Blatt, S.J. (eds) *The Self in Emotional Distress: Cognitive and Psychodynamic Perspectives*, pp. 334–360. London: Guilford Press.

Widiger, T.A., Frances, A., (1987) Interviews and inventories for the measurement of personality disorders. *Clinical Psychology Review* **7**: 49–75.

Widiger, T.A., Frances, A., Warner, L., Bluhm, C. (1986) Diagnostic criteria for the borderline and schizotypal personalities. *Journal of Abnormal Psychology* **95**: 43–51.

Winnicott, D. (1965) *The Maturational Processes and the Facilitating Environment*. London: Hogarth.

Zanarini, M.C., Frankenberg, F.R., Chauncey, D.L., Gunderson, J.G. (1987) The diagnostic interview for personality disorders: interrater and test-retest reliability. *Comprehensive Psychiatry* **28**: 467–480.

Zanarini, M.C., Gunderson, J.G., Frankenberg, F.R. et al. (1989) The revised diagnostic interview for borderlines. *Journal of Personality Disorders* **3**: 10–18.

Zetzel, E. (1968) The so-called good hysteric. *International Journal of Psychoanalysis* **49**: 250–260.

Zilboorg, G. (1941) Ambulatory schizophrenia. *Psychiatry* **4**: 149–155.

Zilboorg, G. (1952) The emotional problem and the therapeutic role of insight. *Psychoanalytic Quarterly* **21**: 1–24.

Zweig-Frank, H., Paris, J. (1991) Parents' emotional neglect and over-protection according to recollections of patients with borderline personality disorder. *American Journal of Psychiatry* **148**: 648–651.

6

Risk Factors for Emergence and Persistence of Psychosis

Jim van Os, Padraig Wright and Robin Murray

INTRODUCTION

Follow-up studies in the functional psychoses mainly serve four purposes. First, they shed light on the natural history of the disorder (natural history studies). Short-term and longer-term follow-up studies can chart the considerable variability in course and outcome, and attempt to distinguish patterns. Second, they identify factors that modify the risk of chronicity and/or treatment response (prediction of outcome studies). These are very important from the clinical point of view, as risk factors for chronicity with high predictive value open the way for preventive measures very early in the course of illness. Third, they assess the predictive validity of diagnostic constructs and/or symptom dimensions (validity studies). In the absence of aetiologically validating criteria for our diagnostic constructs, the establishment of predictive validity is arguably the next important thing, as qualitative differences in course and outcome suggest the need for qualitative differences in approaches to treatment. Fourth, and last, they may provide evidence for contrasting course of illness in high-risk groups (heterogeneity studies). For example, the observation that a risk factor for schizophrenia is also a risk factor for chronicity of disorder, in such a way that it can be distinguished from illness associated with other risk factors, is suggestive of a *discrete effect*, and may lead to reduction of heterogeneity within the functional psychoses.

However, all four approaches are subject to formidable methodological problems. These will therefore first be reviewed below in some detail, before discussing the four uses of longitudinal studies.

INTERPRETING FOLLOW-UP STUDIES OF SCHIZOPHRENIA

Follow-up investigations are 'dirty'. A multitude of factors influence illness course, few of which can be collected, let alone controlled for, by the investigator. Results are therefore easily confounded. Course and outcome are highly dependent on sample selection and attrition, and both generalizability and validity of the findings may be jeopardized. No time is therefore wasted in trying to obtain an understanding of these factors.

Natural History Studies

Interpretation of the many natural history studies is often difficult because of a myriad of factors that are crucial in determining aspects of the results (Vaillant, 1978; Tsuang et al., 1979; Bleuler, 1972, 1978; Bland, 1982; Westermeyer and Harrow, 1988; Bartko et al., 1988; McGlashan et al., 1988; Breier, 1988; Shepherd et al., 1989; An der Heiden and Krumm, 1991; Harding, 1994).

Defining the schizophrenia syndrome

A recent review of the international literature, in which 320 follow-up studies from 1895 to 1992 were surveyed, found that outcome was significantly better in patients diagnosed according to systems with broad criteria or undefined criteria (46.5% and 41.0% were 'improved' respectively), as compared to systems with narrow criteria (27.3% improved). A decline in the reported rate of favourable outcomes over the past decade was also ascribed to shifts in diagnostic criteria (Hegarty et al., 1994). This study highlights the fact that the results of all schizophrenia follow-up studies are highly dependent on the diagnostic construct used. For example, follow-up studies using 'intuitively' defined schizophrenia according to ICD-9 or the older 'broad' concept of DSM-II, on average yield prognostically more favourable results than those using the more restrictive criteria of the later DSM series (Westermeyer and Harrow, 1984).

Indeed, the use of DSM criteria for schizophrenia in follow-up studies has been criticized (Angst, 1988), on the grounds that they select a type of disorder that is already defined in terms of chronicity (i.e. the six months duration criterion). Thus, an element of circularity is introduced: poor outcome disorders have poor outcome.

The use of different diagnostic criteria also has an important influence on the prevalence of important predictors of outcome, which, if results are presented uncontrolled, further complicates the picture. For example, the skewed sex distribution (excess of male patients) found in samples of subjects with 'six-month' DSM-III/IV schizophrenia will be much attenuated in other, less restrictive, schizophrenia constructs (Castle et al., 1993). As female sex is associated with better outcome (see below), the relatively unfavourable outcome in DSM-III/IV schizophrenia as compared to the ICD construct is likely to reflect, at least in part, sex differences in the course of schizophrenia.

Within the series of DSM diagnostic systems, there is likely to be further variation in course and outcome of the schizophrenia construct as criteria are being changed repeatedly. The influence of these changes on results of schizophrenia research has not been investigated, each new version of the DSM series being treated by many as the most 'valid' update in psychiatric classification. The frequent boundary changes, however, are likely to have a subtle, but possibly important, influence on the comparability and generalizability of research results from one DSM generation to the other.

Of course, the real problem is that the validity of the variably defined schizophrenia construct remains uncertain. From the scientific point of view, it is unwise to start with the 'splitting' approach if the diagnostic boundaries remain arbitrarily defined and are subject to frequent boundary changes. Indeed, an American commentator, reviewing the long-term outcome literature, concluded that 'until significant progress is made in reducing the heterogeneity of schizophrenia, its criteria should err in the direction of inclusiveness' (McGlashan, 1988). A more useful approach, therefore, employed by several investigators, is to start out with a 'lumping' approach, and to examine for interaction of effects with diagnostic category. For example, in the Iowa 500 series, all cases of functional psychosis were included, and outcome was compared between various DSM-III categories (Tsuang and Dempsey, 1979) which yielded evidence for an intermediary outcome for schizoaffective disorder, compared to schizophrenia and affective disorder. Another approach is to try to investigate, within a group of patients with functional psychosis, measures of course and outcome in relation to clusters of related

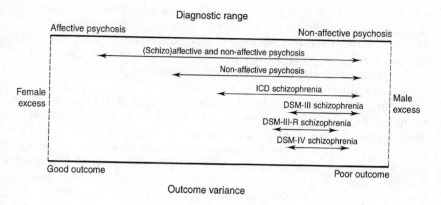

Figure 6.1 Relationship between diagnosis, outcome and gender. Restrictive diagnostic constructs of schizophrenia have less outcome variability, poorer average outcome and a higher male to female ratio than less restrictive constructs. Subtle changes in DSM diagnostic criteria affect outcome comparability across DSM generations.

symptoms (i.e. symptom dimensions), rather than clusters of *cases* (i.e. diagnostic categories). For example, it may be profitable to compare the predictive power of recently identified symptom dimensions (e.g. Liddle et al., 1992) with that of diagnostic categories.

The issues pertaining to diagnostic variation are summarized in Figure 6.1. By including samples with a wide range of clinical expression of psychotic illness, the outcome *variance* found will be greater, and the sex distribution will be less skewed. The advantage of this approach is that within-sample clinical heterogeneity, in terms of either symptom dimensions or diagnostic categories, can be examined more easily than by starting out with narrowly defined cases of schizophrenia at the extreme end of the psychopathological 'continuum' (see below). As research strategies are turning increasingly towards investigation of neural mechanisms of symptom dimensions (e.g. Liddle et al., 1992; McGuire et al., 1993), inclusion of more representative samples (i.e. over the whole continuum of psychosis) also appears the more rational approach.

Assessing course and outcome

Strictly speaking, the term outcome is misleading, as it implies that there is such a thing as an endpoint in the illness process, whereas in actual fact there is a continuous dynamic adaptation between individual, illness, and the environment. Thus, the endpoint implied by the term outcome refers to that of the study rather than the illness course. Here, outcome is used simply to denote the result of the research assessment that took place somewhere during the course of a patient's illness.

In general, outcome studies include a baseline assessment and one or more follow-up assessments. Ideally, the baseline assessment should precede the follow-up assessment, i.e. the study should be prospective. Similarly, serial assessments are desirable so as to be able to build an accurate picture of the patient's illness course. For example, Coryell and colleagues followed a sample of patients over five years using biannual assessments (Coryell et al., 1990a). Very few studies, however, fulfil the criteria of prospective and serial assessments. For example, very long-term follow-up studies (with some exceptions – e.g. Bleuler, 1978), have to depend on retrospective baseline assessments, and serial assessments require complicated statistical analyses. Usually, studies report a baseline assessment and a single follow-up assessment, which consists of cross-sectional and/or retrospective longitudinal assessments. Cross-sectional assessments measure the patient's current state during the follow-up interview, whereas retrospective longitudinal measurements rate, for example, the time spent in hospital or the usual severity of symptoms over a specified period prior to the interview.

In general, the longer the follow-up period, the less representative a single cross-sectional follow-up assessment is likely to be of the patient's illness course, just as a single measurement of temperature is unlikely to tell us much about temperature developments over the last 20 years. Longitudinal assessments have more validity with respect to illness course, but are heavily dependent on the quality of the source of information for the retrospective rating exercise, and the longer the follow-up period, the more contamination by error in the data. Follow-up assessments covering periods of more than five years are likely to be imprecise and require increasingly crude distinctions in order to give some degree of accuracy of variability in course. Instruments have been developed to rate course longitudinally, such as the WHO life chart, which offers a semi-operationalized assessment of social and clinical aspects of illness course (WHO, 1992; see below). For both cross-sectional and longitudinal assessments, informant accounts are crucially important (McGlashan, 1984; An der Heiden and Krumm, 1991).

Outcome of psychiatric illness is multidimensional and difficult to conceptualize in one summary outcome measure (Brown et al., 1966;

Kenniston et al., 1971; Strauss and Carpenter, 1978). Kenniston et al. (1971) drew attention to the fact that, in the same patient, outcome may vary sharply as a function of the outcome measure used: patients may continue to work in spite of severe psychotic symptoms, or alternatively they may be quite isolated while only presenting with mild residual paranoid ideas. Therefore, the use of 'global' outcome measures combining different independent dimensions should be avoided. The usual approach has been to define 'social' and 'clinical' outcomes. Three caveats exist in the adoption of this approach. Firstly, if the outcome measures used are not based on validated instruments, the replicability of results will be jeopardized. Secondly, while the multidimensional approach may reflect clinical reality, the scientific evaluation of putative risk factors for a deteriorated illness course is being made more complex, as multiple testing with a variety of outcome measures is necessary with the inherent problem of false positive results (Type I errors). Thirdly, the decision to define 'social' and 'clinical' outcomes is arbitrary, and when a variety of outcome measures is used, many are likely to be closely interrelated, despite being classified under various social and clinical outcome measures. Therefore, when a collection of outcome measures is used, data reduction may be applied to produce true underlying dimensions of outcome (van Os et al., 1996).

Assessing 'recovery' or 'remission'

The use of dichotomized terms such as recovery or remission is questionable. The psychotic illness process seen in clinical practice is more suggestive of fluctuation along a continuum of illness severity, in comparisons both between and within patients. It may therefore be more useful to rank patients on ordered categories of *operational* measures of illness severity, rather than force a decision about recovery by placing an arbitrary cut-off resulting in loss of information. Bleuler (1978) defined four levels of symptom severity: *most severe, medium severe, less severe* and *cured*. It should be noted that *cured* included those states where psychotic symptoms were still present, although only detectable on detailed psychiatric examination. In Bleuler's 23-year follow-up study, 20% of patients were classified as cured. Care should be taken to compare seemingly similar outcomes across studies. The Iowa 500 follow-up study (Tsuang et al., 1979) reported psychiatric status at 30–40-year follow-up as *no symptoms, some symptoms* and *incapacitating symptoms*. The proportion of patients with *no symptoms* was 20%, similar to

Bleuler's study. However, in the Iowa 500 series a rating of *no symptoms* really meant absence of psychiatric symptoms, and certainly did not include patients with psychotic signs.

The latter example illustrates the limited comparability between studies. In general, measures of course and outcome tend to differ from study to study, and much would be gained if a 'minimal set' (Marengo, 1994) of course parameters were used consistently in the literature. Instruments developed by the WHO (1992) provide semi-operational, multidimensional (social, clinical) measures for course and outcome, which have high face validity. For example, the WHO (1992) modified Bleuler's four categories of symptom severity to give a rating of *usual severity of symptoms* over a limited period (e.g. two years). Similarly, definitions are provided for course type, which are rated as *episodic, continuous, neither episodic nor continuous* and *never actively psychotic in this period* (Table 6.1).

Often measurements of service use are presented, such as time spent in hospital and number of readmissions, which are taken to reflect clinical course and illness severity. Such measures of service use are valuable for economic analyses, but it is not possible to disentangle the administrative, clinical and social factors that determine hospital use (Garmezy, 1970). Better measures include the time patients live *independently*, i.e. outside institutions and supported accommodation (including care provided by relatives at home), or the *relapse rate*, regardless of readmission.

In a recent one-year follow-up study, a combination of *time to first remission* and *level of remission* has been successfully used, with clinical trial instruments such as the Clinical Global Impressions scale (Lieberman et al., 1993). This group introduced a major improvement in outcome methodology, by introducing a standardized antipsychotic treatment protocol over the follow-up period, thus in

Table 6.1 Course type to be rated over a two-year follow-up period as defined in the WHO life chart (WHO, 1992)

Episodic – discrete episodes (none longer than 6 months) with clear periods of remission* in between. At least one remission lasted 6 months or more
Continuous – psychotic* over most of the period. If any remissions, these were brief (none longer than 6 months)
Neither episodic nor continuous – e.g. longest psychotic episode was 12 months and longest remission was 9 months
Never actively psychotic in this period

*Definitions are also provided for 'remission' and 'psychotic'.

fact controlling for treatment administered over the follow-up period (see below). However, the term 'treatment response' to denote outcome variance over one year (Lieberman et al., 1993) is slightly misleading, as variation in outcome may only be partly related to variation in treatment response. For example, their finding that brain pathomorphology predicted level of remission might also have been found if no treatment had been administered at all. The separation of variation due to treatment response and to the underlying illness process itself would require the inclusion of a placebo-medicated control group, which is not feasible for ethical reasons.

Length of follow-up

The length of follow-up varies from one or two years (Johnstone et al., 1990; Jablensky et al., 1992; Lieberman et al., 1993) to two or more decades (Ciompi and Müller, 1976; Ciompi, 1980; Huber et al., 1980; Harding et al., 1987; McGlashan, 1984). The greatest variability in illness is to be found in the first 5–15 years of illness (Strauss and Carpenter, 1977; Bleuler, 1972, 1978), after which less fluctuation in course can be expected, although substantial changes very late in the course may not be infrequent (Bleuler, 1978; Ciompi and Müller, 1976; Harding et al., 1987). Furthermore, with the progression of time, a large group of patients becomes increasingly impaired with each subsequent episode; 35% of patients developed such states of increasing impairment in the first five years of illness in a carefully conducted study of a sample of 49 representative incident cases of schizophrenia (Shepherd et al., 1989). Longer-term studies suggest that this percentage further increases over the next 10 years, but McGlashan (1988) has pointed out that the deterioration then tends to 'bottom out', and is in fact not infrequently followed by a phase of late improvement (Vaillant, 1978; Engelhardt et al., 1982; Harding et al., 1987; Ciompi and Müller, 1976; Bleuler, 1972, 1978). This state of affairs is depicted in Figure 6.2 after Breier et al. (1992). It follows that it is of crucial importance to the result at what point in the illness course the cohort's baseline assessment takes place and for how long the patients are followed up. For example, a follow-up over five years during the 'plateau' phase will reveal little fluctuation; a follow-up very late in the illness may actually show improvement. It is also clear that too large a fluctuation of length of follow-up and/or duration of illness prior to baseline assessment is not to be recommended. If, for example, some patients are first admissions followed for five years and others, within the same sample, are patients with 10-year duration of illness

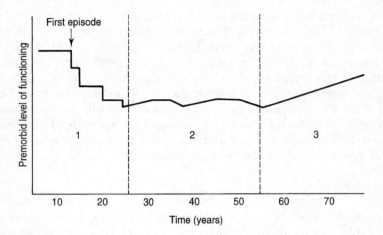

Figure 6.2 Hypothesized 'common' illness course trajectory showing initial stepwise decline with each episode (1), followed by a 'plateau' phase (2) and late improvement (3).

who are followed for 15 years, the resulting mix of follow-up epochs and levels of chronicity will make it very difficult to meaningfully interpret the results.

Controls or no controls?

It is often difficult to compare outcomes across studies, especially natural history studies. For example, being married, having friends or employment are all heavily dependent on the characteristics of the source population. If employment is included among the outcome measures (which it often is), then global outcome will be worse in a study population drawn from an area with high rates of unemployment. Furthermore, it is conceivable that longitudinal variation in psychiatric symptomatology reflects similar, age-related variation in psychological well-being in the normal population. Therefore, results should ideally be compared with a group of psychiatric and non-psychiatric controls. One well-known study (Tsuang and Dempsey, 1979) compared schizophrenic, schizoaffective and affective patients with a group of surgical controls. Thus, outcomes in psychiatric patients could be compared with population baseline values; the rate of 'good' outcome in controls was between 84% and 89%, depending on the outcome measure used.

Sample selection and generalizability of results

The vast majority of studies rely on hospital admission as a selecting criterion. In the case of schizophrenia, this means missing around 10–20% of subjects who will never be admitted, and who might systematically differ on important variables associated with long-term outcome. For example, female patients may be under-represented, given that women have a less deteriorated illness course, and for that reason may be more often treated on an outpatient basis (see also Walker and Lewine, 1993). Studies conducted in private hospitals select individuals from the higher socio-economic classes and/or particular ethnic groups, which also affects generalizability, and results from such institutions do not necessarily apply to all schizophrenic patients. Arbitrary age cut-offs may also jeopardize generalizability (e.g. Ciompi and Müller, 1976; Jablensky et al., 1992).

The issue of generalizability is also important in relation to the length of illness prior to baseline assessment. Some long-term outcome studies followed up patients whose baseline condition was of chronic, severe and persistent illness necessitating very lengthy periods of hospitalization, residing in a rural area (e.g. Harding et al., 1987) or selected for high socio-economic status (e.g. McGlashan, 1984). The findings on the natural history of schizophrenia presented in such studies are only generalizable to similar populations selected for severe disability, area of residence or socio-economic status. For example, in Ciompi and Müller's (1976) study of first admission patients with schizophrenia, followed for an average of 37 years, around 25% of 228 cases had an undulating course type and an outcome of mild or recovered. In the Vermont Longitudinal Research Project, however, which followed 82 schizophrenic patients who were *already* severely disabled at baseline for 20–30 years, this percentage was only 7%. Conversely, the proportion of patients with a more chronic type of course with moderate or severe outcome were 10% and 38% in the Swiss and the American samples respectively (Harding, 1988).

In order to be representative, subjects should ideally be incident cases drawn from a defined geographical area. For example, the WHO Determinants of Outcome Study attempted to identify all cases of non-organic psychosis making a first lifetime contact with a helping agency in 12 areas, and followed 1379 such patients for a period of two years (Jablensky et al., 1992).

In any cohort study, whether retrospective or prospective, the ascertainment of outcome data requires that all subjects are followed into the future, to determine whether they develop the outcome of interest. The major source of bias in cohort studies is failure to obtain adequate information on every study participant, or to collect it in different proportions for those exposed and non-exposed to an important determinant of outcome. For example, differential attrition of individuals with insidious onset of illness and negative symptoms will result in a spuriously high proportion of recovered patients at follow-up; differential attrition of individuals of a particular social class or ethnic group may mean that results are only generalizable to a limited group of patients. To a degree, the likely effect of attrition can be investigated by comparing those who did and did not participate in the study on important baseline variables.

Prediction of Outcome Studies

Prediction of outcome requires careful baseline assessment of predictor variables (exposures). Prospective studies are therefore preferable, with the exception of simple or immutable predictor variables such as age, sex and diagnosis, which can usually be assessed reliably retrospectively. Studies should be carried out blind to index data, to minimize the risk of observer bias.

Specific hypotheses versus general searches for predictors

Studies on prediction of outcome may focus on specific risk factors for chronicity, such as brain abnormalities (e.g. Williams et al., 1985), or try to find predictors among many variables collected at baseline (e.g. McGlashan, 1986a, b). The first approach has some advantages. First, in this way a specific scientific question can be answered. Second, the study can be designed in such a way that information on essential confounders is simultaneously collected, and the most appropriate type of analysis, yielding adjusted estimates of effect size for the specific predictor can be conducted (van Os et al., 1994, 1995, 1996a).

Validity of results

We discussed above the effect of attrition on the generalizability of results in follow-up studies establishing the natural history of disease. Although differential attrition of, for example, female patients may affect generalizability of the study, the study may still be valid for male subjects. In analytic cohort studies, however, where specific hypotheses on associations between predictor variables and outcome are tested, the validity of the results may be seriously affected by losses to follow-up if attrition is related independently to both the predictor variable and other risk factors for the outcome under study. Assume, for example, that the male sex is associated with increased risk of brain abnormality (Lieberman et al., 1992; Castle and Murray, 1991). If, in a study examining the relationship between brain abnormalities and outcome, those lost to follow-up have (i) more brain abnormalities, and (ii) independent of any brain abnormality, better outcome because the majority are females, then a biased estimate of the association between brain abnormality and outcome will result.

Baseline associations or predictors of outcome?

Risk factors for poor social or clinical outcome may in fact be repetitions of associations that were already evident at baseline; these should therefore, where possible, be adjusted for, to assess the true prospective character of risk. For example, evidence of developmental delay in schizophrenic patients may predict high levels of negative symptoms at follow-up, but if a similar association was present at baseline assessment, the statement that developmental delay predicts *subsequent* negative symptoms (i.e. at follow-up) can only be verified by adjusting for baseline level of negative symptoms.

Effect sizes

Rarely are risk factors for poor outcome reported in terms of effect size and confidence intervals, yet if high risk groups are to be targeted for secondary prevention, this is obviously an important issue. The usual practice of reporting only *P*-values has its disadvantages, as *P*-values are dependent on both sample size and effect size, with the result that negative findings are difficult to evaluate. Therefore, it is preferable to report both a measure of effect and an informative measure to evaluate the role of chance such as the range within which the true magnitude of the effect lies with a certain probability (confidence interval).

Confounding

Alternative explanations need to be considered in reporting associations. For example, women are more likely to experience and/or

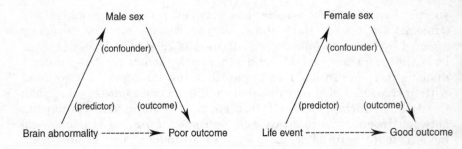

Figure 6.3   Gender may confound many predictor–outcome relationships. Depicted are two popular notions, namely that brain abnormalities and life events are associated with a more and a less deteriorated illness course respectively. However, both associations may be counfounded by gender.

report life events and, in schizophrenia, may be less likely to have brain abnormalities (Bebbington et al., 1993; Castle and Murray, 1991). Therefore, any association between life events or brain abnormalities on the one hand and course and outcome on the other may be confounded by sex. In fact, there is good evidence that sex, social class and ethnicity are all associated with outcome (Bardenstein and McGlashan, 1990; Cooper, 1961; McKenzie et al., 1995). These three variables are likely to be associated also with many biological and social predictor variables, so that a potential confounding mechanism needs to be adjusted for (Figure 6.3). Duration of illness before first treatment may predict poorer outcome (Crow et al., 1986; Jablensky et al., 1992; Loebel et al., 1992). However, none of the studies examining this issue was able to examine the effect of social support, social class or ethnicity (likely to be associated with decreased or delayed access to service and also associated with outcome). A mistake often made is to adjust for confounders only if statistical significance in the association with either the outcome or the predictor variable can be demonstrated. Confounders, however, should be selected and adjusted for *a priori*, on the basis of their potential confounding mechanism, not on statistical significance (Clayton and Hills, 1993). As statistical significance is based on both effect size and sample size, smaller samples are paradoxically much less likely to suffer from confounding if the criterion is based on statistical significance!

Treatment

Treatment is an important factor in prediction of outcome studies. In follow-up studies which examine the natural history of the disorder, treatment may have an important influence on the results. Treatment is a major uncontrolled variable in any 'naturalistic' study, but some (Keller et al., 1983) have argued cogently that treatment becomes an outcome in itself, as it is prescribed in response to the patient's condition and the severity of the underlying illness process, which may not be fundamentally altered by any treatment. In follow-up studies which examine prediction of outcome, the influence of treatment is only important if it is associated both with outcome and, independently, with the exposure under investigation. This may occur under two conditions: (i) clinicians prescribe treatment differentially, and (ii) patients respond to/comply with treatment differentially. However, prescription of treatment is usually according to need, and not to prognosis; differential treatment response/compliance is not really an alternative explanation, but a mediating mechanism, which can subsequently be further investigated.

LONG-TERM OUTCOME

If natural history is defined as the course of disease unmodified by treatment, then our knowledge of the natural history of schizophrenia is largely historical and derives almost exclusively from the period between the development of schizophrenia as a clinical concept at the turn of this century, and the introduction of antipsychotic drugs five decades later. However, it must be borne in mind that serious mental illness has always been 'treated', usually by some form of institutionalization. In considering the outcome of schizophrenia, therefore, it is difficult to disentangle schizophrenia from the response, therapeutic or otherwise, that it elicits. Furthermore, as discussed above, it is important to differentiate between research programmes that recruit schizophrenic patients at diagnosis or first hospitalization, and those that enrol patients during their second or subsequent admissions.

Table 6.2 summarizes some of the literature on long-term outcome of *first admissions*, selected on the basis of criteria discussed above, between the beginning of the century and 1990. The most important conclusions that can be drawn are (McGlashan, 1988):

Table 6.2 Outcome studies in schizophrenia

Reference	Location of study	No. of patients	Mean duration of study (years)	Outcome of study (authors' conclusions and terminology)†
Rosanoff (1914)	New York	169	5	13.6% deceased 23.1% discharged from hospital (of whom 71.8% were not readmitted during the study period) 58.6% chronically hospitalized during the study period
Fuller (1930)	New York	1200	15	25.0% deceased 35.3% discharged from hospital (of whom 52.4% were discharged within the first year after admission) 38.4% chronically hospitalized during the study period
Rupp and Fletcher (1940)	Rhode Island (USA)	641	5–10*	13.9% deceased 27.5% discharged from hospital 53.5% chronically hospitalized during the study period (Tuberculosis was responsible for 48.0% of deaths in the deceased group)
Müller (1951)	Germany	200	30	33.0% 'were recovered or substantially improved' at the time of their discharge from hospital 16.0% 'remained in recovered state throughout follow up period' 17.0% 'showed a phasic recurrent course without change to chronicity' 41.0% 'insidious chronic course, continual need to be in an institution'
Malzberg (1953)	New York	3180	3	59.3% discharged from hospital 16.4% 'recovered' 23.1% 'much improved'
Shepherd (1957)	Buckinghamshire (UK)	137	5	46.8% discharged (1931–1933 cohort; mortality for these patients was 6.3%) 56.8% discharged (1945–1947 cohort; mortality for these patients was 1.7%)
Lehrman (1960)	New York	2941	13–14*	(A reanalysis of the Malzberg (1953) study; Lehrman found that 44.3% of subjects had not been readmitted during the follow-up period, and that 49.9% were out of hospital at the time of follow-up)

Study	Location	N	Years follow-up	Findings
Locke (1962)	Ohio	5781	5	1.6% deceased 70.0% discharged from hospital 22.0% chronically hospitalized during study period
Peterson and Olsen (1964)	Minnesota	177	5	76.0% discharged from hospital 24.0% chronically hospitalized during study period (about a quarter of the cohort were hospitalized at any time during the study)
Wing (1966)	London	111	5	28.0% moderate symptoms during the period of follow-up 48.0% readmitted during the period of follow-up 49.0% functioned adequately outside hospital 38.0% completely asymptomatic in the six months prior to assessment (Wing considered that, overall, about half of the patients had a good outcome and required minimal follow-up care)
Stephens (1978)	Baltimore	349	5–16*	24.0% 'recovered' (includes patients without symptoms and those who are symptomatic but socially independent) 46.0% 'improved' (this category includes patients who are asymptomatic between episodes of schizophrenic relapse, and patients with considerable social impairment, some of whom cannot live independently) 30.0% 'unimproved' (patients in this group are chronically psychotic, and a majority were hospitalized continuously during the study period)
Bland and Orn (1978)	Alberta	43	14	21.0% 'recovered, no social or intellectual deficit' 16.0% 'severe chronic social and/or intellectual deficit' (including 'chronic unremitting institutionalisation') 37.0% 'normal relationships with named persons' 30.0% 'holds job for a number of years … or changes for adequate reasons' 7.0% deceased (Bland and Orn concluded that 60.0% of patients had 'little or no disability', while 20.0% were 'psychiatrically disabled'. Fifty-one percent of the sample had been treated with antipsychotic medication for at least 7 years)

Table 6.2 continued

Reference	Location of study	No. of patients	Mean duration of study (years)	Outcome of study (authors' conclusions and terminology)†
Ciompi (1980)	Lausanne	289	37	27.0% 'remitted completely after one or several acute episodes' (equivalent to Bleuler's recovery category) 46.0% 'developed only slight to moderate residual states' (encompasses Bleuler's mildly and moderately severe end states) 18.0% 'severe chronic phases' (the same as Bleuler's most severe end state) 15.0% employed in full-time posts 39.0% living alone or with relatives (Ciompi viewed outcome as 'favourable' for 49% of the patients he studied, 'unfavourable' for 42.0% (including 24.0% who had 'intermediate', and 18.0% who had severe, outcomes), and 'uncertain or unstable' for 9.0%. However, 61.0% of his sample remained resident in hospital or community institutions, including a proportion of those who experienced a 'favourable' outcome. Overall, Ciompi concluded that 'the large majority of probands were able to spend most of their lives, including the period of advanced age, outside of hospitals')
Gift et al. (1980)	Monroe County	227	2	Gift reported that affective symptoms at onset of schizophrenia had weak prognostic power
Kane et al. (1982)	New York	28	3.5	70.0% relapsed at end of follow-up period (The first year of this study included an antipsychotic/placebo clinical trial; 25.0% of RDC‡ schizophrenic patients treated with antipsychotic relapsed, compared with 85.7% of RDC schizophrenic patients taking placebo)
Salokangas (1983)	Finland	161	7.5–8*	26.0% no symptoms 29.0% occasional mild psychotic symptoms

Study	Location	N	Years	Outcome
Sartorius et al. (1986)	International	1352	2	21.0% neurotic symptoms 24.0% continuous psychotic symptoms 38.9% one episode of psychosis, no or minimal symptoms at follow-up 21.1% periodic relapses
Rabiner et al. (1986)	New York	36	1	39.8% unremitting psychotic symptoms 55.6% 'remission' (no delusions, hallucinations and/or thought disorder for more than 3 months) 22.2% 'relapse' (reoccurrence of delusions, hallucinations and/or thought disorder) 22.2% 'in-episode' (delusions, hallucinations and/or thought disorder present almost continuously during follow-up)
Scottish Schizophrenia Research Group (1989)	Scotland	49	2	37.0% asymptomatic and functioning adequately 38.0% schizophrenic symptoms present at follow-up 47.0% readmitted during follow-up period 23.0% employed at time of follow-up
Beiser et al. (1989)	British Columbia	175	1.5	0.0% 'superior outcome' 2.8% 'working wounded' 41.7% 'walking wounded' 55.6% 'incapacitated'
Shepherd et al. (1989)	London	107	5	1st admission patients – 22.0% had no relapse during follow-up 43.0% remained impaired during follow-up 2.0% deceased 45.0% readmitted during follow-up period 43.0% no social impairment at follow-up 35.0% recurrent psychotic episodes with increasing impairment after each episode 2nd or subsequent admission – 10.0% had no relapse during follow-up 60.0% remained impaired during follow-up

Table 6.2 continued

Reference	Location of study	No. of patients	Mean duration of study (years)	Outcome of study (authors' conclusions and terminology)†
Lieberman et al. (1989)	New York	45	3	11.0% no improvement (improvement defined as a score of 1 or 2 on the Clinical Global Impression scale, and no score greater than 3 on the SADS)
Johnstone et al. (1990)	Harrow, UK	236	2	60.0% relapsed within one year of index admission (In addition to schizophrenia, the sample included subjects with non-affective psychoses)
Salokangas and Stengard (1990)	Finland	227	2	5.0% suicide rate in male patients 0.0% suicide rate in female patients

*Minimum–maximum duration of study.

†Terminology of the original author(s) is indicated by quotation marks; otherwise it is that of subsequent commentators, with an explanatory note in parenthesis where necessary. This technique, rather than arbitrary interpretation by the present authors, is adopted in order to allow comparisons between the individual studies documented in the table.

‡RDC = Research Diagnostic Criteria.

1. Whatever the year, place, length of follow-up, attrition rate and diagnostic criteria used, there is significant variability in long-term outcome.
2. Although there is significant variability, there is no 'cure' for the majority of patients. Illness may often get progressively worse early in the course of the disorder; however, a substantial proportion of patients may experience some late improvement, as discussed earlier.
3. There is a high rate of mortality in patients, most of which, after the decline in tuberculosis earlier this century, is due to suicide: 10–13% of all patients (Roy, 1982; Caldwell and Gottesman, 1990).
4. There is no overwhelming evidence that, with the introduction of antipsychotic medication, the underlying severity of the illness process has been modified, although a small effect cannot be excluded (Wyatt, 1991).

PREDICTIVE VALIDITY

Rightly or wrongly, when psychiatrists use terms like schizophrenia or manic-depressive psychosis, they often take the words to refer to two essentially different concepts. In the context of diagnostic classification, *validation* may be seen as the process of gathering proof that authenticates the fundamental differentness of the diagnostic constructs. The more typical correlates a construct has, the more valid it becomes in the eye of the beholder.

Kendell (1989) has argued that, where psychiatric diagnoses are concerned, *predictive validity*, i.e. the demonstration of a qualitative difference in outcome between two disorders, is the most important of the different forms of validity. In the absence of an aetiologically validated classification, a diagnostic classification with high predictive validity concerning course and treatment response is perhaps for practical purposes not markedly inferior to a truly aetiologically validated classification, or at least arguably constitutes the next best thing.

The question therefore arises whether differences between, for example, schizophrenia and manic-depressive psychosis are *qualitative* and not merely *quantitative*. The literature offers little support for the hypothesis that there are qualitative differences in outcome between schizophrenia and manic-depressive psychosis. What has been demonstrated time and again is that the outcome for schizophrenia is *on average* better than for (schizo)affective disorder, but considerable overlap exists, with many schizophrenic patients showing good outcome and many affective disorder patients having poor outcome (Lee and Murray, 1988). Similarly, many patients with acute onset schizophrenia and initial good outcome will severely deteriorate later in the course of their illness (McGlashan, 1988). Perhaps the strongest argument against qualitative differences between schizophrenia and affective disorder is the fact that intermediary forms of affective and non-affective illness, the so-called schizoaffective disorders (Kasanin, 1933), have an illness course which is also intermediate, i.e. more benign than in schizophrenia, but worse than in affective disorders. For example, Tsuang and Dempsey (1979), in a 30–40-year longitudinal study, showed that outcome for a group of 85 patients exhibiting both affective and schizophrenic features was significantly poorer compared to a group of 325 patients with affective disorders, selected by the criteria of Feighner and colleagues, and significantly better than in a group of 200 schizophrenic patients. Coryell et al. (1990b, c) showed that affective psychotic disorders have a less disabling course than schizoaffective disorders; Grossman et al. (1991) showed that, overall, schizophrenic patients had poorest outcome, followed by schizoaffective patients, bipolar manic, and unipolar depressive patients. Similar findings were reported by Brockington et al. (1980a, b), Marneros et al., (1989, 1990) and Maj and Perris (1990). Longer-term retrospective studies have yielded similar results (reviews by Harrow and Grossman, 1984; Samson et al., 1988). There is further evidence that more acute 'atypical' 'unspecified', 'schizophreniform', 'reactive' and 'delusional' psychoses are more related to affective disorder than to schizophrenia, and occupy a position somewhere between affective and schizoaffective psychosis in terms of outcome, sex distribution, family history and incidence (Robins and Guze, 1970; Fowler, 1978; Murray and O'Callaghan, 1991; Susser and Wanderling, 1994; Tsuang et al., 1976; van Os, 1995).

Thus, rather than discrete qualitative differences in outcome, there appears to be a linear, 'dose–response' relationship between degree of acute onset and/or affective symptomatology and outcome. Kendell and Brockington (1980) specifically tried to disprove the existence of such a linear relationship, but failed. Johnstone et al. (1992) found diagnostic classification only of limited value in predicting outcome in the functional psychoses. In other words, as far as predictive validity is concerned, what appears to have been validated is a psychopathological continuum, and not discrete entities. This conclusion fits well the evidence from studies using other potential validators. For example, there is similar overlap in genetic predisposition between schizophrenia and affective disorder (review by Taylor, 1992). Indeed, one of the conclusions of the Roscommon study, which was one of the very few family studies to use an epidemiological approach to proband sampling, was that 'the familial liability to schizophrenia is, at least in part, a liability to develop psychosis' (Kendler et al., 1993).

There is recent evidence that the psychopathological spectrum in the functional psychoses may be represented inadequately by just one dimension of affective–non-affective symptomatology (Kitamura et al., 1995; van Os et al., 1996a), and the predictive validity of other symptom dimensions also needs to be established. A recent prospective study addressed this issue (van Os et al., 1996a). One-hundred-and-sixty-six patients with at least one psychotic symptom of recent onset underwent detailed assessment of baseline psychopathology. Multivariate analyses established seven psychopathological dimensions, which were examined in relation to four-year course and outcome. Five of these seven syndromes bore differential associations with subsequent treatment and illness course, independent of (i) associations with DSM-IIIR diagnosis, (ii) associations with other prognostic factors and (iii) associations with the baseline values of outcome variables. The most striking associations were shown for an early and insidious onset syndrome with affective flattening, which predicted a more disabled course of illness on three out of four outcome dimensions, and which was commoner in males and single individuals. A second syndrome, characterized by bizarre behaviour, inappropriate affect, catatonia, and poor rapport showed similar, slightly less striking, associations with illness course as well as with poor premorbid social functioning. A third syndrome, characterized by positive psychotic symptoms was to a lesser degree associated with poorer outcome, whereas a fourth syndrome distinguished by affective symptomatology predicted a more benign illness course. A fifth syndrome identified by lack of insight predicted more time in hospital and admission under a section of the Mental Health Act over the follow-up period. Most importantly, perhaps, it was demonstrated that the predictive validity, both in terms of outcome and medical treatment decisions, was considerably higher for the dimensional representation of psychopathology than for (ICD-10 and DSM-III-R) categorical representations (van Os et al., 1996a). These results concur with those of Breier et al. (1991), who reported that the severity of positive and negative symptoms at baseline predicted levels of symptoms and functioning at 2–12-year follow-up in schizophrenia. In particular, negative symptoms at baseline have been associated with poorer outcome (reviewed by Pogue-Geil, 1989), as well catatonia and thought disorder (e.g. Stephens and Astrup, 1963; Bland and Orn, 1980; Tsuang and Winokur, 1974; Tsuang et al., 1981). Similarly, there is a traditional attribution of better prognosis in the presence of an index affective component (reviews by Robins and Guze, 1970; McGlashan, 1988), although not all studies have concurred (e.g. Shepherd et al., 1989).

In summary, quantitative but not qualitative differences in outcome between acute, affective and insidious, non-affective psychotic disorders have been described. What appears most 'valid' is a psychopathological continuum of one or more symptom dimensions. From the scientific point of view, a 'lumping' approach in selecting cases for epidemiological research appears therefore the most logical approach. Of course, the usefulness of diagnostic categories for clinical purposes is a different matter (Kendell, 1993). However, clinical utility should not be confused with scientific validity.

PREDICTION OF OUTCOME

From this follows unavoidably the task so important for clinical and social psychiatry, to search them for symptoms, which from experience will permit predictions regarding the future course and outcome. This will, after all, be the question asked of us.

(Schneider, 1925)

No set of variables has been found that can reliably predict outcome. However, a set of risk factors has emerged. In this section, we will review recent evidence that key demographic, anamnestic and biological variables such as sex, socio-economic status, age and type of onset, country of residence, duration of illness before treatment, substance, use, and expressed emotion are associated with course and outcome. Putative predictors of outcome that have also been associated with risk of *emergence* of disorder, such as life events, familial morbid risk, cerebral ventricle dimensions and early developmental deviance, will be reviewed in the section on heterogeneity of risk. The relationship between the illness manifestations themselves and outcome has been discussed in the section on predictive validity (p. 171).

From the point of view of public health, the identification of factors that mediate the variability in course creates scope for secondary prevention by targeting groups with high risk of continuing social and/or clinical disability. As outlined above, most of the variability in course and outcome takes place relatively early in the illness trajectory (the first 5–15 years), with a high proportion of patients developing progressively greater departure from baseline psychosocial functioning. The challenge for secondary prevention, therefore, lies in altering the course in the early deteriorating phase. We will review first the studies on predictors of outcomes in the early phases. Excellent reviews of predictors for very long-term outcome already exist, and the reader is referred to these (McGlashan, 1988; Angst, 1988). Prediction of suicide has also been the subject of a recent comprehensive review (Caldwell and Gottesman, 1990). Our review will be biased towards those investigations that fulfilled methodological criteria as outlined earlier, especially as regards being prospective and representative, and the quality of exposure assessment.

Sex

The issue of whether or not sex is associated with outcome is of crucial importance (Seeman, 1986; Goldstein, 1988; Childers and Harding, 1990). The sexes are usually combined in a single outcome distribution. There is, however, evidence that outcome may be different across the sexes in first or recent onset representative samples drawn from a defined area using outcome criteria other than just readmission or time in hospital. In such 1–8-year follow-up studies, women have been found, for example, to have a more favourable course pattern, to live more often independently, to be readmitted less, to spend less time in a psychotic state, to be less socially impaired at follow-up, and to spend more time in remission (Salokangas, 1983; Angermeyer et al., 1990; Shepherd et al., 1989; Jablensky et al., 1992; Navarro et al., 1996; Goldstein, 1988). The findings are consistent across cultures, and do not appear to be diagnosis-specific, or related to a particular diagnostic construct of schizophrenia (Navarro et al., 1996; Bardenstein and McGlashan, 1990; Goldstein, 1988; Angermeyer et al., 1990). However, studies that select individuals on the basis of chronicity (e.g. by using criteria from the DSM series) may be less likely to encounter sex differences on a range of measures, as women with a favourable early course will be excluded, resulting in (artificial) homogeneity at the severest end of the spectrum (e.g. Kendler and Walsh, 1995; Goldberg et al., 1995; Childers and Harding, 1990). Furthermore, sex differences in outcome may become more attenuated at longer-term follow-up (Bardenstein and McGlashan, 1990; Lewis, 1992).

Effect sizes range from men being nearly two times more likely to have more than mild social impairment at follow-up and being half as likely to experience a complete remission (Shepherd et al., 1989; our calculation from data provided), being three times more likely to have a non-remitting illness course, and living independently 20% less over the follow-up period (Navarro et al., 1996).

The question arises whether the differences in outcome can be explained by a third variable associated both with sex and outcome, such as substance abuse, age of onset, premorbid adjustment and prevalence of brain abnormality (Castle and Murray, 1991), or whether the differences are *intrinsic* to being female. The lack of diagnostic specificity for the sex–outcome association points in this direction. For example, it may be that in the normal population the life course of men is similarly more often dysfunctional compared to women. If this is the case, then the divergence between the sexes in outcome distribution is immutable and, consequently, separate norms for each sex should be used in reporting outcomes, similar to immutable sex differences in life expectancy at a given age. Alternatively, both intrinsic and confounding mechanisms may contribute to the sex differences in schizophrenia outcomes.

There is evidence that at least a proportion of the differences in outcome variance can be explained by a third variable. Angermeyer et al. (1990) reported that adjustment for age and marital status reduced the effect of sex, although it did not nullify it. Navarro et al. (1996) specifically examined the issue of alternative explanations in a sample of 166 patients with recent onset functional psychotic illness, followed for an average of four years. Women had better outcome, regardless of diagnosis. Adjustment for age and type of onset and diagnosis (females more often presenting with good outcome affective psychosis) reduced the associations between sex and a range of outcome measures by about 20–40%, but did not nullify it. Adjustment for family history, obstetric complications and cerebral ventricle size assessed with CT scanning, only marginally affected the association. Premorbid functioning did not reduce the association, concurring with Goldstein's (1988) finding that premorbid functioning reduced the association between sex and five-year outcome by not more than 13%. Thus, even after adjustment for a range of confounding variables, an effect of sex remained, though much attenuated.

In summary, the finding that women have a less deteriorated illness course is consistent across cultures, diagnostic construct and measures of outcome used. Some of the variation in outcome can be explained by differences in anamnestic variables such as age of onset, marital status and premorbid adjustment, but also differences in clinical expression of the illness itself account for the divergent sex outcome distributions. It cannot be excluded that similar associations between sex and life course exist in the general population, associated with, for example, sex differences in emotional expression or socialization. Thus, the question whether women have different illness characteristics or whether being female confers a relative protection against deteriorated life course in sickness *and* in health must be resolved by controlled studies. The association of sex with both outcome and with many of the other exposures used to predict illness course implies that counfounding by sex should be adjusted for in many instances when testing hypotheses about biological and social predictors of outcome.

Age and Type of Onset

Earlier age of onset and especially insidious types of onset are associated with a more deteriorated schizophrenia illness course (Robins and Guze, 1970; Stoffelmayr et al., 1983; Rabiner et al., 1986; Johnstone et al., 1989; Jablensky et al., 1992; van Os et al., 1994). This finding is not diagnosis-specific, similar findings transpiring in investigations of samples with schizoaffective disorder (e.g. Marneros et al., 1988; Del Rio Vega and Ayuso-Gutierrez, 1990), and affective disorder (e.g. Brodaty et al., 1993; Winokur et al., 1993). The association between age of onset and prognosis has face validity, as the impact of illness is much more damaging in an individual who has not completed the task of social and physical maturation, especially in illnesses which often run a chronic course, such as psychotic disorders. Furthermore, there is some evidence that schizophrenia cases with early age of onset perform less well academically and occupationally *before* illness onset (Johnstone et al., 1989).

Although one recent study reported an effect of age of onset, but not type of onset (Lieberman et al., 1993), it is likely that the effects of early and insidious age of onset are not independent, as they are correlated with each other (van Os et al., 1996a).

Socio-economic Status

Lower social class appears to be associated with poorer outcome in schizophrenia. Cooper (1961) followed a sample of 219 first-admission cases within a defined geographical area in the UK and examined various measures of course and outcome in relation to social class. There was a linear trend in the association between social class and time spent in hospital in the first two and five years of illness. Patients of lower social class were less likely to recover, less likely to respond to rehabilitation, and more likely to be readmitted. Similar findings emerged from a large study in the USA (Myers and Bean, 1968). Three decades later in the UK, McKenzie et al (1995) reported similar findings in the Camberwell Collaborative Psychosis Study which followed 166 subjects of recent-onset psychosis over four years. These authors found that, over three levels of socio-economic status, the risk of non-remitting illness over four years follow-up increased by a factor of 2.4 with each level of social class; the risk of non-recovery over the follow-up period similarly increased by a factor of 2. In this study, the association between social class and outcome was not diagnosis-specific within the functional psychoses. Indeed, similar findings have been reported in a sample of 248 bipolar patients (O'Connell et al., 1991).

Given the public health importance of an association between class and outcome, it is surprising that there has been a great decline in interest in this issue over the last 15 years (Cohen, 1993). Furthermore, socio-economic status is likely to confound many associations between outcomes and social or biological exposures, yet its effect is rarely controlled for.

Developing versus Developed Countries

It has been suggested that comparison of outcome studies across cultures indicates significant variability, with better outcome in non-industrialized societies (Murphy, 1968). However, in view of the multitude of factors influencing course and outcome across studies (discussed above), it is safe to say that the only way to test the hypothesis that outcome of illness is better in developing countries is to conduct a comparative study in a sample of both Western and non-industrialized countries, using the same instruments and sampling techniques. We are therefore dependent on the WHO International Pilot Study of Schizophrenia (IPSS; WHO, 1979) and the later WHO Determinants of Outcome Study (WHO-DOS; Jablensky et al. 1992) for evidence concerning this hypothesis. In the first follow-up study of the IPSS, 609 of 811 prevalent cases of schizophrenia of variable baseline illness chronicity were seen in nine centres worldwide at two years. A much larger number of patients in industrialized countries (11–31%) fell in the 'worst' global outcome group, than in non-industrialized countries (5–15%). However, differential attrition and diagnostic misclassification across centres from industrialized and non-industrialized centres may have contributed to these results (Lin and Kleinman, 1988). In the 10-country WHO-DOS study (Jablensky et al., 1992), nearly 80% of 1379 incident cases were followed up over two years. Again, outcome was superior over two years in developing countries. The comparability of sampling procedures across centres was put in doubt by the widely fluctuating sex ratio across centres (0.5 and 0.7 in Prague and Moscow respectively, versus 2.0 in Nottingham). The divergency in sex ratios cannot possibly represent sex differences in the source populations of the centres, as evidenced by wide fluctuation in the age- and sex-specific incidence rates for both broadly and narrowly defined schizophrenia across centres. The two centres with the lowest attrition rates (6.4% and 5.6%; mean total sample attrition rate: 22%) also had the highest percentages of patients with a course type of *single psychotic episode, complete remission* (54% and 42% respectively), and both these centres were in developing countries. However, this cannot explain why the Nigerian centre, which had a relatively high attrition rate (31%), also had a very high percentage (51%) of patients with the course type of *single psychotic episode, complete remission*. The study also showed that differences in type of onset did not contribute to the observed differences in outcome between developing and developed countries. The follow-up sample from developing countries had significantly more male patients than in developed countries (59% and 49% respectively, $P<0.01$), but this difference would have served only to *obscure* better outcome in developing countries, as women fared significantly better. Indeed, using the WHO-DOS data, Susser and Wanderling (1994) showed that the incidence of non-affective remitting psychosis in developing countries was 10 times the incidence in industrialized parts of the world. Collateral support for better outcome in developing countries was provided by our recent study on outcome of psychosis in a group of both first, and second-generation Afro-Caribbean patients in the UK. Compared to white patients, individuals from the Afro-Caribbean group fared significantly better on a range of outcome measures (McKenzie et al., 1995 – see below). These findings argue against the explanation that outcome is better because vulnerable individuals are less likely to survive and/or procreate in developing countries, leading to an excess of good outcome psychosis in the non-industrialized world.

Duration of Psychosis Before Treatment

In a two-year follow-up of 120 first-admission patients with schizophrenia, who entered a randomized controlled trial of maintenance antipsychotic medication (all patients had received initial treatment for the psychotic episode), duration of illness prior to starting antipsychotic medication was the most important determinant of relapse. Of the patients in whom this interval exceeded one year, all individuals given placebo treatment relapsed, whereas only 18% given active treatment remained relapse-free over the follow-up period (Crow et al., 1986). Similar findings were reported by Rabiner et al. (1986). Both groups of authors suggested that either a third variable, such as insidious onset or lack of social support, or delay in institution of treatment *itself* might account for these results. This is obviously an important issue. If duration before institution of treatment itself has a deleterious effect, then a high proportion of subsequent psychiatric morbidity may be preventable and rigorous early case detecting and treatment programmes would be justified.

As discussed above, delay in coming to medical attention may be associated with a number of factors associated with outcome. Furthermore, informants may give biased accounts if patients had abnormal personalities before the onset of illness. Unless these can be shown not to bias or confound the relationship between duration of psychosis and outcome, no sufficient grounds exist that would justify widespread preventive measures. An earlier study by May et al. (1981) is often cited to support the view that duration of psychosis itself affects outcome. In this study, a large group of first-admission schizophrenic patients (n=228) were randomly assigned to one of five treatment groups. As random allocation is the best way to control for both known and unknown confounders, their results that patients initially treated with antipsychotic drugs did much better in terms of outcome over the subsequent three years than those initially not treated with drugs appears to support the duration hypothesis. However, patients not treated with drugs received other treatments, such as psychotherapy, and the possibility that this treatment had a prognostically unfavourable effect cannot be excluded.

Rabiner et al. (1986) reported on the one-year relapse rates of a group of 64 incident cases of psychosis. Duration of illness was associated with poorer outcome in both affective and non-affective psychosis.

Loebel et al. (1992), in a later study at the same hospital, followed 70 first-admission patients with schizophrenia and schizoaffective disorder who had received standardized pharmacological treatment for up to three years. Duration of illness prior to treatment was significantly associated with time and level of remission, and remained so after adjustment for sex and diagnosis. However, their sample included a mix of ethnic and socio-economic groups whose likely confounding effect was not examined. As explained above, confounding should not be based on statistical significance; if we are to judge the public health importance of untreated duration of psychosis, we need to know the effect size after adjustment for factors that can explain (partly or completely) the association between duration of illness and outcome.

In the WHO-DOS study (Jablensky et al., 1992), duration of illness between onset and initial examination was also associated with four of the seven outcome variables used. Furthermore, the association remained significant after adjustment for setting (developed versus developing country) and type of onset.

In summary, four first-episode studies have concurred in showing that duration of illness prior to treatment is associated with subsequent short-term outcome, regardless of whether duration was measured from first psychotic symptom or from first-ever sign of being unwell. Adjustments have been made for sex, diagnosis and type of onset, but the effects of other important variables such as social class, social support and premorbid abnormalities have not been examined, and it is unclear how much subsequent psychiatric morbidity can be prevented with, if any, each month of untreated psychosis. Therefore, although the association may be genuine, further investigations are needed.

Drug and Alcohol Use

As the prevalence of drug and alcohol use among psychotic patients is high in a variety of countries and settings (15–50% of patients (Bland et al., 1987; McKenna and Paredes, 1992; Strakowski et al., 1993)), even small effects such use may have on subsequent course is of great public health importance. Drug and alcohol use among psychotic patients is more common in male patients (Haas et al. 1990; McGlashan and Bardenstein, 1990) so that the effect of sex must be controlled for in examining associations with course and outcome. Misclassification of exposure status is very high (30% or more) unless laboratory analysis of, for example, urine specimens is used (Shaner et al., 1993). Not only is psychosis often followed by drug abuse, but drug abuse also predisposes to psychosis; diagnostic misclassification may be common if psychosis due to intoxication, withdrawal or concomitant infectious disease is diagnosed as functional psychotic disorder. Subjects may become marginalized through the stigma of using drugs in addition to, or instead of, any deleterious effect on course resulting from the drugs themselves.

It is therefore no wonder that published reports indicate that the relationship between substance use and outcome of psychosis is complicated and inconsistent (Stoffelmeyer and Benijhek, 1989). Nevertheless, they tend to reveal a trend. Reviewing the subject, Turner and Tsuang (1990) concluded that drugs may be precipitating relapse and subsequent readmission among schizophrenic patients who are in remission. The impression that dual-diagnosis patients tend to do worse is confirmed by reports that such individuals make more use of general psychiatric services (Regier et al., 1990), psychiatric emergency services (Schwartz et al., 1972), community services (Pepper et al., 1981), and inpatient services (Safer, 1987). A recent study provided evidence that use of cannabis is associated with more and earlier relapse in recent-onset schizophrenic patients (Linszen et al., 1994). In addition, there was an interaction with intensity of cannabis use, heavy users having poorer outcome: the risk of relapse was 3.4-fold in the group of heavy users (our calculations from the data provided). This study was conducted in a country where use of cannabis is not restricted by legislation and not associated with stigma, and took into account a range of confounding factors, such as sex and use of alcohol and other drugs. As cannabis tends to be the most frequently used drug in many countries, the evidence suggests there is considerable scope for secondary prevention.

Expressed Emotion

The excess risk of relapse over one year associated with 'high' expressed emotion (EE) in the relatives of schizophrenic patients is 2.2 (our calculation from a review of 26 studies involving 1323 subjects by Kavanagh, 1992a). In spite of this relatively modest effect size, the uncertain validity of EE as a concept, and concerns that relapse itself, or severity of illness in the proband determines EE rather than the other way round, the result of clinical trials aimed at modifying relatives' behaviour are encouraging in that it may be possible to reduce the relapse rate associated with EE in the short term by a factor of 2–5 (reviewed by Kavanagh, 1992b). These findings generally apply to samples of patients living with their families, and may not be generalizable to the majority of patients who have other living arrangements such as hostels and supervised residences.

REDUCTION OF HETEROGENEITY

Outcome studies can provide evidence for contrasting course of illness in high-risk groups. 'High-risk' group in this context refers to patients exposed to a risk factor thought to increase the risk of schizophrenia and related psychoses. For example, schizophrenia in a first-degree relative, cerebral ventricle dimensions, life events, ethnic group and childhood developmental deviance have all been shown to increase the risk of schizophrenia *onset* (Shields, 1980; Johnstone et al., 1976; Jones et al., 1994a; Bebbington et al., 1993; van Os et al., 1996). Robins and Guze (1970) identified many of these features also as prognostic features, i.e. as risk factors for *persistence* of illness. The finding that the same risk factor is implicated in both onset and outcome of a disease, in such a way that it can be differentiated from other high-risk groups, is suggestive of the existence of *discrete major effects* (this is not the same as assuming discrete subtypes), and may constitute an important contribution towards elucidating the heterogeneity of underlying mechanisms or possibly even aetiology of functional psychotic illness. It is therefore important to try to integrate conceptually onset and outcome investigations, which may ultimately lead to an empirical model of heterogeneity based on risk factors (Figure 6.4); (Andreasen and Carpenter, 1993).

In this section we will explore the evidence for such discrete effects in the functional psychoses.

Life Events

In spite of the many methodological difficulties in measuring life events, the results of seven studies reviewed by Bebbington and Kuipers (1988) were suggestive of an excess of stressful life events in the three weeks before onset (or relapse) of schizophrenic illness. More recently, support for an association between life events and illness onset has come from three studies which introduced important methodological improvements such as prospective designs, inclusion of appropriate controls, and rating of severity and degree of threat of the life event (Ventura et al., 1989; Malla et al., 1990; Bebbington et al., 1993). The associations between life events and illness onset are not specific to any particular diagnostic category within the functional psychoses, but there is some evidence that the effect sizes are greater in affective illness than in schizophrenia (Paykell, 1978; Brown et al., 1973; Bebbington et al., 1993; Dohrenwend et al., 1995).

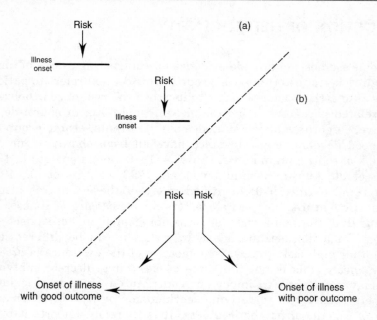

Figure 6.4   Risk factors for emergence of illness also predict persistence of illness. (a) Risk for onset of illness investigated separately from risk for chronicity. (b) Reducing the heterogeneity of psychotic illness: integrating onset and outcome research.

Compared to the increasing sophistication of studies on life events and illness onset, the literature on the relationship between life events and illness outcome has been lagging behind severely. Almost all studies merely used the clinician's impression of stressful life events, some studies reporting a positive association (i.e. better outcome in illness following stressful events – e.g. Vaillant, 1964; Stephens et al., 1966; Day et al., 1987), and other studies reporting inconclusive findings (e.g. Serban, 1975; Cole et al., 1954; Johanson, 1958). Moreover, all these studies may have merely been comparing insidious and acute-onset patients. Insidious onsets can often not be dated with precision, so that no relationship between life events and illness onset can be established. If such cases are rated life event 'negative', the association between life events and outcome may be confounded by type of onset. As women more often report life events (Bebbington et al., 1993) and also have better prognosis, any association must also be controlled for sex.

Harder et al. (1981) prospectively ascertained outcome in 111 first-admission schizophrenic patients (subdivided in three groups of competing definitions of schizophrenia) having assessed at baseline the presence of 'life-events stress' in the previous year with a modified version of the Social Readjustment Rating Scale by Holmes and Rahe. They excluded items that 'were judged to be very likely consequences of the disorder', and excluding events that were 'obviously the result of the patient's pathological condition'. They also weighted the level of stress for recency of occurrence in relation to disease onset. They found that life-events stress was associated with better outcome for two definitions of schizophrenia, but not for the DSM-II definition of the disorder. Although this variability of the findings in relation to definition of illness points to inconsistency, and associations were reported uncontrolled, they remain, nevertheless, suggestive.

In the Camberwell Collaborative Psychosis study, a sample of 59 recent onset psychotic patients with datable onset of illness, half of whom had experienced a life event (LE+) prior to the episode, were assessed with the contextual rating of threat technique developed by Brown and Harris, and followed for four years blind to exposure status. Analyses were adjusted for possible confounding variables, including sex and diagnosis. LE+ patients were nearly 10 times more likely to have a symptom severity of *mild* or *recovered* over most of the follow-up period, and had accordingly spent less time in hospital over the follow-up period. There was an interaction with diagnosis, in that the association was stronger in (but not confined to) the affective psychoses than in schizophrenia (van Os et al., 1994).

The fact that life events, over a number of years of follow-up, predict a less deteriorated illness course needs to be integrated with reports that life events and other stressful factors in the social environment such as 'expressed emotions' (EE) are also associated with increased risk of relapse. The most parsimonious explanation of these findings is to assume that life-event-related illness runs a course of frequent relapses followed by rapid recovery.

Thus, the available evidence suggests that psychotic illness preceded by life events is associated with a less deteriorated illness course. The effect of life events on both onset and outcome appears especially evident at the affective end of the psychopathological continuum in the functional psychoses.

Ethnic Group

An increased incidence of affective and non-affective psychosis ha
been demonstrated in Afro-Caribbeans in several European countrie
(Harrison, 1988; Selten and Sijben, 1994; King et al., 1994; van O
et al., 1996c, 1996d). As discussed above, a number of cross-cultura
studies have shown that the prognosis of psychotic disorders sucl
as schizophrenia is better in non-industrialized countries. Som
researchers have questioned whether Afro-Caribbeans in the Ul
might have a similarly good prognosis and whether the increase
incidence of psychosis in this group might be due to an excess o
good prognosis illness (Littlewood and Lipsedge, 1981).

Follow-up studies set to test this hypothesis have not shown bette
outcome for Afro-Caribbeans when compared to British-born white
or white Europeans (McGovern et al., 1994; Sugarman, 1992
Birchwood et al., 1992). However, this failure may have been due t
a number of methodological flaws. The studies have not controlle
for social class or age of onset of illness, though lower socio-economi
status and early age of onset are related to both ethnic group an
poorer outcome (van Os et al., 1996c; Harvey et al., 1990a). Thus
these factors could mask any better prognosis if they are no
controlled for. McKenzie and colleagues (1995) compared course an
outcome of psychotic illness between two groups of Afro-Caribbear
(n=53) and British-born white individuals (n=60), in a cohort stud
of consecutive admissions, followed up for four years. Subjects wer
patients admitted to two South-London hospitals with a recent-onse
psychotic illness, and the main outcome measures were: illnes
course, self-harm, social disability, hospital use and treatment vari
ables, adjusted for socio-economic origin, sex, age of onset an
diagnosis. The Afro-Caribbean group spent more time recovered ove
the follow-up period (adjusted odds ratio (OR)=5.0), were less likel
to have had a continuous, unremitting illness (adjusted OR=0.3), an
were less at risk of self-harm and suicide (adjusted OR=0.2). Ther
was no evidence for interaction with diagnostic group. However, *post
hoc* analyses revealed that the effect of ethnic group tended to b
stronger in the non-schizophrenic psychoses. These results sugges
that the high incidence observed in UK Afro-Caribbeans is couple
with a less deteriorated illness course in this ethnic group. Exces
exposure to precipitants in the social environment, resulting in goo
prognosis 'reactive' illness may be one explanation. If replicated
these findings have major public health implications.

Cerebral Ventricle Dimensions

That the mean size of the lateral cerebral ventricle is on average larger in schizophrenic patients than in well controls is widely accepted. Jones et al. (1994b) demonstrated a linear trend in the association between lateral ventricle size and onset of schizophrenia, which indicates that risk is not confined to a subgroup with very large ventricles, but rather that ventricular enlargement is best conceived as a continuous risk factor: the larger the ventricles, the greater the risk of schizophrenia. The association does not appear to be entirely specific to schizophrenia, although the association between onset of disorder and cerebral ventricle dimensions appears less strong in the affective psychoses – and also less well investigated (Weinberger et al., 1982; Jones et al., 1994b; Harvey et al., 1990b; Andreasen et al., 1990). However, a recent carefully conducted meta-analysis by Elkis and colleagues (1995) demonstrated that cerebral ventricle size is a risk factor for both affective disorder and schizophrenia, though the effect size is larger in the latter.

The notion that cerebral ventricle dimensions are also associated with illness course speaks to the imagination (Crow, 1980; Murray and O'Callaghan, 1991), but, as with life events, little empirical evidence to support this thesis has been provided. Indeed, there are well over a hundred controlled comparisons investigating cerebral ventricle dimensions as risk factors for *onset* of psychosis, but we were only able to locate four prospective studies (i.e. neuroimaging preceding follow-up) that had specifically addressed the issue of cerebral ventricle size and *persistence* of psychosis (Table 6.3). All studies reported results in the expected direction (poorer outcome in those with larger ventricles or ventricle/brain ratio (VBR). However, two of the studies were very small ($n<25$) to examine effect sizes that are likely to be modest. Three of the studies were uncontrolled, which, given the fact that cerebral ventricle size and the often-used VBR are associated with, for example, age, sex, socio-economic status and ethnic group (Jones et al., 1994b; van Os et al., 1995) suggests that the results may be confounded. The largest study ($n=140$), however, reported that, after adjustment for such confounding factors, cerebral ventricle size was a risk factor for negative symptoms over the follow-up period, attenuated cognitive functioning at follow-up as assessed by the Trails's test and unemployement over the follow-up period. Significant dose–response relationships existed between ventricle size and outcome, and it was shown that the associations were not simply repetitions of associations that could already have

Table 6.3 Review of literature examining ventricular size in relation to outcome of psychotic disorders

Reference	Patient selection	Months of follow-up (SD)	No. of subjects (attrition)	Index diagnosis	Main outcome measures	CT/MRI measure	Adjustment for confounding	Findings
DeLisi et al. (1992)	Incident cases	24 (?)	30 (3%)	DSM-IIIR: schizophreniform (n=19) schizoaffective (n=6) schizophrenia (n=4) atypical (n=1)	Number of admissions, months in hospital, GAS, Strauss Carpenter Scale, BPRS	Ventricular volume, temporal lobe volume (MRI)	No	Ventricular volume correlated with more admissions, more time in hospital, and higher BPRS score
Vita et al. (1991)	Chronic illness	24 (?)	18 (15%)	DSM-III-R chronic schizophrenia	Strauss Carpenter scale, scale for intimacy of interpersonal contacts	VBR, cortical atrophy score (CT)	No	Cortical atrophy, but not VBR, correlated significantly with most outcome measures
van Os et al. (1995)	Recent onset cases	46 (SD=13)	140 (13%)	DSM-III-R psychosis: schizophrenia (n=64) affective (n=36) schizoaffective (n=11) other (n=29)	Usual symptom severity, time living independently, negative symptoms, cognitive functioning employment	Cerebral ventricle dimensions (CT)	Head size, age, sex, class, ethnic group and diagnosis	Cerebral ventricle dimensions continuous risk factor for negative symptoms, cognitive functioning and unemployment
Lieberman et al. (1993)	Incident cases	12	70 (0%)	RDC: schizophrenia (n=54) schizoaffective (n=6)	Time to first remission and level of remission	'Brain abnormality' (mostly enlarged ventricles; MRI)	No	Brian abnormalities associated with both longer time to remission and poorer level of remission

existed at baseline. Effect sizes ranged from being 17 times more likely to be unemployed at follow-up, and nine times more likely to have demonstrated negative symptoms over the follow-up period; effects were stronger in (but not specific to) the DSM-III-R category of schizophrenia (van Os et al., 1995).

In summary, the hypothesized relationship between cerebral ventricle dimensions and outcome has support from four prospective studies. Contrary to life events, there is evidence that the association between ventricle size and outcome is stronger at the non-affective end of the psychopathological continuum of the functional psychoses.

Early Developmental Attenuation

Early developmental deviance is a risk factor for later schizophrenia (Jones et al., 1994a). The specificity of this finding remains in doubt, as evidence has emerged suggesting that individuals with affective disorder and non-schizophrenic psychosis show neurological abnormalities and subtle differences in social and cognitive development, similar to those found in patients with schizophrenia (Rogers, 1990; Done et al., 1994; van Os et al., 1996b).

There is evidence that childhood developmental deficit is not only a risk factor for the *emergence* of psychotic illness, but is also an important risk factor for illness *persistence*. Stoffelmayr et al. (1983) reviewed the early generation of studies relating premorbid adjustment and outcome in schizophrenia, and concluded not only that the two were very strongly related, but also that the strength of the association was largely consistent across studies, most variation being due to random error. However, premorbid adjustment in most of the earlier studies was not assessed in a structured way, from sources of widely varying reliability, and always retrospective. Later studies used better instruments, such as the Premorbid Adjustment Scale (PAS; Cannon-Spoor et al., 1982) which assesses premorbid social and role functioning during childhood, early adolescence, late adolescence and adulthood, but premorbid assessments remained retrospective, with considerable scope for both observation and recall bias, especially in the case of such a remote exposure. Two more recent studies examined schizophrenic patients at their first onset and prospectively investigated premorbid adjustment and course of illness. Rabiner et al. (1986) reported that continual remission after up to one-year follow-up was associated with scores on the Premorbid Asocial Adjustment Scale in a group of 36 schizophrenic patients. Mayerhoff et al. (1994) reported that in a group of 70 first-onset patients, premorbid adjustment measured with the PAS was associated with evidence of 'deficit' syndrome at 6–12 months follow-up. Two prospective 4–6-year studies (Breier et al., 1992; Verdoux et al., 1995) using the Philips scale (Philips, 1953) found that poor premorbid social adjustment was associated with poor outcome, especially in terms of negative symptoms and unemployment. In the study by Breier et al. (1992), premorbid adjustment explained 11% of the variation in negative symptoms at follow-up, and 7% of the variation in quantity of work at follow-up (our calculations from the data provided).

The study of Werry et al. (1991) stands out, as the subjects were incident and representative cases of adolescent-onset psychosis (DSM-III schizophrenia (n=30) and bipolar disorder (n=23)) collected in a defined catchment area, in whom premorbid adjustment could be much more reliably assessed in view of their young age at baseline assessment (mean 13.9 years), and the availability of parental informants. Abnormal premorbid adjustment, using DSM-III-R major divisions of personality disorder on a four-point severity scale, was the best predictor for poor five-year outcome in both schizophrenic and bipolar cases, although *more* so in schizophrenia (diagnostic misclassification was found not to be an issue in this study). Overall, premorbid adaptational functioning explained 7% of occupational functioning, 10% of peer relationships, and 4% of adaptational functioning.

This latter study suggests that the association between premorbid adjustment and outcome is not specific to schizophrenia. Indeed, multiple studies have converged in showing a similar relationship in unipolar, bipolar and schizoaffective disorders (Deister and Marneros, 1993; Brodaty et al., 1993; Scott et al., 1992; Harder et al., 1990; Duggan et al., 1990; Coryell et al., 1990a). However, in a prospective study of a national birth cohort of 5262 individuals, we showed that, although there were no qualitative differences between schizophrenia and affective disorder, even in subjects with severe and chronic depression, associations with indices of early developmental deviance were less strong than in subjects with schizophrenia (van Os et al., 1996b; Jones et al., 1994a).

Familial Morbid Risk

Robins and Guze (1970) suggested that family history might be used to subdivide good and poor prognosis schizophrenia, the former being more likely to be associated with a family history of affective disorder, and the latter with a family history of schizophrenia. Kendler and Tsuang (1988) have reviewed other studies on this topic published between 1931 and 1986. Some showed an association between family history of schizophrenia and poor outcome, and many showed an association between family history of affective disorder and good outcome. However, these studies suffered from many methodological limitations, such as obtaining family history data from case notes or probands, and failure to take into account confounding factors such as family size, age and sex of the relatives in assessing the probands' familial loading for psychiatric disorders (Roy and Crowe, 1994). Weiss et al. (1982) have shown how such methodological problems can lead to biased results. Furthermore, many studies have considered outcome as a unidimensional, global variable, and have not measured outcome in several distinct clinical and social areas of functioning (Strauss and Carpenter, 1978). Samples frequently consisted of a mixture of both recent onset patients and chronic patients, making the outcome findings more difficult to interpret than if homogeneous groups of subjects were studied. Finally, as most of the variability in the course of schizophrenia occurs in the first five years (see above), association with any predictor should be more readily detectable over this period.

Given these methodological limitations, especially as regards assessment and classification of family history, it is not surprising that the literature is inconsistent, some studies demonstrating an association between a positive family history for schizophrenia and poor outcome (McGlashan, 1986a, b; Keefe et al., 1987; Sautter and McDermot, 1994), and others reporting inconclusive findings (Bleuler, 1978; Ciompi, 1980; Huber et al., 1980; Alda et al., 1991).

Two outcome studies took into account some of the confounding factors such as age, sex and family size, in examining the association between familial morbid risk and illness course. Fowler et al. (1972) compared 28 good and 25 poor prognosis schizophrenic patients and interviewed their relatives mostly blind to proband outcome status. Of the 126 first-degree relatives in the poor prognosis group, 13 had schizophrenia; in the good prognosis group the prevalence of schizophrenia was much lower (five out of 137; risk ratio (RR)=0.6; 95% CI=0.5–0.9 – our calculations from the data provided). The risk for affective disorder (bipolar and unipolar depressive disorders) was lower in the poor outcome group, although this just failed to reach statistical significance (RR=0.4; 95% CI=0.2–1 – our calculations from the data provided). Although this study was adjusted for the number of relatives, no adjustment was made for age and sex of the relatives; thus, confounding by age might have operated in producing spurious results. The largest study to date was by Kendler and Tsuang (1988), who examined outcome and familial psychopathology in a sample of 253 DSM-III schizophrenics and their 723 first-degree relatives. Family history was viewed from a cohort perspective, where relatives were regarded as the subjects at risk of developing mental illness, and good or poor outcome in the proband was regarded as an exposure variable. Morbid risk of non-affective psychotic disorder was higher in the relatives of poor-outcome probands, more so at short-term outcome than at long-term outcome, although for both periods this failed to reach statistical significance. Morbid risk of affective illness was significantly higher in relatives of good outcome patients both at short-term and long-term follow-up. A major problem with this study was that information was lost by dichotomizing outcome into good and poor outcome categories, and that short-term outcome (arguably the most sensitive measure) was assessed retrospectively from very old case-note material. Also, the sample was already defined in terms of chronicity at baseline, as the investigators used DSM criteria.

In our own study (Verdoux et al., 1995), we tested for associations between four-year outcome and familial loading for psychotic disorders in a sample of 150 consecutively admitted patients with functional psychosis of recent onset. Information on relatives was obtained through direct interviews of relatives with the Schedule for Affective Disorders and Schizophrenia and with the Family History–Research Diagnostic Criteria method. For each proband, a familial loading score was calculated for (i) broadly defined psychotic disorder, (ii) schizophrenia, and (iii) affective disorder taking into account age, sex and number of relatives. In our sample of psychotic patients, familial loading for *psychotic disorder* predicted persistent negative symptoms over the follow-up period (OR=1.5), and was also associated with more time hospitalized, and more social disability at follow-up, especially in schizophrenia. Greater familial loading for *schizophrenia* predicted a lower likelihood of recovery (OR=2.2), and a greater likelihood of having had persistent negative symptoms over the follow-up period (OR=1.7). All family history–outcome associations had been adjusted for sex and age of onset. No association was found between outcome and familial loading for affective disorder, but the absence of associations may have been due to the fact that we chose a very narrow definition of (hospitalized) affective disorder.

In summary, there is some evidence to suggest that there is a continuum of genetic liability not only to the emergence of psychotic illness, but also the subsequent chronicity of the disorder, more so in schizophrenia than in the non-schizophrenic psychoses. In other words, poor outcome disorders may 'breed true' within families, although in order to examine this further, outcome in the affected relatives of the psychotic probands also needs to be studied.

An Empirical Model of Heterogeneity in the Functional Psychoses Based on Risk Factors for Emergence and Persistence

In the section on predictive validity, we showed that what appears to have been validated across studies is a psychopathological continuum ranging from affective to non-affective psychosis, rather than individual diagnostic categories. Furthermore, the predictive validity of symptom dimensions may be greater than that of diagnostic categories.

In the section on heterogeneity of risk, we showed that various risk factors for emergence of psychosis also influenced outcome, in such a way that two discrete effects are apparent. Life events and ethnic group were associated with good outcome illness, whereas familial morbid risk, early developmental deviance, and cerebral ventricle dimensions predicted a more deteriorated illness course.

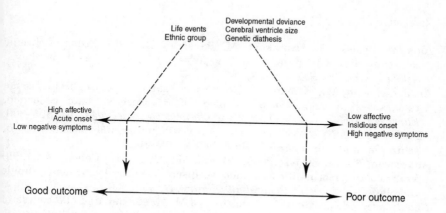

Figure 6.5 Risk factors for emergence and persistence of psychosis interact with psychopathological dimension. The effect of 'constitutional' risk factors is stronger at the insidious onset, non-affective end of the psychopathological continuum, whereas the association with life events and ethnic group is more evident at the affective end of the psychopatho-logical continuum.

There was little evidence that any one risk factor was entirely specific to any diagnostic category within the functional psychoses. However, we have made it clear that the *magnitude* of these risk factors for poor and good outcome illness varies as a function of baseline psychopathology, such that the life events–ethnic group association is more evident at the affective end of the spectrum, and the associations between outcome and familial morbid risk, cerebral ventricle size, and premorbid adjustment at the non-affective end.

These issues are summarized in Figure 6.5. Although this bottom-up empirical model may lack some of the acumen of more comprehensive top-down models that seek to explain the phenomenon of psychosis from beginning to end, they are more flexible and yield more refutable predictions (Murray et al., 1988). Also, the model is more compatible with the search for biological mechanisms of symptom dimensions (e.g. Liddle et al., 1992; McGuire et al., 1993), which are now complementing the traditional approach of comparing diagnostic categories.

Acknowledgements

The authors thank Dr Peter Jones, Dr Pak Sham and Dr Paul Bebbington for their kind help.

References

Alda, M., Zvolsky, P., Dvorakova, M., Paperova, H. (1991) Study of chronic schizophrenics with positive and negative family histories of psychosis. *Acta Psychiatrica Scandinavica* **83**: 334–337.

An der Heiden, W., Krumm, B. (1991) The course of schizophrenia: some remarks on a yet unsolved problem of retrospective data collection. *European Archives of Psychiatry and Clinical Neurosciences* **204**: 303–306.

Andreasen, N.J.C., Carpenter, W.T. (1993) Diagnosis and classification of schizophrenia. *Schizophrenia Bulletin* **19**: 199–214.

Andreasen, N.J.C., Swayze, V.W., Flaum, M., Alliger, R., Cohen, M. (1990) Ventricular abnormalities in affective disorder: clinical and demographic correlates. *Archives of General Psychiatry* **47**: 893–900.

Angermeyer, M.C., Kühn, L., Goldstein, J.M. (1990) Sex and the course of schizophrenia: differences in treated outcomes. *Schizophrenia Bulletin* **16**: 293–307.

Angst, J. (1988) European long-term follow-up studies of schizophrenia. *Schizophrenia Bulletin* **14**: 501–513.

Bardenstein, K., McGlashan, T. (1990) Sex differences in affective, schizoaffective, and schizophrenic disorders. A review. *Schizophrenia Research* **3**: 159–172.

Bartko, J., Carpenter, W., McGlashan, T. (1988) Statistical issues in long-term followup studies. *Schizophrenia Bulletin* **14**: 575–587.

Bebbington, P., Kuipers, L. (1988) Social influences on schizophrenia. In McGuffin, P., Bebbington, P. (eds) *Schizophrenia, The Major Issues*. Oxford: Heinemann.

Bebbington, P., Wilkins, S., Jones, P.B. et al. (1993) Life events and psychosis. Initial results from the Camberwell Collaborative Psychosis Study. *British Journal of Psychiatry* **162**: 72–79.

Beiser, M., Iacono, W.G., Erickson, D. (1989) Temporal stability in major mental disorders. In Robins, L.N., Barrett, J.E. (eds) *The Validity of Psychiatric Diagnosis*, pp. 77–98. New York: Raven Press.

Birchwood, M., Cochrane, R., MacMillna, F. et al. (1992) The influence of ethnicity and family structure on relapse in first-episode schizophrenia. *British Journal of Psychiatry* **161**: 783–790.

Bland, R.C. (1982) Predicting the outcome in schizophrenia. *Canadian Journal of Psychiatry* **27**: 52–62.

Bland, R.C., Orn, H. (1978) 14 year outcome in early schizophrenia. *Acta Psychiatrica Scandinavica* **58**: 327-338.

Bland, R.C., Orn, H. (1980) Prediction of long term outcome from presenting symptoms in schizophrenia. *Journal of Clinical Psychiatry* **41**: 85–88.

Bland, R.C., Newman, S.C., Orn, H. (1987) Schizophrenia: lifetime co-morbidity in a community sample. *Acta Psychiatrica Scandinavica* **75**: 383–391.

Bleuler, M. (1972) *Die Schizophrenen Geistesstörungen im Lichte Langjäriger Kranken – und Familiengeschichten*. Stuttgart: G. Thieme.

Bleuler, M. (1978) *The Schizophrenic Disorders: Long Term Patient and Family Studies*, Clemens, S. (translator). New Haven: Yale University.

Breier, A. (1988) Small sample studies: unique contribution for large sample outcome studies. *Schizophrenia Bulletin* **14**: 589–593.

Breier, A., Schreiber, J., Dyer, J., Pickar, D. (1991) National Institute of Mental Health longitudinal study of chronic schizophrenia. Prognosis and predictors of outcome. *Archives of General Psychiatry* **48**: 239–246.

Breier, A., Schreiber, J.L., Dyer, J. et al. (1992) Course of illness and predictors of outcome in chronic schizophrenia: implications for pathophysiology. *British Journal of Psychiatry* **161** (Suppl. 18): 38–43.

Brockington, I., Kendell, R., Wainwright, S. (1980a) Depressed patients with schizophrenic or paranoid symptoms. *Psychological Medicine* **10**: 665–675.

Brockington, I., Wainwright, S., Kendell, R. (1980b) Manic patients with schizophrenic or paranoid symptoms. *Psychological Medicine* **10**: 73–83.

Brodaty, H., Harris, L., Peters, K., Wihelm, K., Hickie, I., Boyce, P. et al (1993) Prognosis of depression in the elderly. *British Journal of Psychiatry* **163**: 589–596.

Brown, G.W., Bone, M., Dalison, B., Wing, J.K. (1966) *Schizophrenia and Social Care*. London: Oxford University Press.

Brown, G.W., Harris, T.O., Peto, J. (1973) Life events and psychiatric disorders. Part 2: Nature of causal link. *Psychological Medicine* **3**: 159–176.

Caldwell, C.B., Gottesman, I.I. (1990) Schizophrenics kill themselves too: a review of risk factors for suicide. *Schizophrenia Bulletin* **16**: 571–589.

Cannon-Spoor, E., Potkin, S., Wyatt, R.J. (1982) Measurement of premorbid adjustment in chronic schizophrenia. *Schizophrenia Bulletin* **8**: 470–484.

Castle, D., Murray, R. (1991) The neurodevelopmental basis of sex differences in schizophrenia. *Psychological Medicine* **21**: 565–575.

Castle, D., Wessely, S., Murray, R. (1993) Sex and schizophrenia: effects of diagnostic stringency, and associations with premorbid variables. *British Journal of Psychiatry* **162**: 658–664.

Childers, S., Harding, C.M. (1990) Sex, premorbid functioning, and long-term outcome in DSM-III schizophrenia. *Schizophrenia Bulletin* **16**: 309–318.

Ciompi, L. (1980) The natural history of schizophrenia in the long term. *British Journal of Psychiatry* **136**: 413–420.

Ciompi, L., Müller, C. (1976) *Lebensweg und Alter der Schizophrenen. Eine katamnestische Langzeitstudie bis ins Senium.* Berlin–Heidelberg–New York: Springer.

Clayton, D., Hills, M. (1993) Confounding and standardization. In Clayton, D., Hills, M. (eds) *Statistical Models in Epidemiology*, pp. 133–140. Oxford: Oxford University Press.

Cohen, C.I. (1993) Poverty and the course of schizophrenia: implications for research and policy. *Hospital and Community Psychiatry* **44**: 951–958.

Cole, M.E., Swensen, C.H., Pascal, G.R. (1954) Prognostic significance of precipitating stress in mental illness. *Journal of Consulting Psychology* **18**: 171–175.

Cooper, B. (1961) Social class and prognosis in schizophrenia. Part I and Part II. *British Journal of Preventive and Social Medicine* **15**: 17–41.

Coryell, W., Endicott, J., Keller, M. (1990a) Outcome of patients with chronic affective disorder: a five year follow-up. *American Journal of Psychiatry* **147**: 1627–1633.

Coryell, W., Keller, M., Lavori, P. et al (1990b) Affective syndromes, psychotic features, and prognosis. I: depression. *Archives of General Psychiatry* **47**: 651–657.

Coryell, W., Keller, M., Lavori, P. et al (1990c) Affective syndromes, psychotic features, and prognosis. II: mania. *Archives of General Psychiatry* **47**: 658–662.

Crow, T.J. (1980) Molecular pathology of schizophrenia: more than one disease. *British Medical Journal* **280**: 66–68.

Crow, T.J., MacMillan, J.F., Johnson, A.L., Johnstone, E.C. (1986) The Northwick Park study of first episodes of schizophrenia. II: A randomised controlled trial of prophylactic neuroleptic treatment. *British Journal of Psychiatry* **148**: 120–127.

Day, R., Nielsen, J.A., Korten, A. et al (1987) Stressful life events preceding the acute onset of schizophrenia: a cross-national study from the World Health Organization. *Culture, Medicine and Psychiatry* **11**: 123–205.

Deister, A., Marneros, A. (1993) Predicting the long-term outcome of affective disorders. *Acta Psychiatrica Scandinavica* **88**: 174–177.

DeLisi, L.E., Stritzke, P., Riordan, H. et al (1992) The timing of brain morphological changes in schizophrenia and their relationship to clinical outcome. *Biological Psychiatry* **31**: 241–254.

Del Rio Vega, J.M., Ayuso-Gutierrez, J.L. (1990) Course of schizoaffective psychosis: a retrospective study. *Acta Psychiatrica Scandinavica* **81**: 534–537.

Dohrenwend, B.P., Shrout, P.E., Link, B.G., Skodol, A.E., Stueve, A. (1995) Life events and other possible psychosocial risk factors for episodes of schizophrenia and major depression: a case-control study. In Mazure, C.M. (ed.) *Does Stress Cause Psychiatric Illness?* Washington, DC: American Psychiatric Press.

Done, J., Sacker, A., Crow, T.J. (1994) Childhood antecedents of schizophrenia and affective illness: intellectual performance at ages 7 and 11. *Schizophrenia Research* **11**: 96–97.

Duggan, C.F., Lee, A.S., Murray, R.M. (1990) Does personality predict long-term outcome in depression? *British Journal of Psychiatry* **157**: 19–24.

Elkis, H., Friedman, L., Wise, A., Meltzer, H. (1995) Meta-analyses of studies of ventricular enlargement and cortical sulcal prominence in mood disorders. *Archives of General Psychiatry* **52**: 735–746.

Engelhardt, D.M., Rosen, B., Feldman, J., Engelhardt, J.A.Z. (1982) A 15 year follow up of 646 schizophrenic outpatients. *Schizophrenia Bulletin* **8**: 493–503.

Fowler, R.C. (1978) Remitting schizophrenia as a variant of affective disorder. *Schizophrenia Bulletin* **4**: 68–77.

Fowler, R.C., McCabe, M., Cadoret, R., Winokur, G. (1972) The validity of good prognosis schizophrenia. *Archives of General Psychiatry* **26**: 182–186.

Fuller, R.G. (1930) Expectation of hospital life and outcome for mental patients on first admission. *Psychiatric Quarterly* **4**: 295–323.

Garmezy, N. (1970) Process and reactive schizophrenia: some conceptional issues. *Schizophrenia Bulletin* **1**: 30–74.

Gift, T.E., Strauss, J.S., Kokes, R.F., Harder, D.W., Ritzler, B.A. (1980) Schizophrenia: affect and outcome. *American Journal of Psychiatry* **137**: 580–585.

Goldberg, T.E., Gold, J.M., Fuller-Torrey, E.F., Weinberger, D.R. (1995) Lack of sex differences in the neuropsychological performance of patients with schizophrenia. *American Journal of Psychiatry* **152**: 883–888.

Goldstein, J.M. (1988) Sex differences in the course of schizophrenia. *American Journal of Psychiatry* **145**: 684–689.

Grossman, L., Harrow, M., Goldberg, J., Fichtner, C. (1991) Outcome of schizoaffective disorder at two long-term follow-ups: comparisons with outcome of schizophrenia and affective disorders. *American Journal of Psychiatry* **148**: 1359–1365.

Haas, G.L., Glick, I.D., Clarkin, J.F., Spencer, J.H., Lewis, A.B. (1990) Sex and schizophrenia outcome: a clinical trial of an inpatient family intervention. *Schizophrenial Bulletin* **16**: 277–292.

Harder, D., Gift, T.E., Strauss, J.S., Ritzler, B.A., Kokes, R.F. (1981) Life events and two-year outcome in schizophrenia. *Journal of Consulting and Clinical Psychology* **49**: 619–626.

Harder, D., Greenwald, D., Ritzler, B. et al. (1990) Prediction of outcome among adult psychiatric first-admissions. *Journal of Clinical Psychology* **46**: 119–129.

Harding, C.M. (1988) Course types in schizophrenia: an analysis of European and American studies. *Schizophrenia Bulletin* **14**: 633–642.

Harding, C.M. (1994) An examination of the complexities in the measurement of recovery in severe psychiatric disorders. In Ancill, R. (ed.) *Schizophrenia. Exploring the Spectrum of Psychosis*, pp. 153–170. New York: John Wiley.

Harding, C.M., Brooks, G.W., Ashikaga, T., Strauss, J., Breier, A. (1987) The Vermont longitudinal study of persons with severe mental illness, I: methodology, study sample and overall status 32 years later. *American Journal of Psychiatry* **144**: 718–726.

Harrison, G., Owens, D., Holton, A. et al (1988) A prospective study of severe mental disorder in Afro-Caribbean patients. *Psychological Medicine* **18**: 643–657.

Harrow, M., Grossman, L. (1984) Outcome in the schizoaffective disorders: a critical review and reevaluation of the literature. *Schizophrenia Bulletin* **10**: 85–108.

Harvey, I., Williams, M., McGuffin, P., Toone, B. (1990a) The functional psychoses in Afro-Caribbeans. *British Journal of Psychiatry* **157**: 515–522.

Harvey, I., McGuffin, P., Williams, M., Toone, B. (1990b) The ventricle–brain ratio (VBR) in functional psychoses: an admixture analysis. *Psychiatry Research: Neuroimaging* **35**: 61–69.

Hegarty, J.D., Baldessarini, R., Tohen, M., Waternaux, C., Oepen, G. (1994) One hundred years of schizophrenia: a meta-analysis of the outcome literature. *American Journal of Psychiatry* **151**: 1409–1416.

Huber, G., Gross, G., Schüttler, R., Linz, M. (1980) Longitudinal studies of schizophrenic patients. *Schizophrenia Bulletin* **6**: 592–605.

Jablensky, A., Sartorius, N., Ernberg, G. et al (1992) Schizophrenia: manifestations, incidence and course in different culture. A World Health Organization ten-country study. *Psychological Medicine* **20** (Suppl.): 1–97.

Johanson, E.A. (1958) A study of schizophrenia in the male. *Acta Psychiatrica Scandinavica* **125** (Suppl.): 1–56.

Johnstone, E.C., Crow, T.J., Frith, C.D. et al (1976) Cerebral ventricle size and cognitive impairment in chronic schizophrenia. *Lancet* ii: 924–926.

Johnstone, E.C., Owens, D.G.C., Bydder, G.M. et al. (1989) The spectrum of structural brain changes in schizophrenia: age of onset as a predictor of cognitive and clinical impairments and their cerebral correlates. *Psychological Medicine* **19**: 91–103.

Johnstone, E.C., MacMillan, J.F., Frith, C.D., Benn, D.K., Crow, T.J. (1990) Further investigation of the predictors of outcome following first schizophrenic episodes. *British Journal of Psychiatry* **157**: 182–189.

Johnstone, E.C., Frith, C., Crow, T. et al. (1992) The Northwick Park 'functional' psychosis study: diagnosis and outcome. *Psychological Medicine* **22**: 331–346.

Jones, P., Rodgers, B., Murray, R., Marmot, M. (1994a) Child developmental risk factors for adult schizophrenia in the British 1946 birth cohort. *Lancet* **344**: 1398–1402.

Jones, P., Harvey, I., Lewis, S. et al. (1994b) Cerebral ventricle dimensions as risk factors for the functional psychoses. *Psychological Medicine* **24**: 995–1011.

Kane, J.M., Rifkin, A., Quitkin, F., Nayak, D., Ramos-Lorenzi, J. (1982) Fluphenazine vs. placebo in patients with remitted, acute first episode schizophrenia. *Archives of General Psychiatry* **39**: 70–73.

Kasanin, J. (1933) The acute schizoaffective psychoses. *American Journal of Psychiatry* **90**: 97–126.

Kavanagh, D.J. (1992a) Recent developments in expressed emotions and schizophrenia. *British Journal of Psychiatry* **160**: 601–620.

Kavanagh, D.J. (1992b) Interventions for families and social networks. In Kavanagh, D.J. (ed.) *Schizophrenia: An Overview and Practical Handbook* London: Chapman and Hall.

Keefe, R.S.E., Mohs, R.C., Losonczy, M.F. et al. (1987) Characteristics of very poor outcome schizophrenia. *American Journal of Psychiatry* **144**: 889–895.

Keller, M.B., Lavori, P.W., Endicott, J., Coryell, W., Klerman, G.L. (1983) 'Double depression': two-year follow-up. *American Journal of Psychiatry* **140**: 689–694.

Kendell, R.E. (1989) Clinical validity. *Psychological Medicine* **19**: 45–55.

Kendell, R.E. (1993) Diagnosis and classification. In Kendell, R.E., Zealley A.K. (eds) *Companion to Psychiatric Studies*, 5th edn, pp. 277–295. London: Churchill Livingstone.

Kendell, R.E., Brockington, I.F. (1980) The identification of disease entities and the relationship between schizophrenic and affective psychoses. *British Journal of Psychiatry* **137**: 324–331.

Kendler, K.S., Tsuang, M.T. (1988) Outcome and familial psychopathology in schizophrenia. *Archives of General Psychiatry* **45**: 338–346.

Kendler, K.S., Walsh, D. (1995) Sex and schizophrenia. Results of an epidemiologically-based family study. *British Journal of Psychiatry* **167**: 184–192.

Kendler, K.S., McGuire, M., Gruenberg, A.M. et al (1993) The Roscommon family study. I. Methods, diagnosis of probands, and risk of schizophrenia in relatives. *Archives of General Psychiatry* **50**: 527–540.

Kenniston, K., Boltex, S., Almond, R. (1971) Multiple criteria of treatment outcome. *Journal of Psychiatry Research* **8**: 107.

King, M., Coker, E., Leavey, G., Hoare, A., Johnson-Sabine, E. (1994) Incidence of psychotic illness in London: a comparison of ethnic groups. *British Medical Journal* **309**: 1115–1119.

Kitamura, T., Okazaki, Y., Fujinawa, A., Yoshino, M., Kasahara, Y. (1995) Symptoms of psychoses. A factor analytic study. *British Journal of Psychiatry* **166**: 236–240.

Lee, A., Murray, R. (1988) The long term outcome of Maudsley depressives. *British Journal of Psychiatry* **153**: 741–751.

Lehrman, N.S. (1960) A state hospital population five years after admission: a yardstick for further evaluative comparison of follow up studies. *Psychiatric Quarterly* **34**: 658–681.

Lewis, S. (1992) Sex and schizophrenia: vive la différence. *British Journal of Psychiatry* **161**: 445–450.

Liddle, P., Friston, K., Frith, C. et al. (1992) Patterns of cerebral blood flow in schizophrenia. *British Journal of Psychiatry* **160**: 179–186.

Lieberman, J., Jody, D., Geisler, S. et al. (1989) Treatment outcome of first episode schizophrenia. *Psychopharmacology Bulletin* **25**: 92–96.

Lieberman, J.A., Alvir, J., Woerner, M. et al. (1992) Prospective study of psychobiology in first-episode schizophrenia at Hillside hospital. *Schizophrenia Bulletin* **18**: 351–371.

Lieberman, J., Jody, D., Geisler, S. et al (1993) Time course and biologic correlates of treatment response in first episode schizophrenia. *Archives of General Psychiatry* **50**: 369–376.

Lin, K., Kleinman, A.M. (1988) Psychopathology and clinical course: a cross-cultural perspective. *Schizophrenia Bulletin* **14**: 555–567.

Linszen, D.H., Dingemans, P.M., Lenior, M.E. (1994) Cannabis abuse and the course of recent-onset schizophrenic disorders. *Archives of General Psychiatry* **51**: 273–279.

Littlewood, R., Lipsedge, M. (1981) Acute psychotic reactions in Caribbean-born patients. *Psychological Medicine* **11**: 303–318.

Locke, B.Z. (1962) Outcome of first hospitalisation of patients with schizophrenia. *Public Health Reports* **77**: 801–805.

Loebel, A.D., Lieberman, J.A., Alvir, J.M.J. et al. (1992) Duration of psychosis and outcome in first-episode schizophrenia. *American Journal of Psychiatry* **149**: 1183–1188.

Maj, M., Perris, C. (1990) Patterns of course in patients with a cross-sectional diagnosis of schizoaffective disorder. *Journal of Affective Disorders* **20**: 71–77.

Malla, A., Cortese, L., Shaw, T.S., Ginsberg, B. (1990) Life events and relapse in schizophrenia: a one year prospective study. *Social Psychiatry and Psychiatric Epidemiology* **25**: 221–224.

Malzberg, B. (1953) Rates of discharge and rates of mortality among first admissions to the New York civil state hospitals (3rd paper). *Mental Hygiene* **37**: 619–654.

Marengo, J. (1994) Classifying the courses of schizophrenia. *Schizophrenia Bulletin* **20**: 519–535.

Marneros, A., Deister, A., Rhode, A. et al. (1988) Long-term course of schizoaffective disorder. *European Archives of Psychiatry and Neurological Sciences* **237**: 264–275.

Marneros, A., Deister, A., Rohde, A., Steinmeyer, E.M., Jünemann, H. (1989) Long-term outcome of schizoaffective and schizophrenic disorders: a comparative study. *European Archives of Psychiatry and Neurological Sciences* **238**: 118–125.

Marneros, A., Deister, A., Rohde, A. (1990) Psychopathological and social status of patients with affective, schizophrenic and schizoaffective disorders after long-term course. *Acta Psychiatrica Scandinavica* **82**: 352–358.

May, P.R., Tuma, H., Dixon, W.J. (1981) Schizophrenia. A follow-up study of the results of five forms of treatment. *Archives of General Psychiatry* **38**: 776–784.

Mayerhoff, D.I., Loebel, A.D., Alvir, J. (1994) The deficit state in first-episode schizophrenia. *American Journal of Psychiatry* **151**: 1417–1422.

McGlashan, T. (1984) The Chestnut Lodge follow-up study I. Follow-up methodology and study sample. *Archives of General Psychiatry* **41**: 573–585.

McGlashan, T. (1986a) Predictors of shorter-, medium- and longer-term outcome in schizophrenia. *American Journal of Psychiatry* **143**: 50–55.

McGlashan, T.H. (1986b) The prediction of outcome in chronic schizophrenia. IV. The Chestnut Lodge follow-up study. *Archives of General Psychiatry* **43**: 167–176.

McGlashan, T.H. (1988) A selective review of recent North American long-term follow-up studies of schizophrenia. *Schizophrenia Bulletin* **14**: 515–541.

McGlashan, T.H., Bardenstein, K.K. (1990) Sex differences in affective, schizoaffective, and schizophrenic disorders. *Schizophrenia Bulletin* **16**: 319–329.

McGlashan, T.H., Carpenter, W., Bartko, J. (1988) Issues of design and methodology in long-term follow-up studies. *Schizophrenia Bulletin* **14**: 569–574.

McGovern, D., Hemmings, P., Cope, R., Lowerson, A. (1994) Long-term follow-up of young Afro-Caribbean Britons and white Britons with a first admission diagnosis of schizophrenia. *Social Psychiatry and Psychiatric Epidemiology* **29**: 8–19.

McGuire, P.K., Shah, G.M., Murray, R.M. (1993) Increased blood flow in Broca's area during auditory hallucinations in schizophrenia. *Lancet* **ii**: 703–706.

McKenna, A.M., Paredes, A. (1992) Dual diagnosis: empirical and developmental-humanistic approaches. In Galanter, M. (ed.) *Recent Developments in Alcoholism*, pp. 231–239. New York: Plenum Press.

McKenzie, K., van Os, J., Fahy, T. et al. (1995) Evidence for good prognosis psychosis among UK Afro-Caribbeans. *British Medical Journal* **311**: 1325–1328.

Müller, V. (1951) Katamnestiche Erhebungen über den Spontanverlauf der Schizophrenie. *Monatsschrift für Psychiatrie-Neurologie* **122**: 257–276.

Murphy, H.B.M. (1968) Cultural factors in the genesis of schizophrenia. In Rosenthal, D., Kety, S.S. (eds) *The Transmission of Schizophrenia*, pp. 137–153. Oxford: Pergamon Press.

Murray, R.M., O'Callaghan, E. (1991) The congenital and adult-onset psychoses: Kraepelin lost, Kraepelin found. In Kerr A., McClelland, H. (eds) *Concepts of Mental Disorder, a Continuing Debate*, pp. 48–65. London: Gaskell.

Murray, R.M., Lewis, S.W., Owen, M.J. et al (1988) The neurodevelopmental origins of dementia praecox. In Bebbington, P., McGuffin, P. (eds) *Schizophrenia: the Major Issues*, pp. 90–107. Oxford: Heinemann.

Myers, J.K., Bean, L.L. (1968) *A Decade Later: a Follow-Up of Social Class and Mental Illness*. New York: Wiley.

Navarro, F., van Os, J., Jones, P., Murray, R.M. (1996) Explaining sex differences in outcome in the functional psychoses. *Schizophrenia Research* **21**: 161–170.

O'Connell, Mayo, J., Flatow, L., Cuthbertson, B., O'Brien, B.E. (1991) Outcome of bipolar disorder on long-term treatment with lithium. *British Journal of Psychiatry* **159**: 123–129.

Paykell, E. (1978) Contribution of life events to causation to psychiatric illness. *Psychological Medicine* **8**: 245–253.

Pepper, B., Kirschner, M.C., Ryglewicz, H. (1981) The young chronic patient: overview of a population. *Hospital and Community Psychiatry* **32**: 463–467.

Peterson, D.B., Olsen, G.W. (1964) First admitted schizophrenics in drug era. *Archives of General Psychiatry* **11**: 137–144.

Phillips, L. (1953) Case history data and prognosis in schizophrenia. *Journal of Nervous and Mental Disease* **117**: 515–525.

Pogue-Geile, M.F. (1989) The prognostic significance of negative symptoms in schizophrenia. *British Journal of Psychiatry* **7** (Suppl.): 123–127.

Rabiner, C., Wegner, J., Kane, J. (1986) Outcome study of first episode psychosis, I: relapse rate after 1 year. *American Journal of Psychiatry* **143**: 1155–1158.

Regier, D.A., Myers, J.K., Kramer, M. et al. (1984) The NIMH epidemiologic catchment area program: historical context, major objectives and study population characteristics. *Archives of General Psychiatry* **41**: 934–941.

Regier, D.A., Farmer, M.E., Rae, D.S. et al. (1990) Comorbidity of mental disorders with alcohol and other drug abuse. Results from the Epidemiologic Catchment Area (ECA) Study. *Journal of the American Medical Association* **264**: 2511–2518.

Robins, E., Guze, S.B. (1970) Establishment of diagnostic validity in psychiatric illness: its application to schizophrenia. *American Journal of Psychiatry* **126**: 983–987.

Rogers, B. (1990) Behaviour and personality in childhood as predictors of adult psychiatric disorder. *Journal of Child Psychology and Psychiatry* **3**: 393–414.

Rosanoff, A.J. (1914) A statistical study of prognosis in insanity. *Journal of the American Medical Association* **62**: 3–6.

Roy, A. (1982) Suicide in chronic schizophrenia. *British Journal of Psychiatry* **141**: 171–177.

Roy, M.A., Crowe, R.R. (1994) Validity of the familial and sporadic subtypes of schizophrenia. *American Journal of Psychiatry* **151**: 805–814.

Rupp, C., Fletcher, E.K. (1940) A five to ten year follow up study of 641 schizophrenic cases. *American Journal of Psychiatry* **96**: 877–888.

Safer, D.J. (1987) Substance abuse by young adult chronic patients. *Hospital and Community Psychiatry* **38**: 511–514.

Salokangas, R.K.R. (1983) Prognostic implications of the sex of schizophrenic patients. *British Journal of Psychiatry* **142**: 145–151.

Salokangas, R.K.R., Stengard, E. (1990) Sex and short-term outcome in schizophrenia. *Schizophrenia Research* **13**: 333–345.

Samson, J., Simpson, J., Tsuang, M. (1988) Outcome studies of schizoaffective disorders. *Schizophrenia Bulletin* **14**: 543–554.

Sartorius, N., Jablensky, A., Korten, A. et al. (1986) Early manifestations and first-contact incidence of schizophrenia in different cultures: a preliminary report on the initial evaluation phase of the WHO Collaborative study on Determinants of Outcome of Severe Mental Disorders. *Psychological Medicine* **16**: 909–928.

Sautter, F.J., McDermott, B.E. (1994) The short-term course of familial and nonfamilial schizophrenic spectrum disorder. *Journal of Psychiatry Research* **28**: 97–106.

Schneider, K. (1925) Wesen und Erfassung des Schizophrenen. *Zeitschrift für die gesamte Neurologie und Psychiatrie* **99**: 542–547.

Schwartz, D.A., Weiss, A.T., Miner, J.M. (1972) Community psychiatry and emergency service. *American Journal of Psychiatry* **129**: 710–714.

Scott, J., Eccleston, D., Boys, R. (1992) Can we predict the persistence of depression? *British Journal of Psychiatry* **161**: 633–637.

Scottish Schizophrenia Research Group (1989) The Scottish first episode schizophrenia study: V. Two year follow up. *Acta Psychiatrica Scandinavica* 80: 597–602.

Seeman, M.V. (1986) Current outcome in schizophrenia: women vs men. *Acta Psychiatrica Scandinavica* **73**: 609–617.

Selten, J.P., Sijben, N. (1994) First admission rates for schizophrenia in immigrants to the Netherlands. The Dutch National Register. *Social Psychiatry and Psychiatric Epidemiology* **29**: 71–77.

Serban, G. (1975) Relationship of mental status, functioning, and stress to readmission of schizophrenics. *British Journal of Social and Clinical Psychology* **14**: 291–301.

Shaner, A., Khalsa, M.E. Roberts, L. et al. (1993) Unrecognized cocaine use among schizophrenic patients. *American Journal of Psychiatry* **150**: 758–762.

Shepherd, M. (1957) *A Study of the Major Psychoses in an English County.* London: Oxford University Press.

Shepherd, M., Watt, D., Falloon, I. et al (1989) The natural history of schizophrenia: a five year follow-up study of outcome and prediction in a representative sample of schizophrenics. *Psychological Medicine* Monograph Suppl. 15.

Shields, J. (1980) Genetics and mental development. In Rutter, M. (ed.) *Scientific Foundations of Developmental Psychiatry.* London: Heinemann Medical.

Stephens, J. (1978) Longterm prognosis and follow up in schizophrenia. *Schizophrenia Bulletin* **4**: 25–47.

Stephens, J., Astrup, C. (1963) Prognosis in 'process' and 'non-process' schizophrenia. *American Journal of Psychiatry* **119**: 945–953.

Stephens, J., Astrup, C., Mangrum, J.C. (1966) Prognostic factors in recovered and deteriorating schizophrenics. *American Journal of Psychiatry* **122**: 1116–1121.

Stoffelmayr, B., Dillavou, D., Hunter, J. (1983) Premorbid functioning and outcome in schizophrenia: a cumulative analysis. *Journal of Consulting and Clinical Psychology* **51**: 338–352.

Stoffelmeyer, B.E., Benijhek, L.A. (1989) Substance abuse prognosis with an additional psychiatric diagnosis: understanding of the relationship. *Journal of Psychoactive Drugs* **21**: 145–152.

Strakowski, S.M., Tohen, M., Stoll, A.L. et al. (1993) Comorbidity in psychosis at first hospitalization. *American Journal of Psychiatry* **150**: 752–757.

Strauss, J.S., Carpenter, W. (1977) Prediction of outcome in schizophrenia III: five-year outcome and its predictors. *Archives of General Psychiatry* **34**: 159–163.

Strauss, J.S., Carpenter, W. (1978) The prognosis of schizophrenia: rationale for a multidimensional concept. *Schizophrenia Bulletin* **4**: 1978, 56–67.

Sugarman, P.A. (1992) Outcome of schizophrenia in the Afro-Caribbean community. *Social Psychiatry and Psychiatric Epidemiology* **27**: 102–105.

Susser, E., Wanderling, J. (1994) Epidemiology of non-affective acute remitting psychosis vs schizophrenia. *Archives of General Psychiatry* **51**: 294–301.

Taylor, M. (1992) Are schizophrenia and affective disorder related? A selective literature review. *American Journal of Psychiatry* **149**: 22–32.

Tsuang, M.T., Dempsey, G.M. (1979) Long term outcome of major psychoses II. Schizoaffective disorder, compared with schizophrenia, affective disorders, and a surgical control group. *Archives of General Psychiatry* **36**: 1302–1304.

Tsuang, M.T., Winokur, G. (1974) Criteria for subtyping schizophrenia. Clinical differentiation of hebephrenic and paranoid schizophrenia. *Archives of General Psychiatry* **31**: 43–47.

Tsuang, M.T., Dempsey, G.M., Rauscher, F. (1976) A study of 'atypical schizophrenia'. *Archives of General Psychiatry* **33**: 1157–1160.

Tsuang, M.T., Woolson, R.F., Fleming, J.A. (1979) Long term outcome of major psychoses. *Archives of General Psychiatry* **36**: 1295–1301.

Tsuang, M.T., Woolson, R., Winokur, G., Crowe, R. (1981) Stability of psychiatric diagnosis: schizophrenia and affective disorders followed up over a 30- to 40-year period. *Archives of General Psychiatry* **38**: 535–539.

Turner, W.M., Tsuang, M.T. (1990) Impact of substance abuse on the course and outcome of schizophrenia. *Schizophrenia Bulletin* **16**: 87–95.

Vaillant, G.E. (1964) Prospective prediction of schizophrenic remission. *Archives of General Psychiatry* **11**: 509–518.

Vaillant, G.E. (1978) Prognosis and the course of schizophrenia. *Schizophrenia Bulletin* **4**: 20-24.

van Os, J. (1995) *(Genetic) Epidemiology as a Tool to Examine Risk Factors for Onset and Persistence of Illness in the Functional Psychoses.* Maastricht: Maastricht University Press.

van Os, J., Fahy, T., Bebbington, P. et al. (1994) The influence of life events on the subsequent course of psychotic illness. *Psychological Medicine* **24**: 503–513.

van Os, J., Fahy, T., Jones, P. et al. (1995) Increased intra-cerebral CSF spaces predict unemployment and negative symptoms in psychotic illness: a prospective study. *British Journal of Psychiatry* **166**: 150–159.

van Os, J., Fahy, T., Jones, P. et al. (1996a) Psychopathological syndromes in the functional psychoses: associations with course and outcome. *Psychological Medicine* **26**: 161–176.

van Os, J., Jones, P. Lewis, G., Murray, R.M. (1996b) Evidence for similar developmental precursors of chronic affective illness and schizophrenia in a general population birth cohort. *Archives of General Psychiatry* (in press).

van Os, J., Castle, D., Takei, N., Der, G., Murray, R. (1996c) Schizophrenia in ethnic minorities: clarification from the 1991 census. *Psychological Medicine* **26**: 203–208.

van Os, J., Takei, N., Castle, D., Murray, R.M. (1996d) The incidence of mania: time trends in relation to gender and ethnic group. *Social Psychiatry and Psychiatric Epidemiology* **31**: 129–136.

Vaughn, C.E., Leff, J.P. (1976) The influence of family and social factors on the course of psychiatric illness. *British Journal of Psychiatry* **129**: 125–137.

Ventura, J., Nuechterlein, K.H., Lukoff, D., Hardisty, J.P. (1989) A prospective study of stressful life events and schizophrenic relapse. *Journal of Abnormal Psychology* **98**: 407–411.

Verdoux, H., van Os, J., Sham, P. et al. (1995) Does familiality predispose to both emergence and persistence of psychosis? A prospective study. *British Journal of Psychiatry* **163**: 620–626.

Vita, A., Dieci, M., Giobbio, G.M. et al. (1991) CT scan abnormalities and outcome of chronic schizophrenia. *American Journal of Psychiatry* **148**: 1577–1579.

Walker, E.F., Lewine, R.J. (1993) Sampling biases in studies of sex and schizophrenia. *Schizophrenia Bulletin* **19**: 1–7.

Weinberger, D., DeLisi, L., Perman, G. et al. (1982) Computed tomography in schizophreniform disorder and other acute psychiatric disorders. *Archives of General Psychiatry* **39**: 778–783.

Werry, J.S., McClellan, J.M., Chard, L. (1991) Childhood and adolescent schizophrenic, bipolar, and schizoaffective disorders: a clinical and outcome study. *Journal of the American Academy of Child and Adolescent Psychiatry* **30**: 457–465.

Westermeyer, J.F., Harrow, M. (1984) Prognosis and outcome using broad (DSM-II) and narrow (DSM-III) concepts of schizophrenia. *Schizophrenia Bulletin* **10**: 624–637.

Westermeyer, J.F., Harrow, M. (1988) Course and outcome in schizophrenia. In Tsuang M.T., Simpson, J.C. (eds) *Handbook of Schizophrenia*, Rotterdam: Elsevier.

WHO (1979) *Schizophrenia: An International Follow-up Study*. Chichester: Wiley.

WHO (1992) *WHO coordinated Multi-center Study on the Course and Outcome of Schizophrenia*. Geneva: WHO.

Wing, J.K. (1966) Five year outcome in early schizophrenia. *Proceedings of the Royal Society of Medicine* **59**: 17–18.

Williams, A.O., Reveley, M.A., Kolakowska, T., Ardern, M., Mandelbrote, B. (1985) Schizophrenia with good and poor outcome. II. Cerebral ventricular size and its clinical significance. *British Journal of Psychiatry* **146**: 239–246.

Winokur, G., Coryell, W., Keller, M., Endicott, J., Akiskal, H. (1993) A prospective follow-up study of patients with bioplar and primary unipolar affective disorder. *Archives of General Psychiatry* **50**: 457–465.

Wyatt, R.J. (1991) Neuroleptics and the natural course of schizophrenia. *Schizophrenia Bulletin* **17**: 325–351.

7

Neuropathology of Schizophrenia: 1871–1996

Janice R. Stevens

Neuropathological studies of schizophrenia have a long history and still search, so far in vain, for pathognomonic diagnostic features that are either unique to, or are found in, a majority of cases. Atrophic changes in cortex (Alzheimer, 1913; Kraepelin, 1919) and increased ventricular size (Hecker, 1871; Southard, 1915) observed at post mortem in brains of patients diagnosed as dementia praecox were the most common findings reported by neuropathologists at the turn of the last century, and still are the most frequently cited pathology. Unfortunately, such changes are not limited to schizophrenia, nor are they shown by brains of all individuals who have been diagnosed with schizophrenia.

By 1952, when many of the world's leading pathologists gathered at the First International Congress of Neuropathology in Rome, more than 250 articles concerning the neuropathology of schizophrenia (dementia praecox) had already been published. But there was little consensus of opinion among the gathered experts. Although a number of European speakers at the Congress reported cortical atrophy, change in size or appearance of neurones in the cortex, basal ganglia, hypothalamus and basal forebrain of brains from schizophrenic patients, quantitative studies were few, and American and British pathologists remained sceptical that changes reported were more than agonal or post mortem in origin. Interest in the neuropathology of this illness then waned until the introduction of cerebral imaging, which led to new interest in the pathology by psychiatrists, anatomists and pathologists.

In the neuropathology laboratory, new vistas have also opened with the use of histochemical, immunoreactive and molecular methods for identifying specific structural, biochemical and functional disturbances in the brains of patients diagnosed with schizophrenia during life. Strict diagnostic criteria introduced by DSM III-R, IV and ICD-10 have led to study of patient material that is more uniform than in previous times, but this advantage may be offset by the fact that very few cases are now available for post-mortem examination that have never received neuroleptics. These drugs may alter the primary pathology and especially the quantitative studies of ultrastructure, neurotransmitters, enzymes, receptors, and expression of their gene precursors. Parallel studies in experimental animals may solve some of these problems, although rats and humans are not always similar in these domains.

The neuropathologic studies of schizophrenia can conveniently be analysed as follows:

1. Weight and volume.
2. Cerebral ventricles.
3. Cerebral cortex.
4. Corpus callosum and cerebral asymmetry.
5. Basal ganglia.
6. Limbic system: amygdala, hippocampus, cingulate gyrus and hypothalamus.
7. Thalamus.
8. Brainstem.
9. Ultrastructure (electron microscopic studies).
10. The question of gliosis.

WEIGHT AND VOLUME

One of the first psychiatrists to report the weights from a large series of brains from dementia praecox patients was Southard (1914, 1915), pathologist to the State Board of Insanity in Massachussetts, psychiatrist at Danvers State Hospital and Bullard Professor of Neuropathology at Harvard Medical School. Southard reported that the brain weights of patients with severe, chronic dementia praecox were generally equal to or only slightly less than the weights of age matched control brains, and that brain weight was not related to duration or age of onset of the illness. The normal brain weight probably reflected the fact that brains were weighed immediately following removal from the skull and still contained ventricular fluid. So, although Southard reported ventricular enlargement in nearly 40% of the brains examined, it is likely that the weight lost in brain tissue was made up in ventricular cereprospinal fluid (CSF). Johnstone et al. (1994) also reported a small but significant reduction in fixed (but not fresh) brain weight and length of schizophrenic brains compared to age matched controls. Heckers et al. (1991a), however, found no decrease in weight of schizophrenic brains compared to controls.

With respect to volume, reports from brain-imaging studies are also inconsistent, some indicating that brain volume of patients with schizophrenia is normal (Pearlson et al., 1991), or slightly diminished (Zipursky et al., 1994; Flaum et al., 1995). The generally normal brain weight or volume may explain why the size of the skull, which depends on growth of the brain, is not diminished in most schizophrenic patients (Grove et al., 1991) (but see also McNeil et al. (1993) who reported that at birth a significant percentage of future female schizophrenics had a smaller cranial diameter at birth than matched controls). Unless the defects in cerebral morphology of schizophrenia do not involve significant loss of brain substance, the normal skull size and cranial volume of a majority of adults with schizophrenia argue against a major disturbance in brain growth as a common cause of the illness. Alternatively, an early partial obstruction in the CSF pathway could lead to ventricular enlargement, but should increase head size unless there has been compensatory loss of brain tissue. The fact that head size and brain volume are generally normal in adults with schizophrenia suggests that a significant decrease in size of cerebral structures, when present, may represent tissue loss or atrophy, rather than an early developmental anomaly.

CEREBRAL VENTRICLES

Among the earliest published reports of increased ventricular size in schizophrenia were those of Southard (1914, 1915), who reported internal hydrocephalus in nine of 25 autopsied cases of dementia praecox that had been carefully chosen to exclude secondary pathology such as arteriosclerosis, syphilis, or tuberculosis of the central nervous system.

Englargement of the ventricles was more prominent posteriorally than anteriorally, and was most frequent in patients with a diagnosis of catatonia. Ventricular enlargement was also clearly described in a significant number of patients with schizophrenia studied with pneumoencephalography (Jakobi and Winkler, 1927). It seems remarkable now that these important findings had so little influence on psychiatric thought until nearly 50 years later when Johnstone et al. (1976) demonstrated the same finding in a significant number of schizophrenic patients by computed tomography (CT). As CT and magnetic resonance imaging (MRI) became increasingly available, an avalanche of neuroimaging studies followed, which, with a few exceptions usually involving young patients early in their disease, have shown mild to moderate increase in size of the lateral ventricles, the inferior (temporal) horns and the third ventricle (but not the fourth) in 15–20% of patients with schizophrenia compared with sex and age-matched controls. Daniel et al. (1991) pointed out that although a ventricular/brain ratio (VBR) that exceeds the mean of normals by two standard deviations or more was found in only about 20% of schizophrenic patients, the distribution of VBRs is not bimodal but demonstrates a shift upward of the entire cohort, which does not suggest two kinds of schizophrenia, those with and those without ventriculomegaly. When VBRs of monozygotic twins discordant for schizophrenia were compared by CT or MRI, the VBR was generally measurably larger in the affected twins (Reveley et al., 1982; Suddath et al., 1989).

When present, ventricular enlargement in schizophrenia is generally bilateral and diffuse. Third ventricle size correlates strongly with size of the lateral ventricles but is proportionately larger than lateral ventricle increase (Raz and Raz, 1990) and may be found in some patients without lateral ventriculomegaly (Jernigan et al., 1991).

When did the Enlargement of the Ventricles Occur?

On the basis of early pneumoencephalographic (PEG) studies of schizophrenia in the pre-neuroleptic era, Haug (1962) concluded that in about 15% of schizophrenic patients – generally those who had a particularly malignant progressive clinical course, the ventricles enlarged over the first two years of the illness. Southard (1914) also noted that while nine of the 25 brains he examined at post mortem had enlarged ventricles, no patients whose illness was of less than five years duration had an increase in ventricular size, while more than half of patients whose illness was of longer duration had enlarged ventricles. Tanaka et al. (1981) reported significantly larger ventricles and wider sulci in schizophrenics aged 41–60 compared with a younger group (aged 21–40) and age-matched controls, and a positive correlation between third ventricle size and duration of illness. However, without successive measurement of the same cohort under the same conditions, comparison of early and late, more chronic, schizophrenics may give a false impression of progressive enlargement due to the more severe illness in chronic patients compared with patients early in the illness, a third of whom may remit.

Most recent investigations which have measured ventricular size in patients treated with modern neuroleptics, do not find an increase in lateral ventricular size changes over periods of 2–8 years between scans. This finding has been a strong factor leading to the conclusion by many investigators that the ventricular enlargement is present at the onset of the illness and does not increase further (Illowsky et al., 1988; Vita et al., 1988). However, the patients in these studies had been ill for many months to years prior to the first scan. Sequential MRIs carried out at first hospitalization and repeated 1–2 years later on the same cohort of patients also failed to find progressive increase of lateral ventricular size (De Lisi et al., 1991; DeGreef et al., 1991). Although this may suggest that ventricular enlargement predates onset of the illness, as Häfner (1993) points out, most schizophrenic patients have had symptoms for 1–2 years prior to first hospitalization. Treatment given early in the illness or between scans may change the course of pathology as well as the clinical course of the illness (Wyatt, 1991). Does the discrepancy between the progressive clinical and brain pathology reported by early physicians and the static cognitive status and unchanging ventriculomegaly found by recent investigators reflect the effect of neuroleptic treatment, or the fact that the initial imaging studies were made months or years after the first symptoms of the illness?

What is the Significance of the Enlarged Ventricles?

In 1954, more than 20 years before Crow (1980) introduced the heuristic 'positive' and 'negative' symptom dichotomy to psychiatry, Huber (1957) reported that patients with dilated cerebral ventricles had presented with more *defekt* ('negative') symptoms compared to those with smaller ventricles, who demonstrated more *productive* ('positive') signs. Huber also reported ventricles that increased in size over time in cases in which there was progressive clinical deterioration. These findings were supported by Haug (1962) who reported that 28 of his 101 cases who had an 'acute disastrous course' after falling ill in adolescence had increased ventricular volume, in contrast to patients who later recovered from a similar acute psychosis. On the other hand, Lemke (cited in Haug, 1962) repeated the pneumoencephalograms on six of Jacobi and Winkler's cases eight years later and found no evidence of progression of the internal hydrocephalus despite worsening of the clinical state. This led him to conclude that the ventricular enlargement was not evidence of progressive atrophy but was due to a congenital cerebral anomaly.

The importance of ventricular enlargement in the presence of normal skull size is that it means some brain tissue has disappeared or failed to develop. Whether the cause of that loss is degeneration or atrophy associated with, or immediately antecedent to, the onset of the illness or is due to developmental anomalies of brain growth or perinatal brain insult that predispose to development of psychosis 20–30 years later, is clearly an important question. Symmetrical, generally modest enlargement of lateral, third and temporal horns of the ventricles without significant cortical atrophy, as is most commonly reported in schizophrenia, occurs following aqueductal stenosis, encephalitis and brain injury, in many patients with epilepsy and in all the subcortical dementias. Both the older and more recent reports indicate that, in general, enlarged ventricles are less common in schizophrenics with a positive family history of the illness. This makes a purely genetic cause less likely. Enlargement of the ventricles is generally associated with more cognitive disability and a poorer prognosis for recovery. A strong correlation between third ventricle enlargement and cognitive disability was noted by Bornstein et al. (1992). De Quardo et al. (1994) noted that larger ventricles were associated with better premorbid social function and cognitive ability but greater decline in these functions at the time of imaging, a finding that may be more consistent with an atrophic than a developmental process.

The CT and MRI findings on ventricular size have been rather extensively summarized here to complement the post-mortem reports and because ventricular enlargement evident both by post-mortem examination and by brain imaging is the single most replicated neuropathologic finding in schizophrenia. However, the majority of patients with schizophrenia do not show a degree of ventricular enlargement sufficient for their CTs or MRIs to be reported as abnormal by an experienced radiographer without actual measurement and comparison to norms matched for age and gender. Furthermore, since ventricular enlargement also occurs in a large number of other cerebral disorders, both congenital and acquired, large ventricles alone are not useful in making the diagnosis of schizophrenia.

It may also be important to note that patients studied by modern imaging techniques are nearly all under treatment with, or have been previously treated with, neuroleptics. This could change the incidence of ventricular enlargement in two ways. First, neuroleptic treatment slows the course of the illness and keeps most patients out of the hospital most of the time while the earlier post-mortem and PEG studies were made on chronic patients who were often confined in mental institutions for life. If modern neuroleptic treatment actually arrests progression of the illness, the progressive ventricular enlargement reported by earlier investigators in a subset of patients may also be arrested. Secondly, recent imaging and post-mortem studies both suggest that neuroleptic treatment is associated with an increase in the size of the caudate nucleus (Heckers et al., 1991a; Jernigan et al., 1991). It is possible that neuroleptic-induced enlargement of the caudate nucleus, a structure which impinges on the lateral border of the anterior horn of the lateral ventricles, could obscure subtle progression of ventriculomegaly especially of the anterior horns. Although cortical atrophy is generally associated with ventricular enlargement in degenerative disorders such as Alzheimer's disease, in both the post-mortem and imaging studies of patients with schizophrenia, cortical atrophy and ventriculomegaly are not generally present in the same case, nor is there a strong correlation between them in series where both are measured (Raz and Raz, 1990). This fact makes it more likely that the brain tissue loss responsible for lateral ventricle enlargement is subcortical, not cortical.

Among the structures impinging on the ventricles, decrease in volume of which may contribute to ventricular enlargement, are the basal ganglia for anterior horns, thalamus for body of the ventricles, hippocampus and amygdala for inferior horns of the ventricle and medial nuclei of thalamus and hypothalamus for third ventricle. There are also important subcortical fibre bundles such as the fornix and limbic–hypothalamic pathways surrounding the third ventricle that, if atrophic or dystrophic, could contribute to enlargement of the third ventricle.

CEREBRAL CORTEX

The emphasis of both early and recent investigators on both gross and microscopic pathology of schizophrenia has been on the neocortex (Benes et al., 1986). This reflects the conviction that the highest cognitive and social functions of the individual must be represented in this most recently evolved and expanded part of the human brain and that these are most affected in schizophrenia. As with ventriculomegaly, 10–15% of patients with schizophrenia display widened sulci and narrowed gyri, most often in prefrontal or temporal areas at post-mortem examination and by cerebral imaging. However, cortical atrophy does not correlate with ventricular enlargement and is not evident upon visual inspection for the majority of brains of schizophrenic patients.

What is the Cause of Sulcal Widening and Gyral Atrophy in some Cases of Schizophrenia?

Microscopic examinations of cortex by early investigators repeatedly reported disappearance or pathologic appearance of neurones and increase of astroglia, findings suggestive of an ongoing destructive process. However, recent quantitative studies have not reported similar changes when comparisons are made with normal control brains and are conducted by observers 'blind' to the diagnosis. Decreased density of neurones in specific layers of prefrontal cortex have been reported by some investigators (Benes et al., 1986). Selemon et al. (1995) reported *increased* density of neurones, decreased neuropil, and thinning of the cortical mantle in prefrontal area 9 and area 17 (primary visual cortex) of schizophrenic patients compared to control brains. Pakkenberg (1993) found no difference in total neurone numbers in the cortex between schizophrenic patients and controls; Akbarian et al. (1993a, b) reported normal density of neurones in the frontal and temporal cortex of schizophrenics, although the percentage of cells expressing nicotinamide-adenine dinucleotide phosphate-diaphorase (NOS) was reduced. The discrepancies in findings may reflect technical differences in cell enumeration, and also the fact that pooling of brains may mix schizophrenias of different aetiologies. Recent studies using molecular probes for peptides and immunoreactivity of synaptic markers revealed decreases in mRNA for cholecystokinin (Virgo et al., 1995) and synaptophysin (Glantz and Lewis, 1993) in frontal or temporal cortex of schizophrenic brains.

CORPUS CALLOSUM AND CEREBRAL ASYMMETRY

Rosenthal and Bigelow (1972) reported increased thickness of corpus callosum of schizophrenic patients. However, several subsequent studies, including axon counts, showed either slight decreases in size of callosum or no differences from matched controls (Casanova et al., 1989). A number of investigators have reported loss of normal asymmetry of Sylvian fissure or planum temporale in individuals with schizophrenia compared with normal controls (Petty et al., 1995). Crow et al. (1989) proposed that loss of Sylvian fissure asymmetry may be linked to the gene responsible for schizophrenia. Using cerebral imaging, Bartley et al. (1993) did not find altered asymmetry of the Sylvian fissure in schizophrenic brains compared with normals, and Flaum et al. (1995) did not find loss of normal asymmetries of hemispheres, lobar or subcortical structures in schizophrenic brains. Investigations of this important question continue.

BASAL GANGLIA

It is a little curious that so few neuropathologic reports concerning caudate nucleus and putamen appear in recent studies of schizophrenia. Curious because, with the development of the dopamine hypothesis of schizophrenia (Carlsson, 1978), and the discovery that 85% of brain dopamine is contained in these two large nuclei, the focus of neurochemists turned to these regions and the adjacent nucleus accumbens, the 'striatum' for the limbic system. There are many studies indicating increased dopamine and adrenaline content or receptor numbers in the striatum and an equal number that find no such changes when brains from drug-free or drug-naive subjects are examined. As for neuropathology, an early study by Mettler (1955) described acute inflammatory changes in the striatum in cases of malignant catatonia. Bogerts et al. (1985, 1990) described a volumetric reduction in internal pallidum in two separate series of schizophrenic brains. As noted above, several recent neuroimaging studies have reported a measurable increase in volume of the striatum – a finding which has been attributed to the changes in axonal and synaptic organization that occur during treatment with neuroleptics (Heckers et al., 1991a; Jernigan et al., 1991).

Nucleus accumbens, a component of the ventral (limbic) striatum, is a site suspected for schizophrenic pathology because of its position as the dopamine-biased striatal 'filter for the limbic system' (Stevens, 1973). Histologic examination has yielded no evidence for gliosis, neuronal degeneration or other pathologic change in this nucleus. Pakkenberg (1990) however, noted that both the volume and number of neurones were decreased in nucleus accumbens in brains of schizophrenic patients. The increase in dopamine D-2 receptors found in this structure in earlier studies may have resulted from neuroleptic treatment.

LIMBIC SYSTEM: AMYGDALA, HIPPOCAMPUS, CINGULATE GYRUS AND HYPOTHALAMUS

Pierre Paul Broca (1878) is not generally given the credit he deserves for designating the ring of brain tissue that represents the free edge of the cortex on the medial surface of the hemispheres 'le grande lobe limbique'. James Papez (1937) and Paul MacLean (1949) subsequently drew attention to and demonstrated the role of the amygdala and hippocampus, the major subcortical nuclear masses of the limbic system in emotional behaviour. The trajectories of afferent and efferent axons from the amygdala and hippocampus (stria terminalis, fornix) curve around the thalamus *en route* to and from the septum, nucleus accumbens, striatum, hypothalamus, orbital and cingulate cortices. Because the significance of these limbic structures for social behaviour was not recognized until the studies of Papez and MacLean, earlier studies of the neuropathology of schizophrenia were concentrated on the neocortex.

It was not until Bogerts et al. (1985) measured and reported a decrease in size of the hippocampus, parahippocampal gyrus, and amygdala in a number of brains of schizophrenics that the focus of investigation by modern quantitative histologic and imaging techniques turned from lateral ventricles and the neocortex to include examination of limbic structures and the third ventricle. The numerous investigations of the hippocampus and parahippocampal gyrus since that time have reported a relative decrease in size and cell numbers of these and related medial temporal lobe structures in some, but by no means all schizophrenics.

MRI studies have generally confirmed that there is a decreased volume of medial temporal lobe structures bilaterally, sometimes more prominently on the left side. Although difficult to discern by inspection alone when measured on serial MRI slices, the volume of medial temporal structures (amygdala, hippocampus, parahippocampal gyrus) was smaller bilaterally in 13 of the 25 affected twins in the monozygotic twin pairs discordant for schizophrenia studied by Suddath et al. (1989).

The amygdala and hippocampus, the largest structures in the medial temporal lobe, and entorhinal cortex of the parahippocampal gyrus, the covergence site of primary sensory and association cortex on these limbic areas, are of great interest to investigators of schizophrenia because these regions subserve both emotion and memory. How remarkable it is then that these regions stand out in both neuropathologic and brain-imaging studies as uniquely, although not universally, showing a decrease in size in schizophrenia. However, in contrast to temporal lobe epilepsy, in which atrophy, congenital anomalies, neurone loss and gliosis in hippocampal formation are present in 40–50% of cases coming to autopsy, histologic studies of this region in schizophrenia reveal changes that are small and inconsistent. Even in the cases reported by Bogerts et al. (1985), although the decrease in size of the hippocampus was striking in one or two cases, the decreased size of the hippocampus, amygdala or parahippocampal gyrus was not true for every case, but emerged when measurements from all cases were pooled and averaged (see Figure 7.1).

Several investigators have reported decreased numbers of pyramidal neurones in the hippocampus in brains of schizophrenics (Falkai and Bogerts, 1986; Jeste and Lohr, 1989; Benes et al., 1991), but Heckers et al. (1991b) found no decrease in volume and a normal complement of neurones in this structure. Pyramidal cell disorientation as reported by Kovelman and Scheibel (1986) is also disputed (Benes et al., 1991; Christinson et al., 1989; Arnold et al., 1995). Next to Kovelman and Scheibel's report of neurone disorientation and the 'static' enlargement of the lateral ventricles reported by recent MRI studies, Jakob and Beckman's (1986) report of displaced alpha cells in the entorhinal cortex in schizophrenic brains is probably the most important finding that has contributed to the concept of a neurodevelopmental aetiology for schizophrenia. Although initially corroborated by Arnold et al. (1991a), this finding has not been supported by several subsequent studies (Benes et al., 1991; Casanova et al., 1992; Krimer et al., 1995). In view of the rarity in which most histologic findings are replicated in neuropathologic studies of schizophrenia, it is extremely interesting that both Arnold et al. (1995) and Roskiija et al. (1995) have reported a marked decrease in microtubule-associated protein (MAP2) expression by neurones in entorhinal cortex of schizophrenic brains. Associated with dendritic development, the significance of this finding awaits exclusion of neuroleptic effects. Reduced CCK immunoreactivity (Ferrier et al., 1983), reduced mRNA for non-NMDA glutamate receptors in the hippocampus of schizophrenic patients (Harrison et al.,

No.	AGE	AMYG	HIP	ACC	BNST	PVG	CN	PUT	STRI	EXT PALL	INT PALL	GPH	INF HORN
1	26	–		**	–		N		N				N
2	39	N	N	N	–	–		N	N	N	N		
3	44	N	N	N	–	–	N	N	N			–	N
4	19	–	–	N	–		N	N		–	–	–	–
5	59			*	N	N		N	N	N			
6	27			N			N				N		N
7	64	–	–	N	–	N	–		N	–	–	–	–
8	40	–	–	N	–	–	–	–	–	–	–	–	–
9	22	N	N	N	N		N	*	**	N	N	–	N
10	23			N			N	N	N			––	N
11	51			–	N	N	–	–	–	–	–		N
12	74	N	N	–	*	N	–	–	–	–	–		N
13	41			*	*	–	–	–	–	–	–	N	–

▓ 1 standard deviation below control mean
▓ 2 standard deviations below control mean
■ 3 standard deviations below control mean

Figure 7.1   Analysis of volume reduction in specific nuclei of brains of schizophrenic patients measured by Bogerts et al. (1985) identifies anatomic structures falling 1, 2 or 3 standard deviations *below* the mean of control brains, or in the case of inferior horn of lateral ventricle *above* control mean. N, normal; *, **, ***: 1,2,3 SDs above control mean; –, no data. AMYG: amygdala; HIP: hippocampus; ACC: nucleus accumbens; BNST: bed nucleus of stria terminalis; PVG: periventricular grey; CN: caudate nucleus; PUT: putamen; STRI: striatum; EXT PALL: external pallidum; INT PALL: internal pallidum; GPH: gyrus parahippocampus; INF HORN: inferior horn of lateral ventricle. (Adapted from Stevens, J.R. (1986) *Archives of General Psychiatry* **43**: 715–716.)

1991) and a decrease in synaptophysin mRNA in the Ammons horn and subiculum (Eastwood et al., 1995a) support other evidence of some pathologic change in this region.

The cingulate cortex, the largest single structure in the human limbic system, has received particular attention ever since the studies of Southard (1914) who described neuronal loss and satellitosis of glial cells in the cingulate cortex in patients who died with 'acute *dementia praecox*'. Benes (1993) has described decreased density of neurones without increase in glia in specific cortical layers and increased vertical axons in superficial lamina of the cingulate gyrus of schizophrenic brains. Lahti et al. (1995) reported that when the psychotomimetic NMD antagonist ketamine is given to patients with schizophrenia, their psychosis is activated and blood flow in the anterior cingulate cortex is selectively increased.

Summing up, the most frequently reported finding from the host of morphologic studies of limbic structures is that there is modest volume reduction of the parahippocampal gyrus, hippocampus or amygdala in a significant number of patients with schizophrenia compared to controls. However, although many MRI studies support this finding, neither the volume reduction nor evidence for neurone reduction in hippocampus is supported by the only attempt at replication with neuropathologic material (Heckers, 1991b). The same is unfortunately the case for the disarray of hippocampal pyramidal cells reported by Kovelman and Scheibel (1984) and for the anomalous position of alpha 1 cells in the entorhinal cortex reported by Jacob and Beckman (1986). It may be that some schizophrenics show some of these anomalies – others do not, and some normals do. Thus these interesting findings reported in the limbic system are not a sufficient or necessary cause, but may contribute to the illness in specific patients.

THALAMUS

The thalamus borders the third ventricle and body of the lateral ventricles where most of the ventricular enlargement occurs in brains of schizophrenics. As the principal way station between sensory systems and the cerebral cortex, the thalamus is a logical site to search for abnormality in a disorder in which ventricles, especially the third ventricle, are enlarged and profound disturbances in perception are common. Using an unbiased stereologic technique for estimation of neurone numbers, Pakkenberg (1990) reported a significantly decreased neurone count in dorsomedial thalamus, a finding reported many years earlier by Hempel and Treff (as cited in Blinkar and Glezer, 1968) who also reported an increase in glia in this nucleus. A recent MRI study of 102 patients with schizophrenia found a smaller thalamus bilaterally (also bilateral hippocampus, and superior temporal lobe) in schizophrenic patients compared with matched controls (Flaum et al., 1995), supporting an earlier report from this group of volume decrease in the lateral thalamus and adjacent white matter (Andreasen et al., 1994). At the medial border of thalamus bordering the third ventricle are the paraventricular nuclei, located in the area previously shown to be narrowed in schizophrenic brains by Bogerts et al. (1985). Falkai et al. (1991) reported a significant increase in astrocytes in the periventricular area of third ventricle, the periaqueductal area, and in the medial thalamic nuclei bilaterally, findings consistent with earlier reports by Stevens (1982) and Bruton et al. (1990).

BRAINSTEM

The substantia nigra and ventral tegmental area, origins of the nigrostriatal and mesolimbic–mesocortical dopamine pathways, respectively, appear normal in schizophrenic brains. As noted above, histologic examination of the brainstem demonstrated periaqueductal gliosis in a number of schizophrenic patients. Marked gliosis of midbrain tegmentum was seen in a patient with a diagnosis of childhood schizophrenia (Stevens, 1982). Periaqueductal gliosis, enlargement of the third ventricle and reduction in width of the periventricular margin involve nuclei and pathways of the 'reticular activating system', the paramedian collection of neurones, dendrites and axons that extend widely from the brainstem and medial thalamic nuclei to the cortex and are associated with attention and arousal. Disturbance of function in this system could relate to the deficits in attention and thought integration so ubiquitous in schizophrenic patients. In addition, although most modern investigators have focused on area 8 of the neocortex to explain the eye-movement disturbances in schizophrenia, the frequency and type of these disturbances also direct attention to midbrain eye-movement motor nuclei and to the superior colliculus.

ULTRASTRUCTURE ELECTRON MICROSCOPIC STUDIES

Because of the necessity for very fresh brain tissue for electron micro-scopic (EM) study, and because of the difficulty in quantitating changes observed, very few EM studies in schizophrenia are reported. In a study of biopsy material from 'a frontal gyrus' Miyakawa (1972) noted accumulation of a large amount of vesicular material in the axon–oligodendrocyte interface of myelinated fibres. More recently, Ong and Garey (1993), in a qualitative study of a single case, exam-ined a biopsy specimen from the temporal polar cortex from a schizophrenic patient, operated upon for a deep temporal tumour. They reported many unusual asymmetrical synapses with clumped synaptic vesicles, often far from the synaptic thickenings. In system-atic studies comparing ultrastructures from the caudate nucleus and frontal lobe of schizophrenic patients with normal controls, Uranova et al. (1996) reported axonal changes and enlargement of post-synaptic densities in schizophrenic patients. All schizophrenics, however, had received neuroleptic treatment, a factor which itself may change these parameters. Quantitative studies are badly needed, but suffer from the need to prepare tissues within a few hours of death and the need to control for the effect of neuroleptics on axon, dendritic and synaptic morphology.

THE QUESTION OF GLIOSIS

Gliosis, meaning increased glial cells or fibres, is a marker for previous brain injury. Soon after any brain injury, infection, haem-orrhage or infarct, astroglia enlarge and increase in numbers to initiate formation of a glial scar. Months and years after brain injury, the increase in glial cells and protein marking such damage often disappears and a dense network of glial fibrils remains in the area where neurones or axons were destroyed. Glial scarring is absent or much less evident following brain insults that occur prior to birth or following apoptosis, the programmed cell death that occurs during maturation and adult life. Gliosis is thus of considerable importance in distinguishing postnatal brain insults from prenatal abnormality or damage. In their qualitative studies of brains from patients diag-nosed with dementia praecox, both Alzheimer (1913) and Kraepelin (1919) drew attention to enlargement and proliferation of astrocytes and formation of astroglial satellites around neurones showing degenerative changes in superficial layers of the cerebral cortex. Southard (1914, 1915) also emphasized cortical sclerosis (gliosis) in acute cases of short duration. Dide (1934), Winkelman and Book (1949), Morgan and Gregory (1935) and Van der Horst (1952) all published reports of increased glial cells or their processes in the cortex, hypothalamus, hippocampus, striatum or thalamus. Nieto and Escobar (1972), using a special stain to demonstrate glia and their processes, reported widespread gliosis in subcortical structures including the brainstem, reticular formation, hypothalamus, septum, thalamus, hippocampus and periaqueductal grey – findings similar to those reported from examination with Holzer's stain for glial fibrils of brains of schizophrenic patients (Stevens, 1982). Bruetsch (1952) and Fisman (1975) reported glial nodules suggestive of a healing inflammatory process in a significant number of brains examined from patients with schizophrenia. Although Falkai et al. (1991) and Bruton et al. (1990) reported a significant increase in periventricular and periaqueductal gliosis in autopsied schizophrenic brains, most modern quantitative studies do not find increased glial cells in brains of schizophrenic patients. In his delightful autobiography, Meduna (1985) reported that one of the observations leading him to his hypothesis of a biological antagonism between epilepsy and schizophrenia was the abundant gliosis found in the hippocampus in epileptic brains and almost complete absence of gliosis in this structure in schizophrenic patients.

Recent quantitative cytologic studies reporting neuronal loss in cortex, thalamus, nucleus accumbens and hippocampus have emphasized the absence of increased glial cells in these areas. Since gliosis is a sign of previous brain injury and tissue death, these negative reports from recent investigators and the apparent stable size of the enlarged ventricles over time reported in most modern imaging studies have led many investigators to adopt a neurodevelopmental hypothesis of schizophrenia (Murray and Lewis, 1987; Weinberger, 1987).

The variability in reported gliosis over the years could reflect the fact that early and adequate neuroleptic treatment not only ameliorates the disorder but also may retard or prevent neuronal degeneration, progressive ventricular enlargement and associated gliosis. Alternatively, there may be multiple routes to schizophrenia as suggested by the recent splendid study of monozygotic twins discordant with schizophrenia (Torrey 1994). In this study, eight of 27 twin pairs (30%) had some pre- or peri-natal gestational or obstetric complication and early behaviour deviation, and another eight had antecedent head injury or infection affecting the nervous system prior to onset. A final third had neither a history of early nor later brain injury but a positive family history of schizophrenia in a close relative. Many schizophrenic twins had more than one of these potential risk factors.

If there are several routes to schizophrenia, some associated with early brain damage, some with later degeneration and gliosis and some with genetic predisposition, pooling and averaging morphologic and neuropathologic data from a large number of schizophrenic patients who develop the disorder as a result of diverse aetiologies may obscure delineation of a specific neuropathology.

SUMMARY

Summarizing the major replicated findings extracted from several hundred reports of neuropathologic and neuroimaging findings in schizophrenia, it is evident that a variable increase in ventricular size, possible small decrease in brain weight, and less often, a decrease in cortical thickness and gyral width in frontal or temporal lobes have been reported most often, but always in fewer than half of all schizophrenic brains that are studied. In other words, no universal or diagnostic brain lesion has been found. Nor is it clear whether the ventricular and cortical changes reported occur near the onset of the illness, or, as the neurodevelopmental theories propose, occur prenatally or in very early life and thus pre-date the onset of symptoms by many years.

These are disappointing, but not devastating, findings for students of schizophrenic neuropathology. Examination of brains of patients with epilepsy also show specific findings such as medial temporal sclerosis or focal congenital anomalies in only 40–50% of cases, and other evidence of cerebral insult or neoplasm in another 5–10%. Yet when special stains were employed, sprouting of granule cell glutamate axon terminals in dentate gyrus were revealed, a finding that has contributed greatly to understanding of the pathophysiology of seizure disorders (Sutula et al., 1992).

Delineation of the neuropathology of schizophrenia may also be revealed only by special techniques that identify and quantify peptides, structural proteins or molecular markers for specific proteins or receptors, and thus sort out the heterogeneity of schizophrenia. Like epilepsy, schizophrenia appears to be a symptom due to a particular response of the brain to a number of pathologic insults. Faulty pruning of synapses (Feinberg, 1982), or abnormal reinnervation secondary to disturbances in development or injury to the brain (Stevens, 1992) are possibilities. The final answers, however, still elude us.

References

Akbarian, S., Vinuela, A., Kim, J.J. et al. (1993a) Distorted distribution of nicotinamide adenine-dinucleotide phosphate-diaphorase neurons in temporal lobe of schizophrenics implies anomalous cortical development. *Archives of General Psychiatry* **50**: 178–187.

Akbarian, S., Bunney, W.E., Potkin, S.G. et al. (1993b) Altered distribution of nicotinamide-adenine-dinucleotide phosphate-diaphorase cells in frontal cortex of schizophrenia implies disturbances of cortical development. *Archives of General Psychiatry* **50**: 169–177.

Alzheimer, A. (1913) Beiträge zur pathologischen Anatomie der Dementia praecox. *Allgemeine Zeitschift für Psychiatrie und gerichtliche Medizin* **70**: 810–812.

Andreasen, N.C., Arndt, S., Swayze II, V. et al. (1994) Thalamic abnormalities in schizophrenia visualized through magnetic resonance image averaging. *Science* **266**: 294–298.

Arnold, S.E., Hyman, B.T., Van Hoesen, G.W., Damasio, A.R. (1991a) Some cytoarchitectural abnormalities of the entorhinal cortex in schizophrenia. *Archives of General Psychiatry* **48**: 625–632.

Arnold, S.E., Lee, V.M., Gur, R.E. (1991b) Abnormal expression of two microtubule-associated proteins (MAP2 and MAP5) in specific subfields of the hippocampal formation in schizophrenia. *Proceedings of the National Academy of Sciences USA* **88**: 10850–10854.

Arnold, S.E., Franz, B.R., Gur, R.C. et al. (1995) Smaller neuron size in schizophrenia in hippocampal subfields that mediate cortical–hippocampal interactions. *American Journal of Psychiatry* **152**: 738–740.

Bartley, A.J., Jones, D.W., Torrey, E.F. et al. (1993) Sylvian fissure asymmetries in monozygotic twins: a test of laterality in schizophrenia. *Biological Psychiatry* **34**: 853–863.

Benes, F.M. (1993) Neurobiological investigations in cingulate cortex of schizophrenic brain. *Schizophrenia Bulletin* **19**: 537–549.

Benes, F.M., Davidson, J., Bird, E.D. (1986) Quantitative cytoarchitectural studies of the cerebral cortex of schizophrenics. *Archives of General Psychiatry* **43**: 31–35.

Benes, F.M., Sorensen, I., Bird, E.D. (1991) Reduced neuronal size in posterior hippocampus of schizophrenic patients. *Schizophrenia Bulletin* **17**: 597–608.

Bliakov, S.M., Glezer, I.I. (1968) *The Human Brain in Figures and Tables*. New York: Basic Books.

Bogerts, B., Meertz, E., Schonfeldt-Bausch, R. (1985) Basal ganglia and limbic system pathology in schizophrenia. A morphometric study of brain volume and shrinkage. *Archives of General Psychiatry* **42**: 784–791.

Bogerts, B., Falkai, R., Haupts, M. et al (1990) Post mortem volume measurements of limbic system and basal ganglia structures in chronic schizophrenics. Initial results from a new brain collection. *Schizophrenia Research* **3**: 295–301.

Bornstein, R.A., Schwarzkopf, S.B., Olson, S.C., Nasrallah, H.A. (1992) Third-ventricle enlargement and neuropsychological deficit in schizophrenia. *Biological Psychiatry* **31**: 954–961.

Broca, P. (1878) Anatomie comparée des circonvolutions cérébrales. Le grand lobe limbique et la scissure limbique dans le série des mammiféres. *Revue Anthropologique* **1**: 385–498.

Bruetsch, W.L. (1952) Specific structural neuropathology of the central nervous system (rheumatic, demyelinating, vasofunctional, etc.) in schizophrenia. In *Proceedings of the First International Congress of Neuropathology*, Vol. 3, pp. 629–635. Turin, Italy: Rosenberg and Sellier.

Bruton, C.J., Crow, T.J., Frith, C.D. et al. (1990) Schizophrenia and the brain: a prospective clinico-neuropathological study. *Psychological Medicine* **20**: 285–304.

Carlsson, A. (1978) Antipsychotic drugs, neurotransmitters, and schizophrenia. *American Journal of Psychiatry* **135**: 165–173.

Casanova, M.F., Zito, M., Bigelow, L.B. et al. (1989) Axonal counts of the corpus callosum of schizophrenic patients. *Journal of Neuropsychiatry and Clinical Neurosciences* **1**: 391–393.

Casanova, M.F., Zito, M., Altshuler, L. (1992) Normal nucleolar size of entorhinal cortex cells in schizophrenia (letter). *Psychiatry Research* **44**: 79–82.

Christison, G.W., Casanova, M.F., Weinberger, D.R. et al (1989) A quantitative investigation of hippocampal pyramidal cell size, shape and variability or orientation in schizophrenia. *Archives of General Psychiatry* **46**: 1027–1032.

Crow, T.J. (1980) Molecular pathology of schizophrenia: more than one disease process? *British Medical Journal* **280**: 66–68.

Crow, T.J., Ball, J., Bloom, S.R. et al. (1989) Schizophrenia as an anomaly of development of cerebral asymmetry: a postmortem study and a proposal concerning the genetic basis of the disease. *Archives of General Psychiatry* **46**: 1145–1150.

Daniel, D.G., Goldberg, T.E., Gibbons, R.D., Weinberger, D.R. (1991) Lack of a bimodal distribution of ventricular size in schizophrenia: a Gaussian mixture analysis of 1056 cases and controls. *Biological Psychiatry* **30**: 887–903.

DeGreef, G., Ashtari, M., Wu, H.W. et al (1991) Follow up MRI study in first episode schizophrenia. *Schizophrenia Research* **5**: 204–206.

DeLisi, L.E., Hoff, A.L., Schwartz, J.E. et al. (1991) Brain morphology in first-episode schizophrenic-like psychotic patients: a quantitative magnetic resonance imaging study. *Biological Psychiatry* **29**: 159–175.

DeQuardo, J.R., Tandon, R., Goldman, R. et al (1994) Ventricular enlargement, neuropsychological status, and premorbid function in schizophrenia. *Biological Psychiatry* **35**: 517–524.

Dide, M.M. (1934) Les syndromes hypothalamiques et la dyspsychogéneses. *Révue Neurologique* **6**: 941–943.

Eastwood, S.L., Burnet, P.W.J., Harrison, P.J. (1995a) Altered synaptophysin expression as a marker of synaptic pathology in schizophrenia. *Neuroscience* **66**: 309–319.

Falkai, P., Bogerts, B. (1986) Cell loss in the hippocampus of schizophrenics. *European Archives of Psychiatry and Neurological Sciences* **236**: 154–161.

Falkai, P., David, B., Bogerts, B. et al (1991) Quantitative evaluation of astrocyte densities in schizophrenia. *Schizophrenia Research* **4**: 358 (Abs).

Feinberg, I. (1982) Schizophrenia: caused by a fault in programmed synaptic elimination during adolescence? *Journal of Psychiatric Research* **17**: 319–334.

Ferrier, I.N., Roberts, G.W., Crow, T.J. et al (1983) Reduced cholecystokinin-like immunoreactivity in limbic lobe is associated with negative symptoms in schizophrenia. *Life Sciences* **33**: 475–482.

Fisman, M. (1975) The brain stem in psychosis. *British Journal of Psychiatry* **126**: 414–422.

Flaum, M., Swayze, V.W., O'Leary, D.S. et al (1995) Effects of diagnosis, laterality and gender on brain morphology in schizophrenia. *American Journal of Psychiatry* **152**: 704–711.

Glantz, L.A., Lewis, D.A. (1993) Synaptophysin immunoreactivity is selectively decreased in the prefrontal cortex of schizophrenic subjects. *Society for Neurosciences* **19**: 201: 84.10.

Grove, W.M., Lebow, B.S., Medus, C. (1991) Head size in relation to schizophrenia and schizotypy. *Schizophrenia Bulletin* **17**: 157–161.

Häfner, H. (1993) What is schizophrenia? *Neurology, Psychiatry and Brain Research* **2**: 36–52.

Harrison, P.J., McLaughlin, D., Kerwin, R.W. (1991) Decreased hippocampal expression of a glutamate receptor gene in schizophrenia. *Lancet* **337**: 450–451.

Haug, O. (1962) Pneumoencephalographic studies of brain atrophy in mental disease. *Acta Psychiatrica Scandinavica* **38** (Suppl 165): 57–107.

Hecker, E. (1871) Die Hebephrenie: ein Beitrag zur klinischen Psychiatrie. *Archiv für Pathologie und Anatomie Berlin* **52**: 394–429.

Heckers, S., Heinsen, H, Heinsen, Y., Beckman H. (1991a) Cortex, white matter, and basal ganglia in schizophrenia: a volumetric postmortem study. *Biological Psychiatry* **29**: 556–566.

Heckers, S., Heinsen, H., Geiger, B., Beckmann, H. (1991b) Hippocampal neuron number in schizophrenia. A stereological study. *Archives of General Psychiatry* **48**: 1002–1008.

Huber, G. (1957) Pneumoencephalographische und psychopathologische Bilder bei endogenen Psychosen (Monograph aus dem Gasamtgebiete der Neurologie und Psychiatrie 79). Berlin: Springer.

Illowsky, B.P., Juliano, D.M., Bigelow, L.B., Weinberger, D.R. (1988) Stability of CT scan findings in schizophrenia: results of an 8 year follow-up study. *Journal of Neurology, Neurosurgery and Psychiatry* **51**: 209–213.

Jacobi, W., Winkler, H. (1927) Encephalographische Studien auf chronisch Schizophrenen. *Archiv für Psychiatrie und Nervenkrankheiten* **81**: 299–332.

Jakob, H., Beckmann, H. (1986) Prenatal development disturbances in the limbic allocortex in schizophrenics. *Journal of Neural Transmission* **65**: 303–326.

Jernigan, T.L., Zisook, S., Heaton, R.K. et al. (1991) Magnetic resonance imaging abnormalities in lenticular nuclei and cerebral cortex in schizophrenia. *Archive of General Psychiatry* **48**: 881–891.

Jeste, D.V., Lohr, J.B. (1989) Hippocampal pathologic findings in schizophrenia. A morphometric study. *Archives of General Psychiatry* **46**: 1019–1024.

Johnstone, E.C., Crow, T.J., Frith, C.D. et al. (1976) Cerebral ventricular size and cognitive impairment in chronic schizophrenia. *Lancet* ii: 924–926.

Johnstone, E.C., Bruton, C.J., Crow, T.J. et al. (1994) Clinical correlates of postmortem brain changes in schizophrenia: decreased brain weight and length correlate with indices of early impairment. *Journal of Neurology, Neurosurgery and Psychiatry* **57**: 474–479.

Kovelman, J.A., Scheibel, A.B. (1984) A neurohistologic correlate of schizophrenia. *Biological Psychiatry* **19**: 1601–1621.

Kraepelin, E. (1919) *Dementia Praecox and Paraphrenia*. Edinburgh: E. and S. Livingstone.

Krimer, L.S., Herman, M.M., Saunders, J.C. et al. (1995) Qualitative and quantitative analysis of the entorhinal cortex cytoarchitectural organization in schizophrenia. *Abstracts of the Society for Neurosciences* **1**: 239:98.14.

Lahti, A.C., Holcomb, H.H., Medoff, D.R. et al. (1995) Ketamine activates psychosis and alters limbic blood flow in schizophrenia. *Neuroreport* **6**: 869–872.

MacLean, P.D. (1949) Psychosomatic disease and the 'visceral brain'. Recent developments bearing on the Papez theory of emotion. *Psychosomatic Medicine* **11**: 338–353.

McNeil, T.F., Cantor-Graae, E., Nordström, L.G. et al. (1993) Head circumference in 'preschizophrenics' and control neonates. *British Journal of Psychiatry* **162**: 517–523.

Meduna, L.J. (1934) Über experimentelle Campherepilepsie. *Archiv für Psychiatrie und Nervenkrankheiten* **102**: 333–339.

Meduna, L.J. (1985) Autobiography of L.J. Meduna. *Convulsive Therapy* **1**: 43–57.

Mettler, F.A. (1955) Perceptual capacity, functions of the corpus striatum and schizophrenia. *Psychiatric Quarterly* **29**: 89–111.

Miyakawa, T., Sumiyoshi, S., Deshimaru, M. (1972) Electron microscopic study on schizophrenia: mechanisms of pathological changes. *Acta Neuropathologica* **20**: 67–77.

Morgan, L.O., Gregory, H.S. (1935) Pathological changes in the tuber cinereum in a group of psychoses. *Journal of Nervous and Mental Disease* **82**: 286–298.

Murray, R.M., Lewis, S.W. (1987) Is schizophrenia a neurodevelopmental disorder? *British Medical Journal* **295**: 681–682.

Nieto, D., Escobar, A. (1972) Major psychoses. In Minckler, J. (ed.) *Pathology of the Nervous System*, Vol. 3, pp. 2654–2665. New York: McGraw-Hill.

Ong, W.Y., Garey, L.J. (1993) Ultrastructural features of biopsied temporo-polar cortex (area 38) in a case of schizophrenia. *Schizophrenia Research* **10**: 15–27.

Pakkenberg, B. (1990) Pronounced reduction to total neuron number in mediodorsal thalamic nucleus and nucleus accumbens in schizophrenics. *Archives of General Psychiatry* **47**: 1023–1028.

Pakkenberg, B. (1993) Total nerve cell number in neocortex in chronic schizophrenics and controls using optical dissectors. *Biological Psychiatry* **34**: 768–772.

Papez, J.W. (1937) A proposed mechanism of emotion. *Archives of Neurology and Psychiatry* **38**: 725–743.

Pearlson, G.D., Powers, R.E., Barta, P.E. et al. (1991) Mesial temporal volume changes on MRI in schizophrenic and affective patients. *Schizophrenia Research* **4**: 409 (Abs).

Petty, R.G., Barta, P.E., Pearlson, M.B. et al. (1995) Reversal of asymmetry of the planum temporale in schizophrenia. *American Journal of Psychiatry* **152**: 715–720.

Raz, S., Raz, N. (1990) Structural brain abnormalities in the major psychoses: a quantitative review of the evidence from computerized imaging. *Psychological Bulletin* **108**: 93–108.

Reveley, M.A., Clifford, C.A., Murray, R.M. (1982) Cerebral ventricular size in twins discordant for schizophrenia. *Lancet* **i**: 540–541.

Rosenthal, R., Bigelow, L.B. (1972) Quantitative brain measurements in chronic schizophrenia. *British Journal of Psychiatry* **121**: 259–264.

Rosokiija, G., Kaufman, D., Liu, D. et al. (1995) Subicular MAP-2 immuno-reactivity in schizophrenia. *Abstracts of the Society for Neurosciences* (25th Annual Meeting) **3**: 21268, 835.10.

Selemon, L.D., Rajkowska, G., Goldman-Rakic, P.S. (1995) Abnormally high neuronal density in the schizophrenic cortex. *Archives of General Psychiatry* **52**: 805–818.

Southard, E.E. (1914, 1915) On the topographical distribution of cortex lesions and anomalies in dementia praecox, with some account of their functional significance. *American Journal of Insanity* **71**: 383–403 and 603–671.

Stevens, J.R. (1973) An anatomy of schizophrenia. *Archives of General Psychiatry* **29**: 177–189.

Stevens, J.R. (1982) Neuropathology of schizophrenia. *Archives of General Psychiatry* **39**: 1131–1139.

Stevens, J.R. (1992) Abnormal reinnervation as a basis for schizophrenia: a hypothesis. *Archives of General Psychiatry* **49**: 238–243.

Suddath, R.L., Casanova, M.F., Goldberg, T.E. et al. (1989) Temporal lobe pathology in schizophrenia: a quantitative magnetic resonance imaging study. *American Journal of Psychiatry* **146**: 464–472.

Sutula, T.P., Golarai, G., Cavazos, J. (1992) Assessing the functional significance of mossy fiber sprouting. *Epilepsy Research* **7** (Suppl.): 251–259.

Tanaka, Y., Hazama, H., Kawahara, R., Kobayashi K. (1981) Computerised tomography of the brain in schizophrenic patients. *Acta Psychiatrica Scandinavica* **63**: 191–197.

Torrey, E.F. (1994) *Schizophrenia and Manic-Depressive Disorder*. New York: Basic Books.

Uranova, N.A., Orlovskaya, D.D., Casanova, M.F. et al (1996) Ultrastructural morphometric study of glio-synaptic relationships in post mortem caudate nucleus of schizophrenic patients. *Schizophrenia Research* **18**: 181 (Abs).

Van der Horst, L. (1952) Histopathology of clinically diagnosed schizophrenic psychoses or schizophrenia-like psychoses of unknown origin. In *Proceedings of the First International Congress of Neuropathology*, Vol. 3, pp. 648–659. Turin, Italy: Rosenberg and Sellier.

Virgo, L., Humphries, L., Mortimer, A. et al. (1995) Cholecystokinin messenger RNA deficit in frontal and temporal cerebral cortex in schizophrenia. *Biological Psychiatry* **37**: 694–701.

Vita, A., Sacchetti, E., Valvassori, G. et al. (1988) Brain morphology in schizophrenia: a 2–5 year CT scan follow-up study. *Acta Psychiatrica Scandinavica* **78**: 618–621.

Weinberger, D.R. (1987) Implications of normal brain development for the pathogenesis of schizophrenia. *Archives of General Psychiatry*, **44**: 660–669.

Winkelman, N.W., Book, N.H. (1949) Observations on the histopathology of schizophrenia. *American Journal of Psychiatry* **105**: 889–896.

Wyatt, R.J. (1991) Neuroleptics and the natural course of schizophrenia. *Schizophrenia Bulletin* **17**: 325–351.

Zipursky, R.B., Marsh, L., Lim, K.O. et al. (1994) Volumetric MRI assessment of temporal lobe structures in schizophrenia. *Biological Psychiatry* **35**: 501–516.

8

New Pharmacological Treatments in Schizophrenia

Stephen R. Marder and Daniel P. van Kammen

INTRODUCTION

Recent innovations in the prescribing of antipsychotic drugs have led to optimism that the outcome of schizophrenia can be substantially improved. The most dramatic changes have involved the addition of newer drugs that are qualitatively different from older antipsychotics. These newer compounds have advantages compared to conventional compounds in terms of their effectiveness and their side-effect profiles.

Other important innovations in the drug treatment of psychosis do not involve newer drugs, but strategies for improving the use of older compounds. This chapter will first review improvements in the use of conventional drugs and then will discuss clozapine and risperidone, the most recently introduced antipsychotics in the USA. A number of antipsychotics that are currently in development and likely to be approved by the Food and Drug Administration (FDA) in the near future will also be discussed.

NEW APPROACHES TO CONVENTIONAL ANTIPSYCHOTICS

Traditional antipsychotics have a number of important limitations: they have a tendency to cause side-effects – particularly extrapyramidal side-effects (EPS) – at their therapeutic doses, and a substantial proportion of patients – at least 25% of drug-treated schizophrenic patients – have illnesses that are refractory or partially refractory to these drugs. These agents also have a substantial liability to cause tardive dyskinesia and they are relatively ineffective at treating the negative symptoms of schizophrenia. The improvements in the use of these drugs have focused on reducing side-effects by treating patients with the lowest effective dose. While these strategies are helpful, they do not bypass the limitations of these agents.

Dosing Strategies

Finding the best dose of an antipsychotic for acute schizophrenia can be difficult for clinicians. Although titrating dose against side-effects and therapeutic effects is the way clinicians claim they determine dose, this is often problematic with antipsychotics. There is often a delay of days or even weeks between the time a dose is administered and the time that patients demonstrate a therapeutic response. As a result, if a psychiatrist raises the dose of drug at the end of two weeks and the patient responds two days later, he or she may conclude that it was the dosage increase that led to improvement. However, this may confuse a dose effect with a time effect. That is, the patient may have improved if continued on the original dose. This delay in therapeutic response may be the main reason why clinicians – particularly in the United States – tended to treat patients with relatively high drug doses which, in turn, may have led to unnecessary side-effects and diminished effectiveness.

A number of dosage comparison studies have provided valuable information regarding the dose which is likely to be effective for most patients. These studies (reviewed by Baldessarini et al., 1988) indicate that 300 mg or less of chlorpromazine or (5 mg of fluphenazine or haloperidol) is likely to be too low for many psychotic patients. Doses above 1000 mg of chlorpromazine (or 20 mg of haloperidol or fluphenazine) are seldom necessary and may lead to substantial side-effects. Some studies actually suggest that such doses are less effective therapeutically as well. Taken as a group, these studies suggest that treatment with conventional drugs can be improved by judicious choice of drug doses.

Long-term maintenance treatment has also been improved as a result of newer studies that focused on dosing strategies. After patients with schizophrenia have recovered from a psychotic episode and have been stabilized, antipsychotic medications are usually continued with the goal of preventing relapse. This practice is based on the finding that patients who continue to receive antipsychotics while they are stable have much lower relapse rates than patients who receive no medications, or a placebo. However, long-term maintenance is also associated with risks such as drug side-effects or tardive dyskinesia. This had led to a number of studies that have focused on reducing the amount of drug that patients receive without reducing the protection that they receive from the antipsychotics.

Controlled studies have focused on the advantages and disadvantages of lowering the dose of a conventional antipsychotic during maintenance treatment. Studies that lowered doses approximately 80% have found that this reduction is associated with a relatively small but statistically significant increase in the risk of psychotic exacerbations (Kane et al., 1983; Marder et al., 1987; Hogarty et al., 1988). However, there were advantages to the low dose, such as less anxiety and depression, milder side-effects, lower drop-out rates, and decreases in burden on the patient's family. In reviewing these studies, Johnson (1994) has pointed out that patients should have their doses gradually lowered with careful monitoring as the dose is reduced.

Another strategy that has been tested is known as targeted or intermittent treatment. It involves gradually lowering and eventually discontinuing the patient's drug as long as the patient is doing well. Patients are carefully monitored for early signs of worsening and an oral antipsychotic is introduced when patients show prodromal signs of worsening. A number of studies have suggested that this strategy is associated with a relatively high risk of relapse (Carpenter et al., 1987; Jolley et al., 1989; Herz et al., 1991; Gaebel et al., 1993). Because the study by Gaebel et al. (1993) suggested that this strategy is superior to discontinuing medication and waiting until patients show evidence of new psychotic symptoms, it may be appropriate to adapt this method for patients who insist on discontinuing medications or those who are able to detect prodromal signs and willingly resume their medications at an early stage. Van Kammen et al. (1995) have provided a mixed behavioural and biochemical model to predict time-to-relapse in patients who were acutely withdrawn from haloperidol.

Marder and co-workers have proposed a strategy that combines early detection and low-dose treatment. Patients receive a relatively low dose of depot medication such as 5–10 mg of fluphenazine decanoate. Individuals are carefully monitored for symptoms that had preceded earlier relapses. When these prodromal symptoms are identified, the injectable depot drug is supplemented with the oral form (fluphenazine or haloperidol) of the drug. In a double-blind trial, Marder et al. (1994) treated patients with a low dose of fluphenazine decanoate. When subjects fulfilled criteria for a prodromal episode, patients were administered either oral fluphenazine 5 mg b.i.d. or a placebo. Although the risks of a psychotic exacerbation were similar during the first year of the trial, by the second year the risks were significantly reduced in the drug-treated group. This finding suggests that patients and therapists improve over time in their ability to identify periods of increased risk or that the risk decreased significantly after six months.

CLOZAPINE

Clozapine (Clozaril®, Leponex®), a dibenzodiazepine, was originally developed in 1958, but the drug only appeared on the US market in February 1990. Clozapine was found in 1975 to have an excessive risk of agranulocytosis compared to other antipsychotic agents. Subsequent experience indicated that its lymphocytopenia and agranulocytosis could be effectively managed with frequent monitoring. Early studies indicated that clozapine could have a wider therapeutic effect than traditional antipsychotics (Fischer-Cornelissen and Ferner, 1976), which led to further research on clozapine's effectiveness. Those studies documented that clozapine was effective in patients who had not responded well, or not at all, to traditional antipsychotics (Honigfeld et al., 1984; Meltzer, 1989). Negative symptoms in particular seemed to respond as well, while further improvement in positive symptoms continued to be observed beyond what was seen with traditional antipsychotics.

Its weak dopamine and strong serotonin receptor blockade made clozapine the first serotonin–dopamine receptor antagonist (SDA). The challenge that the agent raised to the dopamine hypothesis of antipsychotic drugs also challenged the dopamine hypothesis of schizophrenia. The coming years will bring clinically effective agents that do not have suppressant effects on the white cell system or extrapyramidal or other unpleasant side-effects. These agents will reach a wider group of schizophrenic patients. The high costs of clozapine treatment (which include a weekly blood cell count monitoring system) and its unpleasant side-effects have interfered with a full-scale application. However, the success of clozapine has inspired the development of newer, safer antipsychotic agents.

In spite of their powerful therapeutic effects, antipsychotics do not provide a full symptomatic improvement in all patients. Many schizophrenic patients frequently have lingering positive and negative symptoms, which can substantially impair their adjustment in the community, while others are treatment resistant. The clinician and the patient are left with the sometimes difficult task of weighing clozapine's substantial advantages in some patients against some of the drug's problems which include the risk of dangerous and uncomfortable side-effects such as agranulocytosis, increased seizure risk, sedation, excessive salivation, and weight gain, as well as the need for weekly blood monitoring, and the relatively high cost of the drug. However, the increased clinical response and decreased suicidality, as well as increased compliance through monitoring may set off these costs appreciably (Meltzer and Okayli, 1995; Meltzer and Cola, 1994).

Clozapine is only available in an oral preparation. Similar to other antipsychotics, peak plasma levels are reached approximately two hours following oral administration. Twice-daily dosing will result in steady-state plasma concentrations in less than one week. Clozapine undergoes extensive first-pass metabolism in the liver and gut. Reportedly 80% of administered clozapine appears in the urine or faeces as metabolites. Less than 5% of the parent compound is found unchanged in the urine.

Steady-state plasma concentrations are dose dependent. Thus, a typical daily dose of 300–400 mg (about 5 mg kg^{-1}) is associated with levels ranging between 200 and 400 ng ml^{-1}. The plasma levels of clozapine vary about five- to eight-fold among patients receiving the same daily doses (Perry et al., 1991). Some reports indicate that women have slightly higher and smokers have slightly lower plasma levels (20% to 30%) (Hasagawa et al., 1993). Older adults may have two-fold higher levels than young adults.

Mechanism of Action

Its low propensity to cause EPS, as well as its relatively high $5HT_2$ blockade make this drug an 'atypical' antipsychotic. This is different from conventional antipsychotic medications, all of which cause extrapyramidal side-effects (EPS) as a direct result of their activity at D_2 dopamine receptors in the forebrain. Clozapine in clinically effective doses only occupies 40–50% of D_2 striatal receptor site, with a preference for corticolimbic pathways with activity at a number of other receptors including serotonergic, adrenergic and cholinergic sites. Meltzer (1991) and others have proposed that the differential antipsychotic effect of clozapine is related to its low $D_2/5HT_2$ ratio. Others have focused on its stronger $5HT_3$ blockade, its stronger α_1, α_2, M_1 and H_1 receptor blockade, and its high affinity for the recently discovered D_4 dopamine receptor. Although this D_4 receptor may play a role, it appears that haloperidol has similar strong D_4 receptor blockade. This receptor, however, exists in several polymorphic variants regardless (van Tol et al., 1992). How much this affects drug response independent from diagnosis requires testing. Which of these receptor systems makes the clinical difference between typical and atypical antipsychotics remains unknown at this time.

Treatment Indications

Studies by Kane et al. (1988) have shown that clozapine was more effective than conventional drugs for patients who were treatment refractory. Marder and van Putten (1988) have suggested three populations of schizophrenic patients who are obvious candidates for clozapine: (1) patients with severe schizophrenic symptoms that are poorly responsive or treatment resistant to conventional antipsychotic medications; (2) patients with severe tardive dyskinesia; and (3) patients who are sensitive to severe EPS with traditional agents. Other treatment indications are severe mania and schizoaffective disorders, and in neurological diseases such as idiopathic Parkinson's disease, where they are used as a treatment for psychotic symptoms that are secondary to L-dopa. There is a suggestion that Parkinson's patients respond to relatively low doses of clozapine (doses of 12.5–75 mg). Higher doses, such as 100–250 mg per day may exacerbate the parkinsonian symptoms. Other reports suggest that clozapine may be useful for tremors from Parkinson's disease, alcoholism, and benign essential tremor. More studies are needed to further explore the role of clozapine in the treatment of neurological disorders.

Initiating Treatment

Clozapine should be started with 12.5–25 mg during the day and increased by 25 mg per day every two to three days. The rate of increase is limited by sedation and orthostatic hypotension. There are no dose response studies reported, but in general daily doses between 250 and 500 mg are considered adequate. Doses over 600 mg are seldom indicated. In spite of its low relative potency in many animal studies, clozapine is 1½–2 times more potent than chlorpromazine. Except perhaps for seizures, and possibly early sedation and hypotension, neither clinical nor side-effects are likely to increase in severity with the dose. Discontinuing a traditional antipsychotic to replace it with clozapine can be done abruptly. We recommend, however, that the drug be discontinued over two to four weeks, while the dose of clozapine is increased.

Duration of Treatment

Response in many patients may not be complete before six months or even longer. Reports indicate that clinical improvement may increase over time, thus late response can occur. Schizophrenic patients can be treated safely with clozapine for many years (Juul Povlsen et al., 1985).

Precautions and Adverse Reactions

Although clozapine treatment is associated with a variety of side-effects (Lieberman et al., 1989; Grohmann et al., 1989; Baldessarini and Frankenburg, 1991), the only contraindications to clozapine include a white cell count below 3500, a previous bone marrow disorder, a history of agranulocytosis during clozapine treatment, and the concomitant use of another bone marrow suppressant drug such as carbamazepine because it will be difficult to ascertain whether leucocytopenia or agranulocytosis has been induced. Although the mechanism of action is unknown, there is a slight increase in risk of respiratory depression/collapse if treatment is initiated while patients are taking benzodiazepines (Safferman et al., 1991; Sassim and Grohmann, 1988).

One to two percent of patients receiving clozapine will develop granulocytopenia or agranulocytosis. These patients may have a sudden or a gradual drop in the white blood count. The risk of this adverse effect is greatest during the first three months of treatment (Alvir et al., 1993), but a significant risk remains during the first six months of treatment and perhaps indefinitely. The risk of agranulocytosis increases with age and is higher in females. Agranulocytosis due to clozapine is a potentially fatal condition that requires immediate medical attention. The mortality rate is 1 in 10 000 (Meltzer and Okayli, 1995). Therefore, prior to treating patients with clozapine, clinicians must register patients with the Sandoz company. Moreover, patients are currently required to submit to weekly checks of their white blood counts (WBCs) for as long as they receive the drug and for at least a month after it is discontinued. It is possible that new information about the risk for agranulocytosis over time will result in less frequent monitoring after the first year. After one year of treatment the cumulative incidence is 0.8%. Genetic factors may also play a role.

Current guidelines specify that any fever or sign of infection, e.g. pharyngitis, is an immediate indication for a white blood cell count, particularly in the first 18 weeks of treatment. If the patient has a white cell count below 2000 or a granulocyte count below 1000, clozapine must be discontinued. Patients who develop agranulocytosis should not receive clozapine again. Reports of clozapine re-exposure following haematologic recovery have shown that all such patients again experienced agranulocytosis, but sooner and at lower doses than in their initial treatment. Although a white blood cell count below 3500 is not a proven risk factor, it is suggested that clozapine is administered cautiously in patients with such low levels, because of the difficulty of early identification of agranulocytosis. Similarly, carbamazepine should not be given concomitantly with clozapine.

Several hypotheses about this toxicity have been put forward. A variance in the metabolism of clozapine may lead to the development of toxic metabolites or higher than usual N-desmethylclozapine levels. An alternative hypothesis can be put forward, as has been for other drugs, that neutrophils and their committed stem cell precursors can metabolize clozapine into metabolites that are free radicals, and therefore cytotoxic. This has led to suggestions that the addition of vitamin C or E and other antioxidants (Mason and Fischer, 1992), or trace elements that are cofactors of free-radical scavenger enzymes, such as selenium, zinc and copper (Pippinger et al., 1991), may protect patients who are exposed to clozapine.

Other haematologic changes have been reported with clozapine, such as leucocytosis (0.6%), eosinophilia (1%), leucopenia/neutropenia/decreased white cell count (3%) and rarely, thrombocytopenia. Since 6 February 1990, only a few deaths have been reported to be associated with clozapine-related agranulocytosis and infection. Some of these patients received other medications such as carbamazepine, lithium, and benzodiazepines.

Similar to low potency antipsychotics, clozapine treatment carries the risk of EEG changes and grand mal seizures that are dose dependent. From the initial data it was concluded that in doses over 500 mg the risk of seizures increases considerably, particularly in those with a history of seizures. A pre-existing seizure disorder or head trauma places the patient at a greater risk. The crude rate of seizures is less than 1%.

Several recommendations have been made to lower the risk of seizures, including an EEG before raising the dose over 600 mg per day; combining clozapine with anticonvulsants (e.g. valproate) at doses where a seizure occurred before; monitoring clozapine blood levels; or lowering the dose by 50% after a seizure has occurred, followed by a neurological consultation. It is important to look for other aetiologies in addition to clozapine and avoid combination treatment with other drugs that lower the seizure threshold. Carbamazepine should not be used with clozapine because of its risk of agranulocytopenia and because it may lower blood levels of clozapine. Patients who are on antiepileptic agents may need their doses adjusted according to metabolic changes induced by clozapine administration. Patients who are taking carbamazepine and are candidates for clozapine should preferably be switched to another anticonvulsant. If anticonvulsants are required, the effects on metabolism should be included in the decision about the dose of both clozapine and the drug. Adding benzodiazepines carries a low risk of respiratory depression/arrest (0.31%).

The most frequent cardiovascular side-effects observed are sinus tachycardia and postural hypotension. The tachycardia is probably a direct effect of the vagolytic properties of the drug. It can be present in the supine position, and is therefore not the result of orthostatic changes. Increased pulse rates of 20–25 beats per minute are encountered when clozapine reaches 300 mg per day or more over a seven-day period. Recent data suggest that the prolongation of the QT interval over the square root of the RR interval (seconds) (Bazett formula) that is observed with chlorpromazine, is not observed with clozapine. Reversible non-specific ST-T wave changes, T wave flattening, or inversions (repolarization effects) are seen infrequently and are usually of no clinical significance. These changes are similar with other antipsychotics and are dose dependent. Although some tolerance occurs, it will persist unless the dose is lowered. A β-blocker, such as atenolol or pindolol, may be given depending on the blood pressure. Paradoxically, hypertension has been observed as well (4%).

There is a risk of postural hypotension, progressing to orthostatic collapse, if the initial dose exceeds 75 mg per day. Tolerance often develops over time. It can usually be managed if the initial dose is low, e.g. 25 mg per day, and the dose is gradually increased. When postural hypotension occurs, lowering the dose to the previous level and slower titration will limit the problems. However, 'orthostatic hypotension with or without syncope' can occur with clozapine treatment and may represent a continuing risk in some patients.

Rarely (approximately one case per 3000 patients), collapse can be profound and be accompanied by respiratory and/or cardiac arrest. Orthostatic hypotension is more likely to occur during initial titration in association with rapid dose escalation and may even occur on the first dose. When restarting patients who have had even a brief interval off clozapine, i.e. 36 hours or more since the last dose, it is recommended that treatment be re-initiated at 12.5 mg once or twice daily. Careful monitoring of vital signs is recommended during the first few weeks of treatment.

Sialorrhoea is another uncomfortable but tolerable side-effect, which develops early in treatment. Hypersalivation is most profound during sleep (i.e. decreased swallowing). Patients may complain that their pillow is wet in the morning from excessive salivation. Using a towel over the pillow may be of some help. Although the symptom can be treated with anticholinergics, this is not recommended because of the risk of anticholinergic toxicity. Clonidine (0.1 or 0.2 mg patch once a week) and amitriptyline have been used at bedtime to treat sialorrhoea. Dry mouth, blurring of vision, constipation, and urinary retention are commonly observed antimuscarinic side-effects with clozapine. Other side-effects of the autonomic nervous system, such as increased sweating, have also been reported.

Occasionally benign hyperthermia is observed during the first three weeks of treatment, with a peak incidence on the 10th day (Sandoz NDA, unpublished paper, 1987). The increase in temperature is usually not more than 1–2°F, and spontaneously resolves over a few days with continued treatment without any clinical significance. Occasionally, however, temperature increases above 101°F have been seen, which require temporarily withholding clozapine and frequent haematologic monitoring. Differential diagnoses include drug fever, intercurrent infection, infection secondary to agranulocytosis, dehydration, heat stroke, 'lethal' catatonia, and possibly neuroleptic malignant syndrome (NMS). Patients who develop a high temperature can be given the drug again but with a more gradual increase in dose. If this strategy does not work, clozapine may need to be discontinued.

Mild hypothermia is very frequently observed (87%). Because this effect is observed as frequently as with chlorpromazine, it may well indicate the poikilotherm effect of antipsychotics. It can be treated with benzodiazepines or 500 µg TRH (G. Bissett, personal communication, June 1995).

Weight gain has been reported with clozapine as with most anti-psychotics. The incidence may be higher with clozapine because of its strong $5HT_1$ and histaminic (H_1) receptor affinity. Constipation, most probably due to the antimuscarinic effects of the drug, is the most common gastrointestinal side-effect. It should be treated with stool softeners, laxatives, fibre supplements, and adequate fluid intake. The constipation can progress into intestinal obstruction if not appropriately treated. Nausea (and less frequently vomiting), which occurs sometimes, may be managed by dose reduction. Liver function disturbances are mild and transient. There is so far only one case report of cholestatic jaundice induced by clozapine. Thus, liver function tests should be obtained at baseline and monitored periodically, especially during the initial phase of treatment and after dose increases.

Urogenital effects include enuresis, frequency/urgency, hesitancy, urinary retention, and impotence. So far, there is no report of cloza-pine treatment-associated priapism. Because patients may not share these complaints spontaneously, the clinician should inquire about them. This is particularly important as it may lead to non-compliance, medical complications, and affect the patients' quality of life. Because prolactin levels are less likely to be raised with clozapine than with other antipsychotics, effects of hyperprolactinaemia such as amenor-rhoea, galactorrhoea, or gynecomastia have not been encountered.

Sedation occurs frequently early in treatment and tolerance usually develops after the first few days and weeks. Sedation can be minimized by giving the larger part of the entire dose at bedtime, and by not giving other CNS depressants. The α_1, α_2- and H_1-receptor blocking effects are believed to be the cause. Other CNS effects include dizziness and syn-cope, which may be related to orthostatic hypotension. Confusion and delirium may occur as a result of muscarinic toxicity, because it reverses with intravenous physostigmine and lowering of the dose.

No data on risks during pregnancy or lactation have been reported so far.

Long-term Effectiveness

All of the long-term studies with clozapine have been uncontrolled or retrospective. Nevertheless, they provide further support for the unique properties of clozapine. For example, patients who received clozapine for as long as 13 years were more likely to be discharged and remain out of the hospital. In a European study, patients who received clozapine for at least two years demonstrated an increase in their rate of employment from 3% to 40%. Long-term studies also provide information about the proportion of patients who improve on clozapine after prolonged administration. European studies suggest response rates of 30% to more than 50%. A more recent study by Herbert Meltzer (1995) indicated a response rate of more than 60% after a year of treatment. However, none of these studies included random assignment and controlled comparisons with conventional drug treatment. As a result, the impact of clozapine on the long-term outcome of patients – one of the most compelling questions in the therapeutics of schizophrenia – requires more study.

Comments on Clozapine

Some clinicians point at clozapine's superior effect on negative symptoms, presumably through its serotonergic, noradrenergic or muscarinic and maybe even mixed dopaminergic effects. Although this effect may be real, illness-specific or deficit negative symptoms are difficult to differentiate from drug-induced negative symptoms (with traditional antipsychotics, e.g. akinesia) or those that are secondary to positive symptoms unless the patient is observed under different clinical and medication conditions. Several of the comparison trials used drugs in doses in excess of the recommended doses (e.g. 40 and 60 mg of haloperidol). Therefore, we recommend that patients with such symptoms receive an adequate trial (e.g. six months on the maximum doses tolerated up to 500–750 mg per day) of clozapine (Meltzer, 1995).

Once the appropriate dose has been reached and the patient improves, the medication should be continued probably indefinitely. When the drug is discontinued in a successfully treated patient a rebound worsening is sometimes observed, requiring a tapering of dose and an early addition of the next antipsychotic.

Patients who indeed show remarkable improvement and symptom disappearance will be in need of specific rehabilitation efforts. They may be unable to function in the community without special skill training and stress management. They may need to (re)learn average daily living skills, such as how to deal with interpersonal relationships, appropriate behaviour in social settings, buying groceries and opening a bank account. Living without the feelings of grandiosity and immortality may be difficult to take for some patients. On the other hand, not all patients will respond dramatically to this agent. Families and patients need to be prepared to deal with this disappointment after all the media attention of its success.

RISPERIDONE

Risperidone is the first antipsychotic that is a benzisoxizole derivative. It is characterized by potent central antagonism of both serotonin (particularly $5HT_{2A}$) and D_2 receptors. Risperidone also demonstrates high affinity for α_1 and α_2 receptors but low affinity for β-adrenergic or muscarinic receptors. Preclinical studies indicate that while it is more potent than haloperidol at D_2 antagonism, it is several times less potent than haloperidol at inducing catalepsy (Janssen et al., 1988). This indicates that risperidone should result in substantially less EPS than conventional drugs at the recommended doses. In addition, the activity at $5HT_2$ receptors may result in greater activity against negative schizophrenic symptoms (Bleich et al., 1988).

A number of double-blind trials have compared risperidone with other drugs and placebos (Borison et al., 1992; Marder and Meibach, 1994). In addition to providing evidence regarding the effectiveness of risperidone compared to other drugs, a number of studies have also focused on the dosing of risperidone by comparing a number of fixed doses. This review will first discuss comparisons which permitted the clinician to determine the dose (variable dose studies) and then discuss comparisons which included more than one fixed dose. The advantage of the variable dose studies is that they most closely duplicate a real-life clinical setting in which clinicians individualize treatment. The advantage of fixed dose studies is that they permit comparison of different doses and they eliminate the effect of differences in prescribing habits among clinicians.

Variable Dose Studies

The first published double-blind study of risperidone was a multicentre investigation from Belgium (Claus et al., 1992). Forty-four patients with relatively refractory forms of schizophrenia were assigned to a comparison of risperidone (mean dose, 12 mg) and haloperidol (mean dose, 10 mg). Although the two drugs did not differ significantly in their effectiveness for positive or negative symptoms, there was a tendency for risperidone to be more effective. Risperidone patients were less likely to require antiparkinson medications.

Hoyberg et al. (1993) compared risperidone (mean dose, 8.5 mg daily) and perphenazine (mean dose, 28 mg) in a double-blind study that lasted eight weeks ($N=107$ schizophrenic patients). Although a higher proportion of patients assigned to risperidone (74%) than perphenazine (59%) met improvement criteria for total score on the Positive and Negative Symptom Scale (PANSS), the difference was not statistically significant (ns). For positive symptoms, 69% of risperidone and 73% of perphenazine patients met improvement criteria (ns); for negative symptoms, 76% of risperidone and 53% of perphenazine patients met criteria ($P<0.05$). There were no differences in EPS scores for the two groups.

Fixed Dose Comparisons

The largest risperidone study (Peuskens, 1995) was a multinational study that included 1362 patients who were randomized to a double-blind comparison of 10 mg daily of haloperidol or 1, 4, 8, 12, or 16 mg of risperidone. The 1 mg risperidone dose was considered subtherapeutic and was therefore used as a control. All of the other risperidone doses as well as the haloperidol group demonstrated greater improvement on the total PANSS than the 1 mg risperidone group. The 4 and 8 mg risperidone doses were the most effective, although their advantages over the other conditions were not statistically significant. There was a clear dose-related increase in EPS on risperidone. However, all of the risperidone doses were associated with less EPS than haloperidol. The differences in EPS were statistically significant for all of the risperidone doses with the exception of 16 mg.

The most important placebo-controlled trial was carried out in Canada and the United States. Acutely ill patients with schizophrenia were randomly assigned to groups that received 2, 6, 12, or 16 mg of risperidone, 20 mg of haloperidol or placebo. The results from the US and Canadian studies were very similar. Risperidone at doses above 2 mg and haloperidol 20 mg were consistently more effective for total PANSS and positive symptoms than placebo. The most effective dose of risperidone was 6 mg, which was significantly more effective than haloperidol for both total PANSS and positive symptoms. Risperidone (6 and 16 mg), but not haloperidol, resulted in significant improvements in negative symptoms as measured by the PANSS negative symptoms scale. There were similar results when the proportion of patients meeting criteria for improvement 20% or greater improvement in total PANSS or brief psychiatric rating scale (BPRS) were considered (Figure 8.1).

Risperidone resulted in a dose-related increase in EPS. However, the proportion of patients who required antiparkinson medications

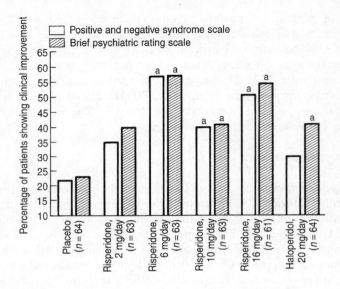

Figure 8.1   Percentage of 378 schizophrenic patients who received placebo, risperidone or haloperidol and showed clinical improvement (20% reduction in total positive and negative syndrome scale and total derived brief psychiatric rating scale scores at end point).[a] [a]$P<0.05$ versus placebo (generalized Cochran–Mantel–Maenszel test, controlled for investigator).

was no greater at the 6 mg dose – the dose at which risperidone was most effective – than on placebo. This observation suggests that patients who are treated with an effective dose of risperidone are less likely to suffer from EPS than patients on high potency drugs such as haloperidol.

Comparisons to Clozapine

Two published studies have compared risperidone with an atypical antipsychotic. The first was carried out by Heinrich et al. (1994) in Germany. Fifty-nine acutely ill patients received 4 mg risperidone, 8 mg risperidone, or 400 mg clozapine daily for 28 days. All three treatment groups improved and there were no significant differences among the groups. The 4 mg risperidone dose was the best tolerated when side-effects were measured. It is important to note that subjects in this study were not selected as being resistant to antipsychotic medications.

Overview of Efficacy

Taken together, these studies indicate that risperidone is an effective antipsychotic that may have advantages over conventional antipsychotics in its side-effect profile and perhaps in its efficacy. The large multicentre studies are most likely to detect differences between risperidone and a comparison drug in efficacy. However, both the 15-nation study and the North American trial compared multiple doses of risperidone to a single dose of a comparator drug. This type of comparison is unfair for obvious reasons. However, a recent met-analysis (Davis, 1994) pooled data from five controlled trials. The results indicated that 53% of risperidone patients met *a priori* criteria for improvement when their dose was greater than 6 mg compared to 40% of individuals who received a conventional antipsychotic ($P<0.001$). Davis also reported that risperidone was 25% better for positive symptoms and 60% better for negative symptoms.

Adverse Effects

As mentioned above, double-blind trials indicate that risperidone results in a dose-dependent increase in EPS. Other common side-effects include sedation, dizziness, constipation, tachycardia, erectile problems in men, weight gain, and decreased sexual interest (Chouinard et al., 1993; Marder and Meibach, 1994). A number of cases of neuroleptic malignant syndrome have been reported on risperidone (Najara and Enikeev, 1995; Lee et al., 1994; Raitasuo et al., 1994; Webster and Wijeratne, 1994). This is not surprising given this drug's substantial antidopaminergic activity. Other cases indicate that risperidone can produce obsessive–compulsive symptoms in some patients (Kopala and Honer, 1994; Remington and Adams, 1994), an observation that has been made with clozapine, another drug with substantial activity at $5HT_{2A}$ receptors (Baker et al., 1992).

Risperidone also results in a substantial rise in plasma prolactin, a direct effect of all drugs with substantial D_2 activity (Bersani et al., 1990). This increase leads to galactorrhoea and menstrual disturbances in some women.

Clinical Use of Risperidone

The results from clinical studies indicate that risperidone is an effective antipsychotic medication that has a relatively mild side-effect profile. In comparison to high potency antipsychotics it results in substantially less EPS without sacrificing effectiveness. Risperidone has not been compared with low potency antipsychotics such as chlorpromazine or thioridazine. Nevertheless, its profile suggests that it will be less sedating and less anticholinergic.

These particular characteristics indicate that risperidone is an appropriate first-line drug for patients with schizophrenia as well as other psychotic disorders when an antipsychotic is indicated. An important limitation is that it is only available as an oral pill. Thus, patients who are likely to do better on a long-acting depot drug – for example, patients with problems in treatment compliance – or patients who are likely to need short-acting injectables may be best treated with a drug that is available for other routes of administration.

It is unclear if risperidone is an appropriate choice for individuals who have failed to respond to a conventional antipsychotic. In the US study (Marder and Meibach, 1994), patients who had been in the hospital for at least six months prior to study tended to have the greatest advantage for risperidone over haloperidol. This suggests that risperidone may be effective for patients with treatment refractory illnesses. Its effectiveness in refractory patients is also supported by a study by Bondolfi et al. (1995).

Olanzapine

Olanzapine or Zyprexa® (Eli Lilly) (Beasley et al., 1996) is a thieno-benzodiazepine that is in the final stages of development. It is an SDA, with specific blockade of $5HT_{2A}$, $5HT_{2C}$, $5HT_3$, α_1, D_2, D_4, M_1 and H_1 receptors. It is the most clozapine-like agent, among those that may soon reach the market, without the typical side-effects. Its side-effects are weight gain, transient sedation and orthostatic hypotension; however, no acute dystonic reactions have been observed, while prolactin is only transiently increased. Negative symptoms improved significantly more with olanzapine than with haloperidol. Studies are underway with treatment-resistant schizophrenic patients. The dose range may be within 10–20 mg per day. Quality of life ratings were higher with olanzapine than with haloperidol.

Sertindole

Sertindole (Serlect®) (Abbott) is an arylpiperidylindole also in the final stages of development. It is an SDA with blockade of $5HT_{2C}$,

$5HT_{2A}$, D_2, α_1 and α_2 receptors. The drug has preferential binding for the mesolimbic dopamine system. Prolactin is only transiently elevated.

Recommended dose range is 12–20 mg per day. The pharmacokinetics are non-linear, so that 24 mg per day produces twice the blood levels of 20 mg. Some patients may require 24 mg per day. It seems to have solid antipsychotic and some antinegative symptom effects without obvious EPS (van Kammen et al., 1996). We expect to learn soon whether sertindole and olanzapine are indeed the low-side-effect challengers to clozapine treatment, as has been hoped. Some patients who did not respond to risperidone responded to sertindole and vice versa. Sertindole has also anti-anxiety effects. It has no extrapyramidal side-effects, but does have some initial autonomic side-effects and in some male patients produces dry ejaculation, which may disappear spontaneously. Although sertindole leads to a lengthening of the QT and QTc interval of the electrocardiogram, the significance of this effect is unclear. Other sexual side-effects affecting libido, ability to experience orgasm or potency are not reported as for the traditional antipsychotics. It has no anti-histaminic or antimuscarinic side-effects. Nasal stuffiness has been reported also.

SEROTONIN DOPAMINE ANTAGONISTS UNDER DEVELOPMENT

Quetiapine

Quetiapine (Seroquel or ICI-204636) (Zeneca) is a dibenzothiazepine derivative with potent activity at $5HT_{2A}$ receptors, but weaker activity at D_1 and D_2 receptors. Studies in monkeys suggest that this drug will have minimal liability for causing EPS (Migler et al., 1993) and that it results in only transient elevations in prolactin (Arvanitis et al., 1995).

Two double-blind trials with quetiapine indicate that it is a promising atypical drug. It is clearly superior to placebo and results in only minimal EPS in patients (Arvanitis et al., 1995). Some of the side-effects include drowsiness, increased heart rate, weight gain and agitation.

Ziprasidone

Ziprasidone (Pfizer) is another antipsychotic with potent antagonist effects at $5HT_{2A}$ and D_2 receptors. A preliminary report from a double-blind study (Ko et al., 1995) indicates that a daily dose of 160 mg of ziprasidone results in clinical improvement without, or with minimal, EPS. Its noradrenaline uptake inhibition may make it of interest in chronic withdrawn schizophrenic patients.

Other Novel SDAs

Several other SDAs (e.g. iloperidone, Hoechst-Marion-Roessel) (Szwerczak et al., 1995) and mazapertine (Janssen) (Reitz and Scott, 1995) are being tested in the clinic, while several other approaches (e.g. D_4 and $5HT_3$ antagonists) are also under study. Mazapertine (Janssen) is a novel potential antipsychotic agent with strong D_2, D_3, $5HT_{1A}$, α_1 and α_2 receptor blockade, which promises a low risk of EPS (Reitz and Scott, 1995). Early studies are underway. Iloperidone (Hoechst-Marion-Roessel) (Szwerczak et al., 1995) has strong D_2, D_3, D_4, $5HT_{2A}$, $5HT_{2C}$ and α_2 receptor blockade, suggesting it to be another interesting potential antipsychotic agent. As with all α_2 antagonists, these drugs need to be started at a low dose because of the risk of orthostatic hypotension.

IS c-*FOS* RELATED TO ANTIPSYCHOTIC EFFECTS?

Induction of immediate early genes such as c-*fos* by antipsychotic drugs may assist in understanding the different profiles of the traditional and atypical agents. Haloperidol induces c-*fos* in the striatum and the nucleus accumbens, while clozapine induces c-*fos* in the medial prefrontal cortex, lateral septal nucleus, the major island of Calleja (D_3 receptor blockade) and the nucleus accumbens but not in the dorsolateral striatum. Olanzapine treatment shows a similar pattern to clozapine but with some c-*fos* induction in the dorsolateral striatum, although this drug has very low EPS liability at the recommended doses. The localization of clozapine- and olanzapine-induced c-*fos* in areas that do not show induction with haloperidol suggests that these areas may be involved in negative symptoms.

IMPACT OF SDAs

The SDAs differ from one another in their clinical profile. These agents are different in their specific affinities, making these drugs potentially more interesting than just another drug with a low $D_2/5HT_2$ receptor blockade ratio. For instance, of the approved SDAs, only risperidone shares α_2 receptor blockade with clozapine; $5HT_{2A}$ receptor blockade varies widely with risperidone, olanzapine, sertindole and ziprasidone showing high affinities, and low affinity in the case of quetiapine. Risperidone has similar D_2 receptor blockade to haloperidol, and haloperidol has similar D_4 receptor affinity to clozapine. Sertindole and ziprasidone have D_2 affinities somewhat less than haloperidol. Quetiapine is remarkably like clozapine in its low D_2 receptor affinity, while olanzapine has higher D_2 affinity than clozapine or quetiapine but less than sertindole and ziprasidone. In addition, ziprasidone is unusual in that it blocks noradrenaline uptake and stimulates $5HT_{1C}$ receptors. It is potentially an interesting drug in patients with emotional withdrawal and amotivational syndromes, who are clinically stable. Because of their $5HT_{2C}$ blockade many of the SDAs may increase weight. Drugs that have a high ratio of $5HT_{2A}/5HT_C$ such as risperidone or iloperidone may have less of a risk of weight gain.

Until more studies in treatment-resistant schizophrenic patients have been published with these newer SDAs, clozapine will remain the drug of choice in these patients. The other SDAs are biochemically different enough that they will become alternatives if someone has not responded to clozapine. These agents are now the first-line drugs, because of their low side-effect profile. A negative response to either clozapine or risperidone does not preclude a positive response with the other.

All of the new agents, because of their lack of, or minimal, EPS and absence of drug-induced negative symptoms, may lead to more successful rehabilitation and better compliance. Because of their lack of muscarinic effects (e.g. cognitive interference) as with clozapine, chlorpromazine, or with anticholinergics, the newer agents (except perhaps olanzapine) may allow for better cognitive rehabilitation. A potential drawback may be that not all patients respond quickly enough to SDAs in the beginning of treatment; benzodiazepines or a more traditional high-potency antipsychotic may need to be added temporarily. That SDAs are unavailable in acute and long-acting injectable or liquid forms limits their uses as first-line drugs as well as in maintenance treatment. At the same time a drug similar to clozapine with fewer side-effects is not a cure-all for schizophrenia either. Clinicians should realize that clozapine does improve about 30% of drug non-responsive patients, still leaving many patients in the non-responsive category. Unrealistic expectations of the newer drugs may lead to disappointments. Pharmaceutical companies are still searching for compounds, which do affect dopamine or serotonin activity. At this time, though, the new drugs that are available promise to be real alternatives to traditional agents. For the first time since the early 1950s, the clinician will be able to tailor a specific antipsychotic to a particular patient's needs.

References

Alvir, J.M.J., Lieberman, J.A., Safferman, A.Z., Schwimmer, J.L., Schoaf, J.A. (1993) Clozapine-induced agranulocytosis incidence and risk factors in the United States. *New England Journal of Medicine* **329**: 162–167.

Arvanitis, L., Miller, B.G., Link, C.G.G., and the US and International SEROQUEL Study Groups (1995) Seroquel (ICI 204 636): a novel, atypical antipsychotic: efficacy and safety results from two phase II, multicenter, placebo-controlled clinical trials (abstract). *Schizophrenia Research* **15**: 142.

Baker, R.W., Chengappa, W., Roy, K., Baird, J.W., Steingard, S. (1992) Emergence of obsessive compulsive symptoms during treatment with clozapine. *Journal of Clinical Psychiatry* **53**: 439–442.

Baldessarini, R.J., Cohen, B.M., Teicher, M.H. (1988) Significance of neuroleptic dose and plasma level in the pharmacological treatment of psychoses. *Archives of General Psychiatry* **45**: 79–91.

Baldessarini, R.J., Frankenburg, F.R. (1991) Clozapine, a novel antipsychotic agent. *New England Journal of Medicine* **324**: 746–754.

Beasley, C.M. Jr, Tollefson, G., Tra, P. et al. (1996) Olanzapine versus placebo and haloperidol: acute phase results of the North American double-blind olanzapine trial. *Neuropsychopharmacology* **14**: 111–123.

Bersani, G., Bressa, G.M., Meco, G., Marini, S. (1990) Combined serotonin-5-HT$_2$ and dopamine-D$_2$ antagonism in schizophrenia: clinical, extrapyramidal and neuroendocrine response in a preliminary study with risperidone (R 64 766). *Human Psychopharmacology Clinical and Experimental* **5**: 225–231.

Bleich, A., Brown, S-J., Kahn, R., van Praag, H.M. (1988) The role of serotonin in schizophrenia. *Schizophrenia Bulletin* **14**: 297–315.

Bondolfi, G., Bauman, P., Patris, M. et al. (1995) A randomized double-blind trial of risperidone versus clozapine for treatment resistant chronic schizophrenia. *American Psychiatric Association Proceedings* NR 486; page 185.

Borison, R.L., Pathiraja, A.P., Diamond, B.I., Meibach, R.C. (1992) Risperidone: clinical safety and efficacy in schizophrenia. *Psychopharmacology Bulletin* **28**: 213–218.

Carpenter, W.T. Jr, Heinrichs, D.W., Hanlon, T.E. (1987) A comparative trial of pharmacologic strategies in schizophrenia. *American Journal of Psychiatry* **144**: 1466–1470.

Chouinard, G., Jones, B., Remington, G., Bloom, D. (1993) A Canadian multicenter placebo-controlled study of fixed doses of risperidone and haloperidol in the treatment of chronic schizophrenic patients. *Journal of Clinical Psychopharmacology* **13**: 25–40.

Claus, A., Bollen, J., De Cuyper, H., Eneman, M. (1992) Risperidone versus haloperidol in the treatment of chronic schizophrenic inpatients: a multicentre double-blind comparative study. *Acta Psychiatrica Scandinavica* **85**: 295–305.

Davis, J.M. (1994) Risperidone: properties, use, efficacy, and side effects. *Directions in Psychiatry* **74**: 1–7.

Fischer-Cornelissen, K.A., Ferner, U.J. (1976) An example of European multicenter trials: multispectral analysis of clozapine. *Psychopharmacology Bulletin* **12**: 34–39.

Gaebel, W., Frick, U., Koepcke, M.W. et al. (1993) Early neuroleptic intervention in schizophrenia: are prodromal symptoms valid predictors of relapse? *British Journal of Psychiatry* **163** (Suppl): 8–12.

Grohmann, R., Ruther, E. Sassim, N., Schmitt, L.G. (1989) Adverse effects of clozapine. *Psychopharmacology* **99** (Suppl): s10–s104.

Hasagawa, M., Gutierrez-Esteinou, R., Way, L., Meltzer, H.Y. (1993) Relationship between clinical efficacy and clozapine plasma concentrations in schizophrenia: effect of smoking. *Journal of Clinical Psychopharmacology* **13**: 383–390.

Heinrich, K., Klieser, E., Lehmann, E., Kinzler, E., Hruschka, H. (1994) Risperidone versus clozapine in the treatment of schizophrenic patients with acute symptoms: a double blind randomized trial. *Progress in Neuropsychopharmacology and Biological Psychiatry* **18**: 129–137.

Herz, M.I., Glazer, W.M., Mostert, A. et al. (1991) Intermittent vs maintenance medication in schizophrenia. *Archives of General Psychiatry* **48**: 333–339.

Hogarty, G.E., McEvoy, J.P., Munetz, M. et al. (1988) Dose of fluphenazine, familial expressed emotion, and outcome in schizophrenia. *Archives of General Psychiatry* **45**: 797–805.

Honigfeld, G., Patin, J., Singer, J. (1984) Clozapine: antipsychotic activity in treatment-resistant schizophrenics. *Advances in Therapy* **1**: 77–97.

Hoyberg, O.J., Fensbo, C., Remvig, J., Lingjaerde, O. (1993) Risperidone versus perphenazine in the treatment of chronic schizophrenic patients with acute exacerbations. *Acta Psychiatrica Scandinavica* **88**: 395–402.

Janssen, P.A., Niemegeers, C.J., Wouters, F.A., Schellekens, K.H. (1988) Pharmacology of risperidone (R 64 766), a new antipsychotic with serotonin-S_2 and dopamine-D_2 antagonistic properties. *Journal of Pharmacology and Exerimental Therapeutics* **244**: 685–693.

Johnson, D.A.W. (1994) Management of depression and negative symptoms. Presented at the *146th Annual Meeting of the American Psychiatric Association*, May.

Jolley, A.G., Hirsch, S.R., McRink, A., Manchanda, R. (1989) Trial of brief intermittent neuroleptic prophylaxis for selected schizophrenic outpatients: clinical outcome at one year. *British Medical Journal* **298**: 985–990.

Juul Povlsen, U., Noring, U., Fog, R., Gerlach, J. (1985) Tolerability and therapeutic effect of clozapine: a retrospective investigation of 216 patients treated with clozapine for up to 12 years. *Acta Psychiatrica Scandinavica* **71**: 176–185.

Kane, J.M., Rifkin, A., Woerner, M. et al. (1983) Low-dose neuroleptic treatment of outpatient schizophrenics. I. Preliminary results for relapse rates. *Archives of General Psychiatry* **40**: 893–896.

Kane, J.M., Honigfeld, G., Singer, J., Collaborative Study Group (1988) Clozapine for the treatment-resistant schizophrenic: a double-blind comparison versus chlorpromazine/benztropine. *Archives of General Psychiatry* **45**: 789–796.

Ko, G., Goff, D., Herz, L. et al. (1995) Status report: ziprasidone (abstract). *Schizophrenia Research* **15**: 154.

Kopala, L., Honer, W.G. (1994) Risperidone, serotonergic mechanisms, and obsessive-compulsive symptoms in schizophrenia. *American Journal of Psychiatry* **151**: 1714–1715.

Lee, H., Ryan, J., Mullett, G., Lawlor, B.A. (1994) Neuroleptic malignant syndrome associated with the use of risperidone, an atypical antipsychotic agent. *Human Psychopharmacology* **9**: 303–305.

Lieberman, J., Kane, J., Johns, C. (1989) Clozapine: guidelines for clinical management. *Journal of Clinical Psychiatry* **50**: 329–338.

Marder, S.R., Meibach, R.C. (1994) Risperidone in the treatment of schizophrenia. *American Journal of Psychiatry* **151**: 825–835.

Marder, S.R., van Putten, T. (1988) Who should receive clozapine? *Archives of General Psychiatry* **45**: 865–867.

Marder, S.R., van Putten, T., Mintz, J. et al. (1987) Low- and conventional-dose maintenance therapy with fluphenazine decanoate: two-year outcome. *Archives of General Psychiatry* **44**: 518–521.

Marder, S.R., Wirshing, W.C., van Putten, T. et al. (1994) Fluphenazine vs placebo supplementation of prodromal signs of relapse in schizophrenia. *Archives of General Psychiatry* **51**: 280–287.

Mason, R.P., Fischer, V. (1992) Possible role of free radical formation in drug-induced agranulocytosis. *Drug Safety* **7** (Suppl): 45–50.

Meltzer, H.Y. (1989) Duration of a clozapine trial in neuroleptic-resistant schizophrenia. *Archives of General Psychiatry* **46**: 672.

Meltzer, H.Y. (1991) The mechanism of action of novel antipsychotic drugs. *Schizophrenia Bulletin* **17**: 263–287.

Meltzer, H.Y. (1995) Clozapine: is another view possible? [editorial]. *American Journal of Psychiatry* **152**: 821–825.

Meltzer, H.Y., Cola, P.A. (1994) The pharmacoeconomics of clozapine: a review. *Journal of Clinical Psychiatry* **55** (Suppl. B): 161–165.

Meltzer, H.Y., Okayli, G. (1995) Reduction of suicidality during clozapine treatment of neuroleptic-resistant schizophrenia: impact on risk–benefit assessment. *American Journal of Psychiatry* **152**: 183–190.

Migler, B.M., Warawa, E.J., Malick, J.B. (1993) Seroquel: behavioral effects in conventional and novel tests for atypical antipsychotic drug. *Psychopharmacology* **112**: 299–307.

Najara, J.E., Enikeev, I.D. (1995) Risperidone and neuroleptic malignant syndrome: a case report [letter]. *Journal of Clinical Psychiatry* **56**: 534–535.

Perry, P.J., Miller, D.D., Arndt, S.V., Cadoret, R.J. (1991) Clozapine and norclozapine plasma concentrations and clinical response of treatment-refractory schizophrenic patients. *American Journal of Psychiatry* **148**: 231–235.

Peuskens, J. (1995) Risperidone in the treatment of patients with chronic schizophrenia: a multinational, multi-centre, double-blind, parallel-group study versus haloperidol. *British Journal of Psychiatry* **166**: 712–726.

Pippinger, C.E., Xianzhong, M., Rothner, A.D. et al. (1991) Free radical enzyme scavenging activity profiles in risk assessment of idiosyncratic drug reactions. In Levy, R.H., Penry, J.K. (eds) *Idiosyncratic Reactions to Valproate: Clinical Risk Patterns and Mechanisms of Toxicity*, pp. 75–88. New York: Raven Press.

Raitasuo, V., Vataja, R., Elomaa, E. (1994) Risperidone-induced neuroleptic malignant syndrome in young patient [letter]. *Lancet* **344**: 1705.

Reitz, A.B., Scott, M.K. (1995) Novel antipsychotics with unique D_2/5-HT$_{1A}$ affinity and minimal extrapyramidal side effect liability. *Advances in Medicinal Chemistry* **3**: 1–55.

Remington, G., Adams, M. (1994) Risperidone and obsessive-compulsive symptoms. *Journal of Clinical Psychopharmacology* **14**: 358–359.

Safferman, A., Lieberman, J.A., Kane, J.M., Szymanski, S., Kinon, B. (1991) Update on the clinical efficacy and side effects of clozapine. *Schizophrenia Bulletin* **17**: 247–261.

Sassim, N., Grohmann, R. (1988) Adverse drug reactions with clozapine and simultaneous application of benzodiazepines. *Pharmacopsychiatrica* **21**: 306–307.

Szwerczak, M.R., Corbett, R., Rush, D.K. et al. (1995) The pharmacological profile of iloperidone, a novel antipsychotic agent. *Journal of Pharmacology and Experimental Therapeutics* **274**: 1404–1413.

van Kammen, D.P., Kelley, M.E. Gurklis, J.A. et al. (1995) Behavioral vs biochemical prediction of clinical stability following haloperidol withdrawal in schizophrenia. *Archives of General Psychiatry* **52**: 673–678.

van Kammen, D.P., McEvoy, J.P., Targum, S.D. et al. (1996) A randomized, controlled, dose-ranging trial of sertindole in patients with schizophrenia. *Psychopharmacology* **124**: 168–176.

van Tol, H.H.M., Wu, C.M., Guan, H.C. et al. (1992) Multiple dopamine D_4 receptor variants in the human population. *Nature* **358**: 149–152.

Webster, P., Wijeratne, C. (1994) Risperidone-induced neuroleptic malignant syndrome [letter]. *Lancet* **344**: 1228–1229.

9

The Pharmacology of Alcohol

Hans Rommelspacher

Only recent developments with some clinical relevance will be presented in this chapter. For more in-depth reading, recent reviews should be consulted (Kranzler, 1995; Rommelspacher, 1995; Schuckit, 1995; Tsai et al., 1995). The term alcohol is used synonymously with ethanol if not stated otherwise. Ethanol is used whenever a chemical reaction is described.

PHARMACOKINETICS OF ETHANOL

Absorption

Alcohol is readily absorbed by diffusion, mainly from the duodenum and jejunum, and to a much lesser extent from the stomach. The intestine is a much more permeable biomembrane than the stomach, with a rate of absorption of $1.78 \, mg^{-1} \, dl^{-1} \, min^{-1}$ (range 0.52–$4.8 \, mg^{-1} \, dl^{-1} \, min^{-1}$). Alcohol is rapidly and uniformly distributed throughout the body water. Alcoholic beverages are, in general, hyperosmolar. Thus, under normal conditions, gastric emptying of the alcohol is delayed until the osmolarity of the gastric content approaches isotonicity (Van Thiel and Gavaler, 1988). When taken at concentrations above 30 mg per 100 ml, ethanol can cause local tissue irritation, superficial erosions, haemorrhages, vasoconstriction and paralysis of smooth muscle of the stomach, leading to a decrease in the rate of absorption of ethanol (Wallgren and Barry, 1970). In a study conducted by Jones et al. (1991) the peak of the blood alcohol concentration (BAC) was reached between 0 and 45 min in 77% of the subjects and within a period of 75 min in 97% ($n=152$). The presence of food in the stomach delays gastric emptying and thus reduces the rate and efficiency of alcohol absorption (Wilkinson et al., 1977). For example in a study by Jones and Jonsson (1994), after an overnight fast ethanol (0.80 g kg^{-1}) was consumed with or without breakfast. The peak BACs were 67 mg% and 104 mg% respectively and the areas under the time/concentration curve (AUC) 241 mg% h^{-1} and 398 mg% h^{-1}, suggesting that the breakfast delays the absorption and in addition boosts the rate of ethanol metabolism. The mean disappearance of the ethanol from blood was calculated to be increased by food by between 36% and 50%.

The mean peak alcohol concentration and the mean AUC were significantly greater in women than they were in men. This difference was due to the difference in the volume of distribution for ethanol between men and women, namely the body water (Widmark, 1932). In men, mean body water expressed as a percentage of body weight ($65\pm2\%$) has been shown to be significantly greater than in women ($51\pm2\%$; Marshall et al., 1983). Whether the pharmacokinetics change during the menstrual cycle remains controversial (Linnoila et al., 1980). Women appear to develop greater degrees of hepatic damage than men, even when their alcohol intake has been related to their lower body weight. A postulated role of the differing vulnerabilities of women and men to alcohol abuse is based on the observation that it is mainly the stomach that is responsible for the first-pass effect of ethanol absorption, and not the duodenum. It has been calculated that 20% of the ingested alcohol can be metabolized in the gastric mucosa (Caballeria et al., 1989). The percentage of metabolized alcohol is higher at low amounts ingested. Furthermore, under conditions of retarded emptying, e.g. by simultaneous food intake or drugs (antihistaminics), the first-pass metabolism in the stomach wall is relatively high. Two types of alcohol dehydrogenase (ADH) isozymes have been detected in the gastric mucosa which are responsible for the first-pass effect (see below; Hernandez-Munoz et al., 1990). The gastric activity of ADH in the mucosa in women has been found to be only 59% of that in men. This difference might contribute to the higher AUCs of women and the greater sensitivity of the liver to chronic ethanol abuse in women (Frezza et al., 1990). However, the first-pass metabolism of ethanol is minimal in the fasting state and lower not only in women than in men, but also in alcoholics than in non-alcoholics. Almost no gastric metabolism is demonstrable in alcoholic women. The lower level of ADH activity might be partly responsible for women's greater susceptibility to gastric ulcers due to the higher concentration of ethanol remaining in the gastric tissues (Lee et al., 1992). Although men in general have a higher level of gastric ADH in the mucosa, the level of this enzyme in men over the age of 50 is not higher than in women (Seitz et al., 1990). In conclusion, gender, lean body mass, age, alcoholism, motility of the stomach and drugs like H_2 receptor blockers which inhibit ADH activity (e.g. cimetidine) all affect the absorption and the extent of first-pass metabolism of ethanol.

Alcohol Dehydrogenase (ADH)

Enzyme characteristics

Human alcohol dehydrogenase (ADH: NAD^+ oxidoreductase, EC 1.1.1.1) constitutes the major oxidative pathway for initial ethanol metabolism. Ethanol is oxidized to acetaldehyde via hydrogen transfer to the cofactor nicotinamide adenine dinucleotide (NAD^+), resulting in conversion to its reduced form, NADH. ADH occurs in the cytosol and is not inducible by substrates. It is universally distributed in living organisms such as animals, plants, and micro-organisms (e.g. *Helicobacter pylori*, which lacks aldehyde dehydrogenase). The enzyme is capable of oxidizing a variety of aliphatic alcohols and a limited number of cyclic alcohols to the corresponding aldehydes. Human ADH consists of two subunits with one active site per unit, and two zinc atoms per subunit. Ethanol can be expected to exhibit combined first-order and zero-order kinetics but it will obey mainly zero-order kinetics at levels above 2 mmol l^{-1}. This means that amounts of alcohol consumed by social drinkers and by alcohol-abusing individuals are converted to acetaldehyde at a constant rate (decrease of the BAC by 0.1 vol% per hour). Only very low amounts are oxidized in a dose-dependent manner. ADH may also play an important role in retinol–retinal interconversion in visual processes. Furthermore, it has been proposed that it may be involved in the metabolism of steroids, bile acids, methanol, ethylene glycol, 1,2-propandiol and cardiac glycosides (Agarwal and Goedde, 1990).

Enzyme classes

Humans produce as many as nine different subunits (α, β_1, β_2, β_3, γ_1, γ_2, π, μ and χ). These polypeptides are encoded by six different genes, two of which are polymorphic. The isozymes have been grouped into class I (α, β and γ) which are mainly expressed in liver, class II (π) observed only in the liver, class III (χ) present in all tissues studied, and class IV (μ) in the gastric mucosa (Bosron et al., 1993; Eklund et al., 1990). Association across the four classes has not been observed except within class I. Eighty to ninety-five percent of the Caucasian populations are homozygous for $\beta_1\beta_1$ and 4–20% carry the β_2 allele, which is mostly coupled with β_1. In contrast, in Oriental populations, approximately the inverse ratio is found. This isozyme composition is called 'atypical'. The β_3 allele is seen in about 25% of Afro-Americans. However, the biological importance of the polymorphism of ADH remains undecided. No heterogeneity is known for the ADH II and ADH III classes (Ehrig et al., 1990).

The class IV isozyme ($\mu=\sigma$-ADH) which is localized in the stomach wall, exhibits a relatively high K_m value for ethanol of 25 mmol l^{-1} and a remarkably high K_{cat} (1500 min^{-1}). High K_m means a low affinity for ethanol, thus the enzyme is active at high concentrations of ethanol. K_{cat} expresses the catalytic activity of the enzyme. This enzyme may be responsible for first-pass ethanol metabolism in the stomach wall (Kedishvili et al., 1995).

Which ADH isozymes are active in the liver? To answer this question one should realize that 1 g l^{-1}(1 per thousand) is equivalent to 17 mmol l^{-1} ethanol. This means that concentrations of ethanol in intoxicated individuals are from 10 to over 20 mmol l^{-1}. The lowest K_m values have the $\beta_1 \beta_1$ (0.049 mmol l^{-1}), the $\beta_2 \beta_2$ (0.94 mmol l^{-1}), the $\gamma_1 \gamma_1$ (1 mmol l^{-1}), and $\gamma_2 \gamma_2$ (0.49 mmol l^{-1}) isozymes. Thus, they are saturated with ethanol for most of the time in contrast to $\alpha \alpha$ (K_m = 4.2 mmol l^{-1}), $\beta_3 \beta_3$ (36 mmol l^{-1}) $\pi \pi$ (34 mmol l^{-1}) and $\chi \chi$ (<1000 mmol l^{-1}) isozymes which are only partially saturated in intoxicated individuals. With regard to the capacity (V_{max}) it can be calculated that the $\beta_2 \beta_2$ and $\beta_3 \beta_3$ isozymes play the major role in the elimination of ethanol (Ehrig et al., 1990). In light of the different affinities of NAD$^+$ to the isozymes, it can be deduced that the β chains contribute most to the observed differences in the metabolism of ethanol. Simulation of the pharmacokinetics of ethanol suggests that the presence of the high V_{max} $\beta_2 \beta_2$ isozyme results in a high elimination rate and the presence of the low V_{max} $\beta_1 \beta_1$ isozyme in a low rate.

The large differences in elimination rates for different phenotypes predicted from simulations are not actually found in drinking experiments. In Orientals and Caucasian populations about 50% and 4–20% of individuals respectively express the β_2 chain. However, the mean alcohol elimination rate in the former is only about 20% higher than that in the latter, suggesting that other factors such as the rate of NADH reoxidation, which is necessary to provide the enzyme with the required status of the coenzyme, the often observed zinc deficiency (Bode et al., 1988) or ethanol distribution phenomena contribute essentially.

The major rate-limiting step of the elimination of ethanol is the amount of ADH and/or the rate of NADH reoxidation. The aldehyde dehydrogenase (ALDH) activity is not rate-limiting provided the individual expresses the ALDH 2 isozyme with the low affinity for acetaldehyde (see below).

Other Alcohol-metabolizing Enzymes (MEOS, Catalase)

The microsomal ethanol-oxidizing system (MEOS) is the major non-ADH pathway of alcohol oxidation in the liver (the enzyme occurs in a variety of other organs including the brain). The enzyme(s) is NADPH and oxygen dependent and belongs to the cytochrome P-450 superfamily. The products of the reaction are acetaldehyde, water, and NADP. The activity of the MEOS per gram liver tissue in humans has been estimated to be about 0.023 µmol acetaldehyde generated per minute, as compared to a total ADH activity of about 2.6 µmol. The contribution of MEOS is thus small, but its activity can be induced by chronic alcohol intake (5–6-fold in rats). The P-450 cytochrome isozyme with the highest affinity for ethanol has been designated CYP2E1, and is followed by that termed the CYP1A1 type. CYP2E1 can be induced by several different conditions such as starvation, high-fat feeding and diabetes. Induction not only leads to increased formation of acetaldehyde but may also play an important role in the hepatotoxicity of a number of drugs, carcinogens, and xenobiotics by way of an increased metabolism of these compounds (e.g. isoniazide, phenylbutazone, acetaminophen, meprobamate, pentobarbital, aminopyrine, tolbutamide, propranolol, and rifampicin; Lieber, 1984). Oxygen radicals are generated during the oxidation process of ethanol to acetaldehyde by CYP2E1. Under conditions whereby the enzyme is induced, those molecules may contribute to the hepatotoxicity of ethanol (oxidative stress) mainly if the cellular defence mechanisms are weakened (e.g. by chronic ethanol abuse). An indicator for the augmented hepatocellular vulnerability would be the level of glutathione and of L-cysteine (Wlodek and Rommelspacher, 1994).

The half-life of the induced CYP2E1 is in the order of 6 h or less in rats. The induction of the enzyme occurs by two different mechanisms dependent on the concentration of ethanol. Moderate ethanol levels result in a greater availability due to stabilization, whereas high levels (>0.25%) are able to invoke activation of the CYP2E1 gene (Roberts et al., 1994).

Another of the enzymes involved in ethanol metabolism is catalase. Much of the catalase in the liver is located in the peroxisomes. The reaction of the enzyme is based on the transfer of two protons from the ethanol to H_2O_2 resulting in the formation of $2H_2O$ and acetaldehyde. It is generally accepted that the contribution of catalase to ethanol oxidation is minimal.

In summary, in Caucasians the capacity of all enzymes involved in ethanol metabolism is about $0.1 \, g \, kg^{-1} \, h^{-1}$, whereas in Orientals it is somewhat higher ($0.13 \, g \, kg^{-1} \, h^{-1}$; Agarwal and Goedde, 1990). Thus, the polymorphism of ADH seems to be compensated by the other metabolic pathways.

Aldehyde Dehydrogenase (ALDH)

Enzyme characteristics

The removal of aldehydes is mediated by a number of unspecific enzymes such as aldehyde oxidase, xanthin oxidase and aldehyde dehydrogenase. The major pathway of acetaldehyde in the human liver and other organs is catalysed by the NAD^+-dependent aldehyde dehydrogenase (ALDH, aldehyde: NAD^+ oxidoreductase, EC 1.2.1.3.).

At least four isozymes coded by different gene loci have been detected in humans (Goedde and Agarwal, 1987). A structurally based classification similar to that of ADH has been proposed. The known ALDH sequences can be grouped into three distinct, but related, structural families, classes 1, 2 and 3. The class 1 isozymes are localized in the cytosolic fraction, whereas the class 2 isozymes are found in the mitochondria. Class 3 has been detected in rat hepatoma cells. The structural genes of human classes 1 and 2 ALDH have been assigned to chromosomes 9 and 12, respectively (Hsu et al., 1986).

The cytosolic class 1 ALDH has a K_m value of 30 µmol l^{-1} for acetaldehyde, the mitochondrial class 2 ALDH of 3 µmol l^{-1}. The cytosolic ALDH is inhibited by disulphiram, the mitochondrial isozyme only by high concentrations of disulphiram. Disulphiram binds to the cysteine at position 302 which is an essential residue at the active centre of the cytosolic enzyme.

The Oriental variance of human class 2 ALDH

ALDH 2 (mitochondrial) inactive individuals suffer from the so-called flush reaction. This is characterized by cutaneous vasodilatation, drowsiness, headache, palpitation, increased heart rate and nausea after ethanol ingestion. A structural mutation is responsible for the inactivity of the enzyme. The active and inactive enzymes differ by a single amino acid (glutamate to lysine exchange at position 487). The subunits generated from the typical ALDH 2 and atypical ALDH 2 allele combine randomly to tetramers. Tetramers with at least one inactive subunit are enzymatically less active.

Organ distribution

The liver has by far the highest capacity to metabolize acetaldehyde among all tissues. It contains the low K_m isozyme ALDH 2 and the high K_m isozymes ALDH 1, 3 and 4. Both ALDH 1 and 2 isozymes have been detected in soluble and particulate fractions of human autopsy liver material. The cytosolic fractions both showed strong ALDH 1 and ALDH 2 bands. The mitochondrial fraction was composed of a very strong ALDH 2 and a very weak ALDH 1 band. Thus, the assignment of ALDH 2 to the mitochondrial (low K_m) class and the classification of ALDH 1 (high K_m) as the cytosolic enzyme is a simplification (Agarwal and Goedde, 1990).

Human stomach extracts show considerable ALDH activity. The presence of classes 1, 2, 3, 4 or 5 have been reported. Stomach ALDH showed less affinity for acetaldehyde than the liver extract.

ALDH classes 1 and 2 have been found in human placenta. Calculations based upon *in vitro* activity determinations indicate that the enzyme activity may be too low to prevent the placental passage of normal concentrations of blood acetaldehyde produced by maternal ethanol metabolism. Thus, increased blood acetaldehyde concentrations resulting from acute alcohol intoxication may readily reach the fetus (Meier-Tackmann et al., 1985).

ALDH has been found to be the most important enzyme for the metabolism of biogenic amine neurotransmitter aldehydes (products of the reaction of monoamine oxidase). In all brain regions investigated, the total aldehyde-oxidizing capacity of brain tissue was twice as high for acetaldehyde as for the dopamine-derived aldehyde. Most of the activity was found in the mitochondrial and microsomal fractions. Both a low K_m ALDH and a high K_m ALDH have been described without further classification (Hafer et al., 1987).

A considerable acetaldehyde-oxidizing capacity has been demonstrated in erythrocytes. A single high K_m enzyme has been identified (ALDH 1), which is identical with the cytosolic enzyme of the liver (Agarwal et al., 1989).

At least three ALDH isozymes (ALDH 1, 2, 3) have been detected in human skin biopsy material and fibroblasts. High amounts of ALDH 1 and a low amount of ALDH 2 isozyme have been found in hair follicles (Agarwal and Goedde, 1990).

The flushing reaction

The incidence of alcohol flushing among Orientals is much higher than in Caucasians, e.g. around 50% versus 5–10%. It is interesting that in a Japanese sample the frequency of the atypical ADH 2 was found to be higher in alcohol flushers than in non-flushers (Shibuya et al., 1989). As described above, the atypical ADH 2 isozyme is highly prevalent among Orientals and has a high conversion capacity of ethanol to acetaldehyde.

Functionally, in individuals lacking mitochondrial ALDH (ALDH 2) isozyme activity, product inhibition of ADH by acetaldehyde can be expected. Thus, the elimination rate of ethanol is lower than in individuals with normal ALDH 2. In this situation, the capacity to oxidize acetaldehyde to acetate appears to become partially rate-limiting.

A large study in Japanese individuals with ALDH 2 deficiency demonstrated that the prevalence of the deficient phenotype is about 50% in non-alcoholics but only 9% in alcoholics (Shibuya and Yoshida, 1988). Drinking frequency decreased in the following order: typical homozygote, heterozygote, atypical homozygote (Takeshita et al., 1994). The alcohol metabolism is more strongly affected in atypical homozygous individuals than in heterozygous (Enomoto et al., 1991). No Japanese or Chinese alcoholic was ever found with an atypical homozygous genotype. Thus, atypical homozygous individuals are protected against alcoholism. The underlying mechanism is presumed to be the aversiveness of the excessive acetaldehyde concentrations generated in these individuals which are almost in the order of magnitude of those of disulphiram-treated alcoholics. In contrast to these unequivocal findings, the genotype with heterozygous ALDH 2 does probably not protect from alcoholism which is in contradiction to earlier studies. Only 86% of Japanese with inactive ALDH 2 always flushed and 47% of the homozygous active genotype experienced flushing (Higuchi et al., 1992). There is no empirical evidence that flushing *per se* is intrinsically aversive. Euphoria was also experienced by flushers in laboratory settings. Increased blood and urinary catecholamines were observed in flushing individuals with a high blood acetaldehyde concentration. The acetaldehyde levels never reached those of atypical homozygous individuals. The flushing subjects reported overall more intense, but not less pleasant reactions to alcohol than non-flushing subjects (Wall et al., 1992). These and other studies, including animal experiments, demonstrate that low doses of acetaldehyde are reinforcing.

A sample of 1225 Japanese individuals were investigated for their flushing frequency defined as 'always', 'sometimes' and 'never'. The 'sometimes' flushing men were 1.7 times more likely than the 'never' flushers and three times more likely than the 'always' flushers to abuse alcohol. An even more dramatic difference was observed in Japanese women, with the 'sometimes' flushers posing a risk 2.8 times that of the 'never' flusher and 7.8 times that of the 'always' flushers. The flushers included both ALDH 2-active and -inactive phenotypes (Higuchi et al., 1992a). In conclusion, these and other studies suggest that slight flushing increases the risk of alcohol abuse. Furthermore, the contribution to the risk of alcohol abuse of the atypical high-capacity ADH and of other classes of ALDH remains to be elucidated. Whether the heterozygous individuals have a higher risk of alcohol-related diseases, e.g. liver cirrhosis, that may also be different from those of subjects with typical ALDH, is not clear.

THE EFFECTS OF ETHANOL

Central Nervous System

Ethanol has a biphasic effect on the central nervous system (CNS). Low doses induce a stimulation resulting from depression of inhibitory control mechanisms, whereas higher doses induce depression of CNS functions. Individual sensitivity differs, possibly partly as a result of genetic factors (Schuckit, 1994). Memory, concentration and insight are dulled and then lost. The personality becomes expansive and vivacious, and uncontrolled mood swings and emotional outbursts may be evident. Despite the fact that ethanol does not activate a specific receptor mechanism it becomes increasingly evident that it acts by interfering at protein–protein interaction sites and possibly at interfaces between proteins and the phospholipid bilayer of the neuronal cell membranes. Thus, it can be expected that ethanol preferentially affects complex protein–protein interactions in the course of transmembrane signal transduction and ion channel opening.

GABA-ERGIC MECHANISMS

GABA and benzodiazepine agonists appear to be fairly inactive in modulating voluntary ethanol intake (Beaman et al., 1984; Daoust et al., 1987; Smith et al., 1992). The GABA$_A$ antagonists picrotoxin and bicuculline diminish some ethanol induced behaviours, such as motor impairment, sedation/hypnosis and anxiolysis (Häkkinen and Kulonen, 1976; Liljequist and Engel, 1982, 1984; Dar and Wooles, 1985; Dudek et al., 1989; Hellevuo et al., 1989; Becker and Anton, 1989; Hinko and Rozanov, 1990). GABA$_A$ antagonists and benzodiazepine inverse agonists reduce alcohol drinking (June et al., 1991). Such findings suggest that GABA$_A$ responses are involved in ethanol-drinking behaviour. Furthermore, substances which are anxiogenic, like the benzodiazepine inverse agonist, reduce alcohol drinking in rodents. On the other hand, GABA$_A$ activation might be a part of the mechanism sustaining and prolonging the drinking bouts, possibly by inhibition of satiety mechanisms. It is well established that benzodiazepine agonists increase food intake and inverse agonists reduce it (Cooper, 1987). In alcohol withdrawal studies it has been shown that some symptoms can be effectively alleviated by GABA$_A$ agonists (Gonzales and Hettinger, 1984; Frye et al., 1986) suggesting that GABAergic mechanisms are involved in physical dependence.

In Vivo Studies

Blunted responsiveness of brain glucose metabolism in recently detoxified alcoholics shown by positron emission tomography scanning with 18F-FDG (fluorodeoxyglucose) following a loading dose of lorazepam has been explained by diminished GABA-benzodiazepine receptor function. Reduced responsiveness to lorazepam has been found primarily in the basal ganglia, thalamus and orbitofrontal cortex, and not in the occipital cortex or cerebellum. Some of these areas form part of the neuronal circuit that regulates the initiation and termination of behaviours. When disrupted, this system can lead to the emergence of compulsive repetitive behaviours. Decreased response to inhibitory neurotransmission has been seen as partly responsible for the lack of control and compulsive alcohol intake seen in alcoholics.

One major advance in the understanding of the molecular action of ethanol was the discovery of the benzodiazepine receptor partial inverse agonist RO 15-4513. The imidazobenzodiazepine reversed the reduction of rat locomotor activity caused by ethanol. No reversal of the ethanol effect in the rotating rod test (assessment of complex motor co-ordination) was observed, whereas the impairment of performance on the horizontal wire (simple motor co-ordination) was blocked by low doses (mice, ED_{50} 0.84 mg kg^{-1} p.o.). The lethal effects of high doses of ethanol were not affected (Bonetti et al., 1989). These findings are compatible with the postulate of multiple mechanisms of action of ethanol. RO 15-4513 binds with a strong affinity to cerebellar granule cells (diazepam insensitive, Sieghard et al., 1987). The binding depends on the expression of the α_6 subunit, which is unique to the granule cells in the cerebellum and contains an arginine residue instead of a histidine at position 100. The histidine is crucial for the binding of benzodiazepines (BZ) to α_1, α_3 and α_5 subunits (diazepam-sensitive) (Lüddens et al., 1990). α_6 subunit-containing recombinant receptors belong to the GABA$_A$ receptors most sensitive to GABA itself. It has been estimated that α_6 subunit-containing receptors are more than 10 times as sensitive to GABA than, for example, α_1 subunit-containing receptors (Korpi and Lüddens, 1993). In vitro investigation of the BZ agonist-insensitive site is hampered by the high endogenous concentrations of GABA, which tend to desensitize the α_6 subunit-containing receptors.

In Vitro Studies

The pharmacological actions of ethanol at the receptor level emerge at about 5–10 mmol l^{-1} and often peak at about 50 mmol l^{-1} (Mehta and Ticku, 1988; Aguayo, 1990; Engblom and Äkerman, 1991). The modulation of the binding of several ligands on the GABA$_A$ receptor occurs only at very high concentrations (100 mmol l^{-1}) as in the case of the convulsant site (Malminen and Korpi, 1988). It therefore seems unlikely that the actions of ethanol would be based simply on specific modulation of the binding of any natural ligand to GABA$_A$ receptors. Ethanol does not consistently facilitate the depressant effect of GABA in biochemical experiments (Harris and Sinclair, 1984; Palmer and Hoffer, 1990). The reason is unknown and may depend on the concentrations of endogenous substances and/or endogenous modulating mechanisms such as phosphorylation or dephosphorylation. In addition, neurosteroids (steroids produced in the brain) appear to induce rapid changes in sensitivity after stimulation by ethanol.

Low ethanol concentrations probably affect $GABA_A$ receptors by inducing phosphorylation coupled to the alternatively spliced long form of the γ_2 subunit. The eight additional amino acids of this subunit form an extra consensus sequence for protein kinase C in the putative intracellular loop (Wafford and Whiting, 1992). Many studies have demonstrated that the phosphorylation of the γ_2 subunit by stimulation of protein kinase C is not the only mechanism by which ethanol potentiates the action of GABA.

The partial BZ antagonists are anxiogenic and are too non-specific, as they bind with strong affinity to several forms of $GABA_A$ receptors. New compounds with a stricter subtype selectivity would be worth investigating. For instance, $GABA_A$ receptor-mediated modulation of the monoaminergic neurones takes place via receptors containing more α_3 than α_1 subunits (Fritschy et al., 1992), whereas the α_1 subunit is much more frequent elsewhere in the brain. It is the α subunit variant that determines the efficacy of the allosteric interaction with benzodiazepine receptor ligands at the $GABA_A$ receptor, one example being the greater efficacy of triazolam than dizepam at $\alpha_1/\beta_{2,3}/\gamma_2$ receptors, whereas the reverse is true at $\alpha_3/\beta_{2,3}/\gamma_2$ receptors. Therefore, ligands specific for the α_3 subunit-containing receptors might be used to alter specifically the function of monoaminergic neurones, which are part of the neurobiological basis of ethanol and drug misuse (see the dopamine section) and the physical symptoms of withdrawal.

GLUTAMATERGIC MECHANISMS

Receptors of the excitatory amino acids glutamate and aspartate mediate fast excitatory neurotransmission in the CNS. Glutamate receptors can be classified into two major families: the cation-channel-coupled class and the metabotropic G-protein-phospholipase-coupled class. The cation-channel-coupled class is subdivided into NMDA and non-NMDA (kainate, AMPA) receptors. The NMDA type receptors are the target of ethanol, which affects glutamatergic transmission in three ways: by interfering with fast excitatory neurotransmission, by promoting excitotoxicity and by impairing neurodevelopment.

Low concentrations of ethanol (5–20 mmol l^{-1}) inhibit both pre- and post-synaptic NMDA receptors. The inhibition is reversed by glycine in cerebellar granule cells, which is a necessary coactivator of the NMDA receptor (Rabe and Tabakoff, 1990). These findings suggest that ethanol competes with glycine to the glycine-binding site. However, others have found that glycine seems to be limited to only some NMDA subtypes since such an interaction has not been observed in the cerebral cortex (Gonzales and Woodward, 1990). In line with these effects of acute ethanol, two recent studies demonstrated that $2\,g\,kg^{-1}$ ethanol provided protection against NMDA-induced convulsant activity (Kulkarni et al., 1990) and cytotoxicity (Chandler et al., 1991).

Chronic attenuation of glutamatergic neurotransmission by ethanol results in compensatory upregulation of NMDA receptors. As a consequence, ethanol withdrawal seizures are blocked by NMDA antagonists. Similar upregulation of NMDA receptors in the locus coeruleus enhances the activity of noradrenergic neurones, thus accounting for the autonomic instability and behavioural agitation seen in alcohol withdrawal. Psychotic symptoms may be explained by the activation of dopaminergic mechanisms. However, the glutamate-mediated increased release is presumably only one of several mechanisms for the pathogenesis of psychotic symptoms.

Little is known about the role that zinc deficit plays in the changes of NMDA receptor activity in chronic alcoholics. Zn^{2+} has an inhibitory effect on NMDA receptor function (Peters et al., 1987).

The upregulation of NMDA receptors renders the central nervous system more vulnerable to excitotoxic insults due to the increase of calcium influx. Comparable mechanisms play a role in hippocampal dysregulation in fetal alcohol syndrome and the damage to the mamillary bodies and several regions in the brainstem and thalamus observed in Wernicke–Korasakoff syndrome (Tsai et al., 1995).

The impaired cognition and blackouts that occur in chronic ethanol abuse may be explained by acute attenuation of NMDA transmission by ethanol. NMDA transmission in the hippocampus is essential for long-term potentiation, a cellular analogue of memory acquisition. The cerebral cortex contains abundant NMDA receptors, which serve an integral role in corticocortical and corticofugal transmission. NMDA receptor supersensitivity may thus account for the diffuse cerebral atrophy seen in chronic alcoholism.

The glutamate-induced impairment of the various cerebral functions could be prevented and treated by NMDA receptor antagonists and compounds which inhibit the propagation of the NMDA receptor-elicited signals. One such compound is acamprosate (calcium acetyl-homotaurinate), which is used to prevent relapse in weaned alcoholics. However, acamprosate does not seem to attenuate ethanol-induced neurodegeneration (see below).

EFFECTS OF ETHANOL ON SEROTONERGIC MECHANISMS

Preclinical studies have demonstrated that enhancement of serotonin (5-hydroxytryptamine, 5HT) function reduces alcohol consumption. Agonists of the $5HT_{1A}$ receptor subtype (ipsapirone, buspirone, 8-OH-DPAT) attenuate ethanol intake in genetically heterogeneous rats (Svensson et al., 1989; Kostowski and Dyr, 1992; Meert, 1993). However, buspirone was without important effects on the high-alcohol-preferring Wistar rats. The $5HT_{1C}/5HT_2$ agonist DOI (1-[2,5-dimethoxy-4-iodophenyl]-2-aminopropane) and the mixed $5HT_{1B}/5HT_{1C}$ agonists m-CPP (1-[3-chlorophenyl]piperazine) and TFMPP (m-trifluoromethyl-phenylpiperazine) reduced alcohol intake in rats (Sellers et al., 1992). The $5HT_2/5HT_{1C}$ receptor antagonist ritanserin failed to alter ethanol consumption (Svensson et al., 1993), whereas others have found reduced ethanol intake (Meert, 1993).

Ethanol potentiates the function of $5HT_3$ receptors at low concentrations (EC_{50} 30 mmol^{-1}). However, this effect is somewhat inconsistent, which may be due to subtle differences in receptor/channel state or post-translational modification (Lovinger and Zhou, 1994). Several studies have been conducted to investigate the role of $5HT_3$ receptors in ethanol consumption. Antagonists selectively atten-uate increases of dopamine levels in the nucleus accumbens produced by ethanol (Carboni et al., 1989) and reduce ethanol intake in the continuous access two-bottle choice test (Fadda et al., 1991). The authors suggest that $5HT_3$ antagonists do not affect ethanol-seeking behaviour, but terminate responding due to an attenuation of ethanol-induced increases in mesolimbic dopamine. In contrast to the above-mentioned findings, ethanol consumption in Wistar rats was not altered by the $5HT_3$ antagonists ondansetron and granisetron (Svensson et al., 1989). Others have pointed out that only low doses (0.001 mg kg^{-1}) of the $5HT_3$ antagonist ICS 205-930 reduce rats' pref-erence for ethanol, while high doses do not (0.1 mg kg^{-1}) (Kostowski et al., 1993).

Platelet 5HT levels are decreased in alcohol-abusing and -dependent patients on the day of acute withdrawal and after two weeks of abstinence (Bailly et al., 1993). Smoking alcoholics have higher levels than non-smoking alcoholics. Smoking alcoholics with antisocial personality have very high levels (more than twice that of non-alcoholics; Rommelspacher and Schmidt, unpublished). Whether this reflects the situation in the brain is not clear.

A deficiency in brain serotonin function could result from a reduced availability of its precursor tryptophan. Tryptophan hydroxylase, the rate-limiting enzyme in the biosynthesis of 5HT is not saturated with tryptophan in the brain (Badawy et al., 1993). In healthy human volunteers, ethanol acutely lowers circulating tryptophan availability to the brain, thus reducing cerebral 5HT synthesis, possibly by enhancing the activity of the tryptophan-metabolizing enzyme, the tryptophan pyrrolase in the liver. In abstaining alcoholics, tryptophan degradation seems to be even greater, causing a decrease in tryptophan availability to the brain. It is, however, unclear whether this decrease and higher liver tryptophan pyrrolase activity in abstinence, which is likely to be associated with it, are due to previous long-term alcohol consumption, or whether they are inherent biological determinants of a low brain 5HT in alcoholism. The latter possibility is supported by the role played by the human tryptophan pyrrolase gene in alcoholism. Activity or expression of liver tryptophan pyrrolase and/or their induction by glucocorticoids may be important biological determinants of disposition to alcohol consumption (Badawy et al., 1993). These findings are also important because it has been postulated that a subgroup of alcoholics with impulse control disorders have low brain 5HT levels. Several studies have been carried out in humans with compounds that enhance 5HT function. When used in combination with relapse prevention psychotherapy, fluoxetine failed to prevent relapse in alcoholics with mild to moderate alcohol dependence and no comorbid depression (Kranzler et al., 1995).

ROLE OF THE DOPAMINERGIC SYSTEM

The dopamine mesolimbic system is a central feature of the neurobiological basis of reward-motivated behaviour. In animal studies, ethanol, opiate, nicotine, cocaine and amphetamine administration activate the system which consists of neurones of the ventral tegmental area which project to forebrain structures, mainly the nucleus accumbens, olfactory tubercle, frontal cortex, amygdala and septal area. The mesolimbic dopaminergic system appears to act as a modulator and gating mechanism for signals mediating basic biological drives (e.g. eating, sexual behaviour) and motivational variables. These signals are thought ultimately to be translated into motor acts.

Dopamine seems to be involved in the incentive aspects of reward and therefore in the mechanism of acquisition and reacquisition (relapse). Once acquired, maintenance of self-administration relates not only to incentive but also, and particularly, to the consumatory properties of the stimulus which might be independent of dopamine (Di Chiara and North, 1992; Herz and Shippenberg, 1989; Koob, 1992). The activity of the mesolimbic dopaminergic neurones is regulated by the tonically active endogenous opioid system, with μ-receptors mediating activation and kappa-receptors inhibiting neuronal activity (Spanagl et al., 1992). It has recently been shown that Δ9-tetrahydrocannabinol stimulates the mesolimbic dopaminergic neurones in male rats (Navarro et al., 1993).

Ethanol-induced release of dopamine seems to be an indirect effect involving endogenous δ-opioid mechanisms in the ventral tegmental area (Widdowson et al., 1992).

Others have postulated that the ethanol effects are mediated by central nicotinic acetylcholine receptors (Blomqvist et al., 1993).

Alcoholics who relapsed within 3 months after withdrawal showed significantly less dopamine-receptor response during early withdrawal (Dettling et al., 1995). The findings suggest that alcoholics with reduced dopamine responsivity have an increased risk of relapse.

ROLE OF THE β-CARBOLINES AND TETRAHYDROISOQUINOLINES

The biosynthesis of the so-called condensation products utilizes neurotransmitters such as dopamine and serotonin as precursors. Since the first steps of the biosynthesis of morphines in the opium poppy are identical with that of the condensation products, the hypothesis was put forward that the products represent morphine-like compounds in mammals. It has been shown that the β-carbolines (BCs) and the tetrahydroisoquinolines (TIQs) have low affinities for opioid receptors considering the low natural concentrations of these compounds in mammals (Rommelspacher et al., 1994). It should be of interest to reveal the role of the BCs and TIQs in the pathogenesis of drug dependence as the plasma levels of some BCs and TIQs are elevated even during long-term abstinence (Rommelspacher et al., 1991). The changes in the concentrations seem to be specific for alcoholism and drug dependence as no changes have been detected in patients with anxiety syndromes and Parkinson's disease. They act as neuromodulatory compounds by inhibiting the enzyme monoamine oxidase subtype A (May et al. 1991) and by activating specific receptors (Pawlik and Rommelspacher, 1988; Rommelspacher et al., 1995) which stimulate the release of dopamine in the nucleus accumbens (Sällström Baum et al., 1995). Thus, the enhanced levels in alcoholics and heroin addicts (Stohler et al., 1995) could activate craving processes.

THE PHARMACOLOGY OF ALCOHOL WITHDRAWAL

Clinical Picture

The physiological symptoms of withdrawal appear when individuals abusing alcoholic beverages regularly and heavily reduce or cease drinking. Approximately one half or more of the patients may exhibit some level of autonomic nervous system dysfunction, including sweating, an increase of heart rate, increases in respiratory rate, and mild elevations in body temperature. Also seen in 50% or more of patients are signs of increased deep tendon reflex activity and tremor. Gastrointestinal symptoms including anorexia or nausea and vomiting are seen in one third to one half, while emotional complaints including dysphoria are seen in 75% or more (Schuckit, 1995).

There are several conditions involved in the much rarer severe alcohol withdrawal syndromes. First, fewer than 5% of alcohol-dependent men and women experience one or more grand mal convulsions. It is estimated that alcohol withdrawal is the most common reason for an acute seizure observed in an emergency room. These convulsions are most likely to be observed within the first 24 to 48 hours of abstinence, usually involve one, or at most several, seizures, and rarely progress to status epilepticus or a condition of repeated difficult-to-control seizures. A second period of increased risk for seizures occurs four to six days after the withdrawal from alcohol drinking. These seizures are usually not observed in clinical practice since anticonvulsant medication is usually administered before and during this period.

The second variant of severe alcohol withdrawal is described as alcohol withdrawal delirium, also known as delirium tremens (DT). This clinical condition is characterized by severe overactivity of the autonomous nervous system (i.e. pulse rates of 120 per minute or more, marked elevation in blood pressure, marked increase in respiratory rate, hyperthermia, etc.), an intensification of the usual hand tremor observed during withdrawal, and severe confusion. In the context of any state of severe confusion, especially with associated agitation, hallucinations are relatively common. These are usually visual or tactile in nature and are likely to disappear rapidly as the state of confusion lifts. Once DT begins, it is likely to continue for roughly five days. Following acute withdrawal a condition is observed that might be described as protracted abstinence syndrome (Schuckit, 1995).

Pathobiochemistry of Withdrawal Seizures

Glutamatergic mechanisms seem to play an eminent role in the pathogenesis of seizures during the first risk period (24–48 hours of withdrawal). The number of NMDA receptors is increased in several brain regions as a result of the alcohol abuse. This is possibly attributable to the development of mechanisms that compensate for inhibiting actions of ethanol (Figure 9.1). Changes in the composition of NMDA receptor subunits (fewer glycine-binding subunits) have been assumed to be caused by chronic ethanol ingestion. It is not known whether these changes have functional consequences (Hoffman, 1995). A greater than normal number of active NMDA receptors stimulate brain neurones after elimination of the 'ethanol-block' in the course of withdrawal. It is therefore interesting that the time course for withdrawal seizures parallels the changes in NMDA receptors in the hippocampus of ethanol-fed mice (Gulya et al., 1991).

During the alcohol withdrawal state, the synaptic release, uptake, and tissue concentrations of glutamine are increased. However, regional variations in these effects are observed, and also in their degree (Keller et al., 1983). Dopamine and noradrenaline release is known to be regulated by presynaptic (NMDA) receptors. It is the upregulation of NMDA receptors in the locus coeruleus and the decrease of α_2-adrenergic receptors that accounts for the autonomic instability and behavioural agitation observed in alcohol withdrawal (Engberg and Hajos, 1992; Matussek et al., 1984). In addition,

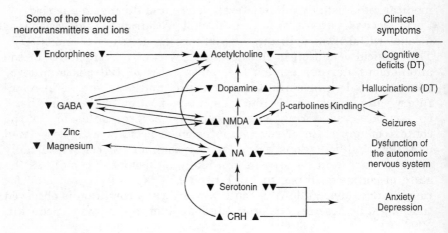

Figure 9.1 Adaptation dynamics of neuronal mechanisms during alcohol withdrawal. The solid triangles before the terms indicate the status during early withdrawal (24–48 h), the triangles after the terms the status a few days later. The arrows demonstrate the interactions between the mechanisms and point to the clinical consequences. Because of the complicated interactions, only the main lines of evidence are presented.

the concentration of magnesium and zinc, natural inhibitors of the NMDA receptor, are often low, which would facilitate the activation of the receptors. Furthermore, repeated withdrawal from ethanol induces kindling processes in the amygdalae and the ventral tegmentum which involve glutamatergic mechanisms (Ballenger and Post, 1978; McCowan and Breese, 1990). Thus repeated withdrawal increases the risk of seizures (Becker and Hale, 1993).

There is substantial evidence that downregulation of GABA$_A$ receptor function as well as upregulation of voltage-dependent calcium channels may also contribute to the symptoms of withdrawal. It is interesting that the required dosages for sedatives, e.g. benzodiazepines, are unusually high during withdrawal (Nolop and Natow, 1985).

It seems that the restitution dynamics vary among the transmitter systems. This may explain the occurrence of a second phase of increased risk of seizures (4–6 days after cessation of drinking). For example, the normalization of glutamatergic mechanisms proceeds faster than the restitution of GABAergic mechanisms. Additional factors must be involved. It has been observed that the natural proconvulsant β-carbolines increase during the first week of withdrawal (Spies et al., 1996; Wodarz et al., 1996). Activating peptides as corticotropine-releasing hormone might also contribute to an increased susceptibility.

The possible contribution of other neurotransmitters in the acute phase of withdrawal as well as a late stage (days 4–6) is depicted schematically in Figure 9.1. The state of the neurotransmitters is indicated by solid triangles. For example, the concentration of endorphines is decreased during the early and late withdrawal period. The arrow indicates that consecutively cholinergic mechanisms are disinhibited. The increased activity of cholinergic mechanisms is caused by the lowered GABA activity and the increased noradrenergic activity as well. In the later period of withdrawal, the cholinergic activity is rather reduced, which may contribute to cognitive deficits observed during delirium tremens (DT). The scheme gives an idea of the complexity of interactions and the dynamics of changes.

Medications

The following proposals for medication are dictated by the aetiological mechanisms presented in the above section. Even alcoholics who are apparently at low risk are assumed to be possibly deficient in folic acid, thiamine, and perhaps niacin. In the absence of stigmata of severe vitamin deficiencies, these problems are usually easily corrected with giving multiple vitamins, including folic acid and thiamine orally for a period of weeks (Schuckit, 1995).

The magnesium deficiency should be treated by substitution therapy (Flink, 1986). A mild zinc deficiency has also been described which can develop with an associated decrease in sexual functioning, decreased night vision, altered protein metabolism, diarrhoea, skin lesions, and a decrease in mental functioning (McClain et al., 1986).

Again, the dosage of benzodiazepines required is high. Sellers and colleagues recommend 20 mg diazepam by mouth every 2 hours up to a maximum of 100 mg on day 1. This dosage is subsequently decreased by 25–50% over the following few days (Sellers and Naranjo, 1986). Additional medication has been described in several monographs.

Another GABAergic compound of interest for drug dependence is gammahydroxybutyric acid (GHB). It occurs naturally in brain neurones and activates GABAergic mechanisms. GHB has been successfully used to alleviate withdrawal syndrome in alcoholic patients (Gallimberti et al., 1992). Preliminary results indicate that it may prove useful in the treatment of opiate withdrawal symptoms as well (Cibin et al., 1993).

Abecarnil, an anxioselective and anticonvulsant β-carboline which acts at benzodiazepine receptors might prove useful in the prevention of withdrawal seizures. It has agonistic and partial agonistic effects on the α_1 subunit with some lower affinity to the binding sites on the α_3 subunit (Stevens et al., 1990).

PHARMACOTHERAPY OF ALCOHOLISM

Until recently, the advances in the pharmacotherapy of alcoholism depended on the availability of medications for other clinical uses. There were two main reasons for this. Firstly, the preclinical findings about the pathobiochemistry of alcoholism were not sufficient to develop a theoretical rationale for specific medications and secondly, the risk of unwanted side-effects was high in long-term treatment with newly developed drugs. Other factors were the lack of interest of the pharmaceutical industry, and in many European countries, the dominance of psychotherapy and pedagogical traditions which prevented the acceptance of alcoholism as a disease with a neurobiological basis instead of a personality problem. Animal studies on the effects of a variety of drugs on alcohol consumption have increasingly set the stage for clinical trials in alcoholism.

In the context of a more rational approach to drug developments, Meyer (1989) has elaborated six major areas in which initiatives in the pharmacotherapy of alcoholism are most promising. These include the alleviation of the symptoms of protracted abstinence, the reduction of the desire to drink as part of a general effect on oral consumption behaviour, the remediation of alcohol induced cognitive impairment, the blocking of alcohol-reinforcing effects, the production of aversive reactions as a consequence of alcohol consumption, and the treatment of psychopathology that is comorbid with alcoholism. Other efforts of researchers in the field focus on matching psychotherapy and pharmacotherapy to specific patient characteristics (e.g. typology) to enhance treatment outcome.

Most of the experience with medication for the detoxified alcoholic has been gained with disulphiram (Antabus). The drug binds irreversibly to aldehyde dehydrogenase. As a result, after drinking alcoholic beverages, acetaldehyde builds up in the body. The intensity of the physical reaction depends both on the blood alcohol concentration (BAC) and on some as yet poorly understood individual characteristics of the patient. Without the intake of alcohol, the alcoholic individual experiences no negative effects of disulphiram (tiredness, sleepiness, dizziness, poor memory, headache, unpleasant taste, gastrointestinal disturbances and rush were assessed; Branchey et al., 1987). On the other hand, possible craving attacks are not prevented by the medication. The physical sensations following consumption of alcohol include facial flushing, palpitations, tachycardia, difficulty in breathing, a possibly serious fall in blood pressure, nausea and vomiting. The most usual reaction begins within minutes to half an hour after drinking and may last 30–60 minutes. Once it has begun, no antagonist therapy is available. Most authors advocate supportive care, antihistamines and antiemetics. Although a relatively healthy individual is likely to tolerate the acetaldehyde-induced symptoms well, they can be quite dangerous for individuals with a history of serious heart disease, stroke, serious hypertension or diabetes. Acetaldehyde binds irreversibly to proteins. Haemoglobin is a well-investigated example (Itälä et al., 1995). Other proteins with free amino- or thiol-groups are also attacked by acetaldehyde with possible toxic damage of liver tissue. Consequently, liver enzymes are elevated in those alcoholic subjects who drink alcohol despite treatment with disulphiram. The increase is correlated to drinking status but not to the dose of disulphiram (Iber et al., 1987) which is somewhat surprising.

Controlled trials comparing a group taking disulphiram with a drug-free control group have shown a higher rate of abstinence with disulphiram. Other studies comparing disulphiram with a placebo have shown a certain superiority of the active drug (Chick et al., 1992). A difficulty with disulphiram is the need to take the drug daily. Investigators are currently working on the development of a long-asting implant. There may be a subgroup of alcoholics who are more responsive to this drug, e.g. those with high levels of functioning and enhanced levels of motivation or those who in the past have maintained abstinence only with disulphiram (Fuller et al., 1986).

OTHER DRUGS OF POSSIBLE USE IN ALCOHOLIC REHABILITATION

In 1992 two placebo-controlled treatment trials indicated that the potent opiate receptor antagonist naltrexone (Trexam) appears to add a significant new potential for alcohol rehabilitation. In one study in which 50 mg of naltrexone were administered per day for 12 weeks to 70 alcohol-dependent outpatient men, no differences were found between the experimental groups as regards the proportion that returned to heavy drinking, but the rate of continued heavy drinking was significantly lower in the individuals on naltrexone (Volpicelli et al., 1992). In the second study, 97 alcoholic men and women received 50 mg per day naltrexone or placebo. From the results it appears that those receiving the active drugs had less severe alcohol-related problems, including better abstention rates, fewer drinking days and fewer relapses (O'Malley et al., 1992).

The effectiveness of naltrexone as an adjunct in alcoholism treatment was demonstrated in consecutive human studies. However, previous animal experiments suggest that the effect of naltrexone might not generalize to long-term conditions (Kornet et al., 1991). In 1995 naltrexone was approved by the FDA (Revia). Safety data indicate that serious side-effects are uncommon. The most common side-effect was nausea, which was usually mild and transient and reported in about 10% of patients. The label contains a boxed warning with detailed information regarding the risk of hepatotoxicity when naltrexone is administered in doses in excess of the recommended dose.

Naltrexone is rapidly and completely absorbed after oral administration but undergoes substantial first-pass extraction and metabolism in the liver (80–90%). Naltrexone has a half-life of about 10 h and a low terminal elimination phase half-life of 96 h (Verebey et al., 1976).

Another potential drug for relapse prevention is acamprosate (Campral), a derivative of homotaurine. The drug has been approved as an adjunct for alcoholism treatment by the French government authorities. Its superiority over placebo has been demonstrated in a multinational trial including several thousand alcoholics. The treatment period lasted 12 months, with a catamnestic observation period of another 12 months. The mechanism of action is elusive. Neurophysiological experiments have provided some evidence of an antiglutamatergic action. The drug is well tolerated. Liver and kidney functions were not disturbed, the effects of alcohol were not increased and neither a pharmacological dependence nor drug interactions were reported (Sass et al., 1996). In contrast to several other medications, acamprosate seems to be specific for alcoholism since the drug has neither antidepressant, neuroleptic, nor tranquillizing properties.

Another treatment strategy derives from animal studies which indicate that drugs which can increase the amount of the brain neurotransmitter serotonin may be associated with a decrease in ethanol intake (Sellers et al., 1992). There is considerable evidence that some alcoholic individuals may have lowered central serotonin neurotransmission (Le Marquand et al., 1994). These results are bolstered by limited clinical studies with serotonin-enhancing anti-depressants, e.g. zimelidine (Zalmid) and fluoxetine (Prozac), which found similar changes among alcoholics. It is important to remember, however, that there is no convincing evidence that antidepressants in general are effective in altering the alcohol intake pattern. No superiority over placebo was found in a recent study with fluoxetine (Kranzler et al., 1995a).

Serotonin-receptor antagonists reduce the preference for alcohol in laboratory rats. One example is the $5HT_2$-receptor blocker amper-ozide (Myers, 1994), another ritanserin (Meert and Janssen, 1991). However, all studies in alcoholic individuals failed to demonstrate a superiority of serotonin antagonists over placebo.

A number of additional potential treatments are also of interest but require further evaluation. Examples include the potential importance of angiotensin-converting enzyme inhibitors, the potential usefulness of dopamine agonists such as bromocriptine (Parlodil) and lisuride (Sitland-Marken et al., 1990), and the possible usefulness of thyroid hormones in alcoholic rehabilitation. The most promising leads to date relate to acupuncture, a treatment of established importance in opiate withdrawal, but even here, larger, better-controlled trials are required before any general recommendation can be made (Schuckit, 1995).

References

Agarwal, D.P., Goedde, H.W. (1990) *Alcohol Metabolism, Alcohol Intolerance and Alcoholism*. Berlin, Heidelberg, New York: Springer-Verlag.

Agarwal, D.P., Goedde, P., Goedde, H.W., Hempel, J. (1989) Aldehyde dehydrogenase from human erythrocytes: structural relationship to the liver cytosolic enzyme. *Enzyme* **42**: 47–52.

Aguayo, L.G. (1990) Ethanol potentiates the GABA_A-activated C1-current in mouse hippocampal and cortical neurones. *European Journal of Pharmacology* **187**: 127–130.

Badawy, A.A., Morgan, C.J., Thomas, R. (1993) Tryptophan and 5-hydroxy-tryptamine metabolism in alcoholism. In Taberner, P.V., Badawy, A.A. (eds) *Advances in Biomedical Alcohol Research*, pp. 231–235. Oxford: Pergamon Press.

Bailly, D., Vignan, J., Racadot, N. et al. (1993) Platelet serotonin levels in alcoholic patients: changes related to physicological and pathological factors. *Psychiatry Research* **47**: 57–68.

Ballenger, J.C., Post, R.M. (1978) Kindling as a model for alcohol withdrawal syndromes. *British Journal of Psychiatry* **133**: 1–14.

Beaman, C.M., Hunter, G.A., Dunn, L.L., Reid, L.D. (1984) Opioids, benzodiazepines and intake of ethanol. *Alcohol* **1**: 39–42.

Becker, H.C., Anton, R.F. (1989) The benzodiazepine receptor inverse against RO 15-4513 exacerbates, but does not precipitate, ethanol withdrawal in mice. *Pharmacology, Biochemistry and Behaviour* **32**: 163–167.

Becker, H.C., Hale, R.L. (1993) Repeated episodes of ethanol withdrawal potentiate the severity of subsequent withdrawal seizures: an animal model of alcohol withdrawal 'kindling'. *Alcoholism: Clinical and Experimental Research* **17**: 94–98.

Blomqvist, O., Engel, J.A., Nissbrandt, H., Soderpalm, B. (1993) The mesolimbic dopamine-activating properties of ethanol are antagonized by mecamylamine. *European Journal of Pharmacology* **249**: 207–213.

Bode, J.C., Hanisch, P., Henning, H. et al. (1988) Hepatic zinc content in patients with various stages of alcoholic liver disease and in patients with chronic active and chronic persistent hepatitis. *Hepatology* **8**: 1605–1609.

Bonetti, E.P., Burkhard, W.P., Gabl, M. et al. (1989) RO 15-4513: Partial inverse agonism at the BZR and interaction with ethanol. *Pharmacology, Biochemistry and Behaviour* **31**: 733–749.

Bosron, W.F., Ehrig, T., Li, T.-K. (1993) Genetic factors in alcohol metabolism and alcoholism. *Seminars in Liver Disorder* **13**: 126–135.

Branchey, L., Davis, W., Lee, K.K., Fuller, R.K. (1987) Psychiatric complications of disulfiram treatment. *American Journal of Psychiatry* **144**: 1310–1312.

Caballeria, J., Frezza, M., Hernandez-Munoz, R. et al. (1989) Gastric origin of the first-pass metabolism of ethanol in humans: effect of gastrectomy. *Gastroenterology* **97**: 1205–1209.

Carboni, E., Elio, A., Frau R., Di Chiara, G. (1989) Differential inhibitory effects of a 5-HT$_3$ antagonist on drug-induced stimulation of dopamine release. *European Journal of Pharmacology* **164**: 515–519.

Chandler, L.J., Summers, C., Crews, F.T. (1991) Ethanol inhibits NMDA-stimulated excitotoxicity. *Alcoholism: Clinical and Experimental Research* **15**: 323.

Chick, J., Gough, K., Falkowski, W. et al. (1992) Disulfiram treatment of alcoholism. *British Journal of Psychiatry* **161**: 84–89.

Cibin, M., Pagnin, P., Sabbion, P.P. et al. (1993) Gammahydroxybutyrate for the treatment of opiate withdrawal symptoms. *Neuropsychopharmacology* **9**: 77–82.

Cooper, S.J. (1987) Bidirectional changes in the consumption of food produced by β-carbolines. *Brain Research Bulletin* **19**: 347–358.

Daoust, M., Saligant, C., Lhuintre, J.P. et al. (1987) GABA transmission but not benzodiazepine receptor stimulation, modulates ethanol intake by rats. *Alcohol* **4**: 469–472.

Dar, M.S., Wooles, W.R. (1985) GABA mediation of the central effects of acute and chronic ethanol in mice. *Pharmacology, Biochemistry and Behavior* **22**: 77–84.

Dettling, M., Heinz, A., Dufen, P., Rommelspacher, H. et al. (1995) Dopaminergic responsivity in alcoholism: trait, state, or residual marker? *American Journal of Psychiatry* **152**: 1317–1321.

Di Chiara, G., North, R.A. (1992) Neurobiology of opiate abuse. *Trends in Pharmacological Science* **13**: 185–193.

Dudek, B.C., Phillips, T.J. (1989) Genotype-dependent effects of GABAergic agents on sedative properties of ethanol. *Psychopharmacology* **98**: 518–523.

Ehrig, T., Bosron, W.F., Li, T.K. (1990) Alcohol and aldehyde dehydrogenase. *Alcohol and Alcoholism* **25**: 105–116.

Eklund, H., Muller Willer, P., Horjales, E. et al. (1990) Comparison of three classes of human liver alcohol dehydrogenase. Emphasis on different substrate binding pockets. *European Journal of Biochemistry* **193**: 303–310.

Engberg, G., Hajos, M. (1992) Ethanol attenuates the response of locus coeruleus neurones to excitatory amino acid agonists *in vivo*. *Naunyn Schmiedeberg's Archives of Pharmacology* **345**: 222–226.

Engblom, A.C., Akerman, K.E.O. (1991) Effect of ethanol on γ-amino-butyric acid and glycine receptor-coupled Cl-fluxes in rat brain synaptoneurosomes. *Journal of Neurochemistry* **57**: 384–390.

Enomoto, N., Takase, S., Yashara, M., Takada, A. (1991) Acetaldehyde metabolism in different aldehyde dehydrogenase-2 genotypes. *Alcoholism: Clinical and Experimental Research* **15**: 141–144.

Fadda, F., Garau, B., Marchei, F., Columbo, G., Gessa, G.L. (1991) MDL 7222, a selective 5-HT$_3$ antagonist, suppresses voluntary ethanol consumption in alcohol-preferring rats. *Alcohol* **26**: 107–110.

Flink, E.B. (1986) Magnesium deficiency in alcoholism. *Alcoholism: Clinical and Experimental Research* **10**: 590–594.

Frezza, M., Diladova, C., Pozzato, G. et al. (1990) High blood alcohol levels in women. The role of decreased gastric alcohol dehydrogenase activity and first-pass metabolism. *New England Journal of Medicine* **322**: 95–99.

Fritschy, J.M., Benke, D., Mertens, S. et al. (1992) Five subtypes of type A γ-aminobutyric acid receptors identified in neurons by double and triple immunofluorescence staining with subunit-specific antibodies. *Proceedings of the National Academy of Sciences, USA* **89**: 6726–6730.

Frye, G.D., McCown, T.J., Breese, G.R., Peterson, S.L. (1986) GABAergic modulation of inferior colliculus excitability: role in the ethanol withdrawal audiogenic seizures. *Journal of Pharmacology and Experimental Therapeutics* **237**: 478–485.

Fuller, R.K., Branchey, L., Brightwell, D.R. et al. (1986) Disulfiram treatment of alcoholism: a veterans administration cooperative study. *Journal of the American Medical Association* **256**: 1449–1455.

Gallimberti, L., Ferri, M., Ferrara, S.D., Fadda, S., Gessa, G.L. (1992)

Gamma-hydroxybutyric acid in the treatment of alcohol dependence: a double-blind study. *Alcoholism: Clinical and Experimental Research* **16**: 673–676.

Goedde, H.W., Agarwal, D.P. (1987) Polymorphism of aldehyde dehydrogenase and alcohol sensitivity. *Enzyme* **37**: 29–44.

Gonzales, L.P., Hettinger, M.K. (1984) Intranigral muscinol suppresses ethanol withdrawal seizures. *Brain Research* **298**: 163–166.

Gonzales, R.A., Woodward, J.J. (1990) Ethanol inhibits *N*-methyl-D-aspartate-stimulated [^{3}H]norepinephrine release from rat cortical slices. *Journal of Pharmacology and Experimental Therapeutics* **253**: 1138–1144.

Gulya, K., Grant, K.A., Valverius, P., Hoffman, P.L., Tabakoff, B. (1991) Brain regional specificity and time course of changes in the NMDA receptor–ionophore complex during ethanol withdrawal. *Brain Research* **547**: 129–134.

Hafer, G., Agarwal, D.P., Goedde, H.W. (1987) Human brain aldehyde dehydrogenase: activity with DOPAL and isozyme distribution. *Alcohol* **4**: 413–418.

Häkkinen, H.M., Kulonen, E. (1976). Ethanol intoxication and γ-aminobutyric acid. *Journal of Neurochemistry* **27**: 631–633.

Harris, D.P., Sinclair, J.G. (1984) Ethanol–GABA interactions of the rat Purkinje cell. *General Pharmacology* **15**: 449–454.

Hellevuo, K., Kiianmaa, K., Korpi, E.R. (1989) Effect of GABAergic drugs on motor impairment from ethanol, barbital and lorazepam in rat lines selected for differential sensitivity to ethanol. *Pharmacology, Biochemistry and Behavior* **34**: 399–404.

Hernandez-Munoz, R., Caballeria, J., Baraona, E. et al. (1990) Human gastric alcohol dehydrogenases: its inhibition by H_2-receptor antagonists, and its effect on the bioavailability of ethanol. *Alcoholism: Clinical and Experimental Research* **14**: 946–950.

Herz, A., Shippenberg, T.S. (1989) Neurochemical aspects of addiction: opioids and other drugs of abuse. In Goldstein, A. (ed.) *Molecular and Cellular Aspects of the Drug Addiction*, pp. 111–141. Berlin, Heidelberg, New York: Springer-Verlag.

Higuchi, S., Muramatsu, T., Shigemorik, K. (1992) The relationship between low K_m aldehyde dehydrogenase phenotype and drinking behavior in Japanese. *Journal of Studies on Alcohol* **53**: 170–175.

Higuchi, S., Parrish, K.M., Dufour, M.C., Towle, L.N., Harford, T.C. (1992a) The relationship between three subtypes of the flushing response and DSM-III alcohol abuse in Japanese. *Journal of Studies on Alcohol* **53**: 553–560.

Hinko, C.N., Rozanov, C. (1990) The role of bicuculline, aminooxyacetic acid and gabaculline in the modulation of ethanol-induced motor impairment. *European Journal of Pharmacology* **182**: 261–271.

Hoffman, P.L. (1995) Effects of alcohol on excitatory amino acid receptor function. In Kranzler, H. (ed.) *The Pharmacology of Alcohol Abuse*, pp. 75–102. Berlin, Heidelberg, New York: Springer-Verlag.

Hsu, L.C., Yoshida, A., Mohandas, T. (1986) Chromosomal assignment of the genes for human aldehyde dehydrogenase-1 and aldehyde dehydrogenase 2. *American Journal of Human Genetics* **38**: 641–648.

Iber, F.L., Lee, K., Lacoursiere, R., Fuller, R. (1987) Liver toxicity encountered in the veteran administration trial of disulfiram in alcoholics. *Alcoholism: Clinical and Experimental Research* **11**: 301–304.

Itälä, L., Seppä, K., Turpeinen, U., Sillanaukee, P. (1995) Separation of hemoglobin acetaldehyde adducts by high-performance liquid chromatography–cation-exchange chromatography. *Analytical Biochemistry* **24**: 323–329.

Jones, A.W., Jonssen, K.A. (1994) Food-induced lowering of blood ethanol profiles and increased rate of elimination immediately after a meal. *Journal of Forensic Science* **39**: 1084–1093.

Jones, A.W., Jonssen, K.A., Neri, A. (1991) Peak blood-ethanol concentration and the time of its occurrence after rapid drinking on an empty stomach. *Journal of Forensic Science* **36**: 376–385.

June, H.L., Lummis, G.H., Colker, R.E., Moore, T.O., Lewis, M.J. (1991) RO 15-4513 attenuates the consumption of ethanol in deprived rats. *Alcoholism: Clinical and Experimental Research* **15**: 406–411.

Kedishvili, Bosron, W.F., Stone, C.L. et al. (1995) Expression and kinetic characterization of recombinant human stomach alcohol dehydrogenase. *Journal of Biological Chemistry* **270**: 3625–3630.

Keller, E., Cummins, J.T., Hungen, K.V. (1983) Regional effects of ethanol on glutamate level, uptake and release in slice and synaptosome preparations from rat brain. *Substance and Alcohol, Actions and Misuse* **4**: 383–389.

Koob, G.F. (1992) Drugs of abuse: anatomy, pharmacology and function of reward pathways. *Trends in Pharmacological Science* **13**: 177–184.

Kornet, M., Goosen, C., Van Ree, J.M. (1991) Effect of naltrexone on alcohol consumption during chronic alcohol drinking and after a period of imposed abstinence in free-choice drinking rhesus monkeys. *Psychopharmacology* **104**: 367–376.

Korpi, E.R., Lüddens, H. (1993) Regional γ-aminobutyric acid sensitivity of t-butylbicyclophosphoro-[^{35}S]thionate binding depends on γ-amino-butyric acid$_A$ receptor subunit. *Molecular Pharmocology* **44**: 87–92.

Kostowski, W., Dyr, W., (1992) Effects of 5-HT$_{1A}$ receptor agonists on ethanol preference in the rat. *Alcohol* **9**: 283–286.

Kostowski, W., Dyr, W., Krzascik, P. (1993) The abilities of 5-HT$_3$ receptor antagonist ICS 205-930 to inhibit alcohol preference and withdrawal seizures in tats. *Alcohol* **10**: 365–373.

Kranzler, H.R. (ed.) *The Pharmacology of Alcohol Abuse*. Handbook of experimental pharmacology Vol. 114, Berlin, Heidelberg, New York, London: Springer-Verlag.

Kranzler, H.R., Burleson, J.A., Korner, P. et al. (1995) Placebo-controlled trial of fluoxetine as an adjunct to relapse prevention in alcoholics. *American Journal of Psychiatry* **152**: 391–397.

Kulkarni, S.K., Mehta, A.K., Ticku, M.K. (1990) Comparison of anticonvulsant effect of ethanol against NMDA-, kainic acid- and picrotoxin-induced convulsions in rats. *Life Sciences* **46**: 481–487.

Lee, L., Schmidt, K.L., Tornwall, M.S., Henagan, J.M., Miller, T.A. (1992) Gender differences in ethanol oxidation and injury in the rat stomach. *Alcohol* **9**: 421–425.

Le Marquand, D., Pihl, R. D., Benkelfat, C. (1994) Serotonin and alcohol intake, abuse and dependence: clinical evidence. *Biological Psychiatry* **36**: 326–337.

Lieber, C.S. (1984) Alcohol and the liver: 1984 update. *Hepatology* **6**: 105–116.

Liljequist, S., Engel, J.A. (1982) Effects of GABAergic agonists and antagonists on various ethanol-induced behavioral changes. *Psychopharmacology* **78**: 71–75.

Liljequist, S., Engel, J.A. (1984) The effects of GABA and benzodiazepine receptor antagonists on the anti-conflict actions of diazepam or ethanol. *Pharmacology, Biochemistry and Behavior* **21**: 521–525.

Linnoila, M., Erwin, C.W., Ramm, D., Cleveland, W.P., Brendle, A. (1980) Effects of alcohol on psychomotor performance of women: interaction with menstrual cycle. *Alcoholism: Clinical and Experimental Research* **4**: 302–305.

Lovinger, D.M., Zhou, Q. (1994) Alcohol potentiation of the function of recombinant 5-HT$_3$ receptors expressed in mammalian cells. *Alcoholism: Clinical and Experimental Research* **18**: 483.

Lüddens, H., Protchett, D.B., Kohler, M. et al. (1990) Cerebellar GABA$_A$ receptor selective for a behavioural alcohol antagonist. *Nature* **346**: 648–651.

Malminen, O., Korpi, E.R. (1988) GABA/benzodiazepine receptor/chloride ionophore complex in brains of rat lines selectively bred for differences in ethanol-induced motor impairment. *Alcohol* **5**: 239–249.

Marshall, A.W., Kingstone, D., Boss, M., Morgan, M.Y. (1983) Ethanol elimination in males and females: relationship to menstrual cycle and body composition. *Hepatology* **3**: 701–706.

Matussek, M., Ackenheil, M., Herz, A. (1984) The dependence of the clonidine growth hormone test on alcohol drinking habits and the menstrual cycle. *Psychoneuroendocrinology* **9**: 173–177.

May, T., Rommelspacher, H., Pawlik, M. (1991) [^{3}H]Harman binding experiments. I. A reversible and selective radioligand for monoamine oxidase subtype A in the CNS of the rat. *Journal of Neurochemistry* **56**: 490–499.

McClain, C.J., Antonow, D.R., Cohen, D.A., Shedlofsky, S.I. (1986) Zinc metabolism in alcoholic liver disease. *Alcoholism: Clinical and Experimental Research* **10**: 582–589.

McCowan, I.J., Breese, G.R. (1990) Multiple withdrawals from chronic ethanol 'kindles' inferior collicular seizure activity: evidence for kindling of seizures associated with alcoholism. *Alcoholism: Clinical and Experimental Research* **14**: 394–399.

Meert, T.F. (1993) Effects of various serotonergic agents on alcohol intake and alcohol preference in Wistar rats selected at two different levels of alcohol preference. *Alcohol* **28**: 157–170.

Meert, T.F., Janssen, P.A.J. (1991) Ritanserin: a new therapeutic approach for drug abuse. Part I: effects on alcohol. *Drug Development Research* **24**: 235–249.

Mehta, A.K., Ticku, M.K. (1988) Ethanol potentiation of GABAergic transmission in cultured spinal cord neurons involves γ-aminobutyric-acid$_A$-gated chloride channels. *Journal of Pharmacology and Experimental Therapeutics* **246**: 558–564.

Meier-Tackmann, D., Korenke, G.C., Agarwal, D.P., Goedde, H.W. (1985) Human placental aldehyde dehydrogenase: subcellular distribution and properties. *Enzyme* **33**: 153–161.

Meyer, R.E. (1989) Prospects for a rational pharmacotherapy of alcoholism. *Journal of Clinical Psychiatry* **50**: 403–412.

Myers, R.D. (1994) New drugs for the treatment of experimental alcoholism. *Alcohol* **11**: 439–451.

Navarro, M., Fernandez-Ruiz, J.J., De Miguel, R. (1993) An acute dose of Δ^9-tetrahydro-cannabinol affects behavioral and neurochemical indices of mesolimbic dopaminergic activity. *Behavioural Brain Research* **57**: 37–46.

Nolop, K.B., Natow, A. (1985) Unprecented sedative requirements during delirium tremens. *Critical Care Medicine* **13**: 246–247.

O'Malley, S., Jaffe, A.J., Chang, G. et al. (1992) Naltrexone and coping skills therapy for alcohol dependence. *Archives of General Psychiatry* **49**: 881–887.

Palmer, M.R., Hoffer, B.J. (1990) GABAergic mechanisms in the electrophysiological actions of ethanol on cerebellar neurones. *Neurochemical Research* **15**: 145–151.

Pawlik, M., Rommelspacher, H. (1988) Demonstration of a distinct class of high-affinity binding sites for [^{3}H]norharman ([^{3}H]β-carboline) in the rat brain. *European Journal of Pharmacology* **147**: 163–171.

Peters, S., Koh, J., Choi, D.W. (1987) Zinc selectively blocks the action of N-methyl-D-aspartate on cortical neurons. *Science* **236**: 589–593.

Rabe, C.S., Tabakoff, B. (1990) Glycine site directed agonists reverse ethanol's action at the NMDA receptor. *Molecular Pharmacology* **38**: 753–757.

Roberts, B.J., Shoaf, S.E., Jeong, K.S., Song, B.J. (1994) Induction of CYP2E1 in liver, kidney, brain and intestine during chronic ethanol administration and withdrawal: evidence that CYP2E1 possesses a rapid phase half-life of 6 hours or less. *Biochemical and Biophysical Research Communications* **25**: 1064–1071.

Rommelspacher, H. (1995) Recent developments in the neurobiology of alcoholism and drug dependence with focus on the contributions of European laboratories. *European Addiction Research* **I**: 20–25.

Rommelspacher, H., Schmidt, L.G., May, T. (1991) Plasma norharman (β-carboline) levels are elevated in chronic alcoholics. *Alcoholism: Clinical and Experimental Research* **15**: 553–559.

Rommelspacher, H., May, T., Salewski, B. (1994) Harman (1-methyl-β-carboline) is a natural inhibitor of monoamine oxidase type A in rats. *European Journal of Pharmacology* **252**: 51–59.

Rommelspacher, H., Sällström Baum, S., Klinker, F. (1995) β-carbolines stimulate benzodiazepine-independent receptor mechanisms. *Society of Neuroscience* **21**: 634.1.

Sällström Baum, S., Hill, R., Rommelspacher, H. (1995) Norharman-induced changes of extracellular concentrations of dopamine in the nucleus accumbens of rats. *Life Sciences* **56**: 1715–1720.

Sass, H., Soyka, M., Mann, K., Zieglgänsberger, W. (1996) Relapse prevention by acamprosate: results from a placebo-controlled study on alcohol dependence. *Archives of General Psychiatry* **53**: 673–680.

Schuckit, M. (1994) Low level of response to alcohol as a predictor of future alcoholism. *American Journal of Psychiatry* **151**: 184–189.

Schuckit, M. (1995) *Drug and Alcohol Abuse*. London: Plenum Medical.

Seitz, H.K., Egerer, G., Simanowski, U.A. (1990) High blood alcohol levels in women. *New England Journal of Medicine* **323**: 58.

Sellers, E.M., Naranjo, C.A. (1986) New strategies for the treatment of alcohol withdrawal. *Psychopharmacology Bulletin* **22**: 88–92.

Sellers, E.M., Higgins, G.W., Sobell, M.B. (1992) 5-HT and alcohol abuse. *Trends in Pharmacological Science* **13**: 1369–1375.

Shibuya, A., Yoshida, A. (1988) Genotypes of alcohol-metabolizing enzymes in Japanese with alcoholic liver disease: a strong association of the usual Caucasian aldehyde dehydrogenase gene (ALDH 2/2) with the disease. *American Journal of Human Genetics* **43**: 744–748.

Shibuya, A., Yasunami, M., Yoshida, A. (1989) Genotype of alcohol dehydrogenase and aldehyde dehydrogenase loci in Japanese alcohol flushers and nonflushers. *Human Genetics* **82**: 14–18.

Sieghard, W., Eichinger, A., Richards, J.G., Möhler, H. (1987) Photoaffinity labeling of benzodiazepine receptor proteins with the partial inverse agonist [^{3}H]RO 15-4513: a biochemical and autoradiographic study. *Journal of Neurochemistry* **48**: 46–52.

Sitland-Marken, P.A., Wells, B.G., Froemming, J.H., Chung-Chou, C., Brown, C.S. (1990) Psychiatric applications of bromocriptine therapy. *Journal of Clinical Psychiatry* **51**: 68–82.

Smith, B.R., Robidoux, J., Amit, Z. (1992) GABAergic involvement in the acquisition of voluntary ethanol intake in laboratory rats. *Alcohol and Alcoholism* **27**: 227–231.

Spanagl, R., Herz, A., Shippenberg, T.S. (1992) Opposing tonically active opioid systems modulate the mesolimbic dopaminergic pathway. *Proceedings of the National Academy of Sciences, USA* **89**: 2046–2050.

Spies, C., Rommelspacher, H., Winkler, T. et al. (1996) β-Carbolines in chronic alcoholics following trauma. *Addiction Biology* **1**: 93–103.

Stevens, D.N., Schneider, H.H., Kehr, W. et al. (1990) Abecarnil, a metabolically stable anxioselective beta-carboline acting at benzodiazepine receptors. *Journal of Pharmacology and Experimental Therapeutics* **253**: 334–343.

Stohler, R., Rommelspacher, H., Ladewig, D. (1995) The role of beta-carbolines (harman/norharman) in heroin addicts. *European Psychiatry* **10**: 56–58.

Svensson, L., Engel, J.A., Harris, E. (1989) Effects of 5-HT receptor agonist 8-OH-DPAT on ethanol preference in the rat. *Alcohol* 6: 17–21.

Svensson, L., Fahike, C., Hard, E., Engel, J.A. (1993) Involvement of the serotonergic system in ethanol intake in the rat. *Alcohol* 10: 219–224.

Takeshita, T., Morimoto, K., Mao, X., Hasimoto, T., Furuyama, J. (1994) Characterization of the three genotypes of low K_m aldehyde dehydrogenase in a Japanese population. *Human Genetics* 94: 217–223.

Tsai, G., Gastfriend, D.R., Coyle, J.T. (1995) The glutamatergic basis of human alcoholism. *American Journal of Psychiatry* 152: 332–340.

Van Thiel, D.H., Gavaler, J.S. (1988) Ethanol metabolism and hapototoxicity: does sex make a difference? In Galanter, M. (ed.) *Recent Developments in Alcoholism*, pp. 291–304. New York: Plenum.

Verebey, K., Volavka, J., Mulé, S.J., Resnick, R.B. (1976) Naltrexone: disposition, metabolism, and effects after acute and chronic dosing. *Clinical Pharmacology and Therapeutics* 20: 315–328.

Volpicelli, J.R., Alterman, A.I., Hayashida, M., O'Brien, C.P. (1992) Naltrexone in the treatment of alcohol dependence. *Archives of General Psychiatry* 49: 876–880.

Wafford, K.A., Whiting, P.J. (1992) Ethanol potentiation of GABA$_A$ receptors requires phosphorylation of the alternatively spliced variant of the γ_2-subunit. *FEBS Letters* 313: 113–117.

Wall, T.L, Thomasson, H.R., Schuckit, M.A., Ehlers, C.L. (1992) Subject feelings of alcohol intoxication in Arians with genetic variations of ALDH 2 alleles. *Alcoholism: Clinical and Experimental Research* 16: 991–995.

Wallgren, H., Barry, H. (1970) Absorption, diffusion and elimination of ethanol. Effect on biological membranes. In Tremolières, J. (ed.) *International Encyclopedia of Pharmacology and Therapeutics* Vol. 1, pp. 161–188. New York: Pergamon.

Widdowson, P.S., Holman, R.B. (1992) Ethanol-induced increase in endogenous dopamine release may involve endogenous opiates. *Journal of Neurochemistry* 59: 157–163.

Widmark, E.M.P. (1932) *Die theoretischen Grundlagen und die praktische Verwendung der gerichtsmedizinischen Alkoholbestimmung.* Berlin: Urban und Schwarzenberg.

Wilkinson, I.K., Sedman, A.J., Sakmar, E., Lin, Y.L., Wagner, J.G. (1977) Fasting and non-fasting blood ethanol concentration following repeated oral administration of ethanol to one adult. *Journal of Pharmacokinetic Biopharmacology* 5: 41–52.

Wlodek, L., Rommelspacher, H. (1994) Ethanol-induced changes in the content of thiol compounds and of lipid peroxidation in livers and brains from mice: protection by thiazolidine derivatives. *Alcohol and Alcoholism* 29: 649–657.

Wodarz, N., Wiesbeck, G.A., Rommelspacher, H. (1996) Excretion of β-carbolines harman and norharman in 24-h urine of chronic alcoholics during withdrawal and controlled abstinence. *Alcoholism: Cervical and Experimental Research* 20: 709–710.

10

Pharmacotherapy of Sexual Dysfunction

Angelos Halaris

Sexual dysfunction can present in a variety of ways and may accompany a variety of medical, psychiatric and psychological conditions. The prevalence of sexual dysfunction is very high but it cannot be accurately determined for a variety of reasons. For one, subjects who suffer from such dysfunction, especially women, are still reluctant to come forward and discuss such a problem with their physician. Many will spend a lifetime enduring the problem, such as decreased sexual desire, anorgasmia or dyspareunia, out of a sense of shame, embarrassment or guilt. Cultural and societal attitudes, even in western countries, very often stigmatize those who 'have a sexual problem'. Then there are many physicians, including family physicians, psychiatrists, gynaecologists and urologists who never resolved their own sense of discomfort in discussing sexual matters with their patients. If they do inquire into this sphere during history taking, they are very often at a loss diagnosing the problem correctly and suggesting the proper treatment approach to their patient. A high percentage of all physicians, independent of specialization, do not possess the skills to facilitate the expression of such personal and intimate matters by their patients. As a result, patients will either avoid the presentation of their sexual problems, or they may mask the real complaint with another, more socially acceptable physical complaint for which there usually is no pathology to be uncovered. This situation partly relates to inadequate preparation of medical students and resident physicians in the recognition and treatment of sexual dysfunction and partly, but equally importantly, to lack of instruction in how to elicit an appropriate sexual history from the patient. Many medical school curricula do not offer any instruction at all in these matters, or, if they do, it is mostly theoretical and not patient oriented.

Although it is being increasingly recognized that sexual dysfunctions are exceptionally common, well designed studies of prevalence are notably lacking. Indeed, the entire literature on any aspect of sexual dysfunction is sparse as compared to a host of other medical and psychiatric conditions which afflict a vastly smaller percentage of the population. Compare, for instance, the literature on depressive illness. In any given year the number of articles which appear in the world literature is at least one hundred-fold greater than the number of articles on sexual function and dysfunction. I do not believe there is any other aspect of daily human function (and associated dysfunction) that has received such disproportionately low attention as the disorders of sexual function. In a widely cited study on the prevalence of sexual disorders, Frank et al. (1978) reported that 63% of the women and 40% of the men surveyed had experienced a specific sexual problem. When asked whether they had 'general sexual difficulties', 77% of the women and 50% of the men admitted to such. What is striking about this study is that the couples these authors surveyed were allegedly well adjusted with a high degree of marital satisfaction. Masters and Johnson (1970) reported that sexual problems can be found in half of all marriages, and other investigators have found that 75% or more of all couples seeking marital therapy experience some type of sexual dysfunction as their core problem (Greene, 1970; Sager, 1974).

During the past few years there has been an interest in the biology of sexual function and dysfunction among human subjects. Since it has been increasingly recognized that certain pharmacologic agents can induce certain types of sexual dysfunction, such as erectile dysfunction, inhibition of ejaculation or anorgasmia, efforts have been made to search for agents which may correct, or at least improve certain types of dysfunction. Our understanding of the complex central and peripheral mechanisms of human sexual response is still woefully inadequate. Consequently, the development and use of pharmacologic agents to correct sexual dysfunction is still in its infancy. Nevertheless, some noteworthy approaches are already available to the general physician. As we advance our expertise and sophistication in understanding the complex interactions between emotional parameters and organic responses in the area of sexual function, more targeted interventions will be discovered.

In this chapter I will attempt to summarize those areas for which pharmacotherapeutic approaches hold some promise to provide at least partial relief, even when the cause or the underlying problem may not be readily apparent. I will use the classification of sexual dysfunction as presented by Halvorsen and Metz in their classic two-part article (1992a,b). According to this classification, there are four major categories: (a) disorders of sexual desire; (b) disorders of sexual arousal; (c) orgasmic disorders; and (d) sexual pain disorders. Each of these categories comprises a number of specific disorders. The specific disorders can be primary or secondary to another cause or factor. These factors can be organic or psychogenic in nature but quite often a combination of factors is present. One hallmark of sexual disorders is that in most instances they tend to assume a chronic course often due to a sense of shame in seeking help or due to an underlying chronic condition such as depression. Acute disturbances are usually drug-induced and, in most instances, will reverse themselves upon discontinuation of the agent, if this is possible. Often, however, this is ill-advised and the patient may have to tolerate the 'side-effect' of sexual dysfunction in order to reap the therapeutic benefit of the drug being consumed because an overriding medical or psychiatric condition necessitates such administration. The final section of this chapter will provide an overview of drug-induced sexual dysfunction.

DISORDERS OF SEXUAL DESIRE

Hypoactive Sexual Desire Disorder

Perhaps the most common sexual dysfunction is hypoactive sexual desire disorder or decreased libido. In western societies this is the most frequent complaint patients present to their family physician if they are comfortable discussing this issue. The degree to which individuals are comfortable to discuss a sexual matter with their physician, or to respond truthfully to a survey even when anonymity is guaranteed, is a main reason why the determination of incidence and prevalence rates for this dysfunction is so difficult to obtain accurately. Another reason is that there is a very wide range in what constitutes normal sex drive across the population. For example, there are individuals for whom having intercourse once or twice a year is satisfactory whereas others may wish or require a frequency of once or twice a day. Many factors influence the intensity and preferred frequency of intercourse, such as partner availability and partner responsivity, age, presence, intensity and duration of stress factors in an individual's life, pregnancy, and nutritional status, to mention only the most common ones. In spite of these confounding factors, the incidence of hypoactive sexual desire in the adult population of the United States has been estimated to be as high as 50% (Frank et al., 1978; Segraves and Segraves, 1991) while the prevalence over one's entire adult life is most certainly much higher. Approximately 70% of those individuals seeking help for this problem are women (LoPiccolo and Friedman, 1988).

Before considering any type of therapeutic intervention, the physician must carefully and thoroughly consider all possible organic factors which could account for the presence of hypoactive sexual desire. A careful medical, psychiatric and sexual history is essential. Attention must be paid to changes in intensity of sexual desire, interpersonal issues, relationship and marital issues, history of alcohol or other substance use or abuse, medication use and life stressors. Reversible organic causes of decreased libido include endocrine factors, pituitary and hypothalamic factors, psychiatric conditions including chemical dependence and drug-induced dysfunction. Irreversible causes include neurologic hepatic and renal disease or terminal illness of any origin (Alexander, 1993). Of the psychiatric conditions which are commonly accompanied by decreased libido (although at times no change or even increased libido may occur) depression is most frequent. Anxiety disorders, in more severe forms, may also lead to a decrease in sexual interest, and obsessive–compulsive disorder often detracts from sexual interest as the patient becomes increasingly preoccupied with obsessive thoughts or compulsive acts. Schizophrenic patients are known to experience fear of intimacy and a primary hypoactive sexual desire disorder may be related to the basic psychopathology of this condition. Antipsychotic medication is generally associated with hypoactive sexual desire and with erectile dysfunction and anorgasmia. However, it is likely that decreased libido may well be a primary symptom of schizophrenic illness. Alcohol use eventually blunts sexual desire and often leads to problems of arousal, mainly erectile dysfunction, which may secondarily lead to decreased libido. Chemical dependency of most any kind eventually depresses sexual desire.

There are certain primary sexual disorders which may lead to depressed sexual desire. Such conditions include erectile dysfunction, retarded or premature ejaculation, female arousal dysfunction (with failure to lubricate), female orgasmic inhibition, dyspareunia and vaginismus (Alexander, 1993). These conditions must be recognized with careful history taking and physical examination and every effort should be made to correct them, if at all possible. Hypoactive sexual desire can then be viewed as an avoidant defence mechanism to protect the patient from experiencing either painful intercourse or embarrassment. Ultimately avoidant behaviour leads to the loss of the desire to engage in sexual intercourse.

Diminished libido is a main feature of major depressive disorder. Upon successful antidepressant drug treatment the expectation is that the patient should gradually return to a normal frame of mind and should resume normal functions and normal patterns of behaviour, including the resumption of sexual activity. Unfortunately, however, in spite of overall improvement, the patient frequently continues to complain of diminished libido and/or difficulties with sexual arousal. This is usually due to the fact that most anti-depressant agents can cause sexual dysfunction as a side-effect. As Segraves (1993) correctly points out, 'it is extremely difficult to disentangle whether the complaint is part of the syndrome being treated or the result of treatment itself'. Here again, taking careful history and ascertaining the extent of overall recovery from depression is critical in making the distinction whether decreased libido is related to inadequate resolution of depression or whether it is a side-effect of the agent used. Tricyclic antidepressants, monoamine oxidase inhibitors, antipsychotic agents (at times used in combination with antidepressants), lithium salts, atypical antidepressants, serotonin reuptake inhibitors and benzodiazepines can all cause inhibition of sexual desire (Harrison et al., 1986; Jacobsen, 1992; Segraves, 1993).

If it has been determined that low libido is a side-effect of the medication used in the treatment of depression, then several options should be considered before discontinuing the agent and/or switching to another antidepressant. Often tolerance to this (and other) side-effects does develop, and, if the patient is willing to wait it out for a few weeks, then this should be the first step. The dose could also be reduced somewhat as long as the therapeutic effect is not being jeopardized. Switching from a tertiary to a secondary tricyclic may alleviate the side-effect (Schubert, 1992). Addition of yohimbine at a dose of 6 mg t.i.d. may reverse low libido, as described by Jacobsen in the case of fluoxetine-induced low libido (Jacobsen, 1991). Substitutions with bupropion may be another approach, as described by Gardner and Johnston (1985). Lastly, the most recently introduced antidepressant into the US market, nefazodone, is claimed to cause no sexual dysfunction. If this is borne out with wider use of the agent, then most certainly this would be a useful choice.

If hypoactive sexual desire is not associated with depressive or dysthymic disorder, is not caused by substance abuse or any other reversible organic condition and is not secondary to another sexual dysfunction, then a careful assessment of its nature must be undertaken before any pharmacotherapeutic intervention is decided upon. Psychological factors, relationship issues and the course of the problem must be carefully and compassionately explored. If it is determined that psychotherapy is the treatment of choice, it should be recommended strongly. However, the results may be slow in coming and therefore pharmacotherapy may be attempted in the interim. Yohimbine has been claimed to enhance libido through central mechanisms possibly involving the noradrenergic system. However, there are no well controlled studies documenting its efficacy in the treatment of low libido. Administration of androgenic compounds (e.g. methyltestosterone, fluoxymesterone, testosterone enanthate) can increase sexual desire in hypogonadal men and in women with low sexual desire. In women the virilizing effects must be taken into consideration. In men with normal levels of testosterone, the benefits are questionable. Lastly, hyperprolactinaemia is associated with inhibition of sexual desire and administration of bromocriptine mesylate to reduce serum levels to normal range is acceptable as long as the origin of the prolactin elevation has been ascertained.

It is quite clear from the above that our armamentarium in dealing with hypoactive sexual desire disorder is very limited. This is due to the fact that the basic neurophysiology and neurochemistry mediating sexual desire is largely unknown. 'Sex drive' is a complex phenomenon that awaits to be elucidated. Until we succeed in clarifying the neuronal circuits responsible for mediating sexual desire, we will not be able to understand exactly what goes wrong when sexual desire is diminished. Specific and reliable pharmacotherapeutic interventions may not become available until the basic mechanisms and the pathophysiology of sexual desire have been elucidated.

Sexual Aversion Disorder

A related disorder, recognized separately in DMS-IV (American Psychiatric Association Press, 1994), is sexual aversion disorder. This entity could be viewed as an extreme form of hypoactive sexual desire disorder, but it is characterized by aversion and active avoidance of genital sexual contact with a sexual partner. The disturbance must cause marked distress or interpersonal difficulty, as defined by DSM-IV. The causes of this disorder can be varied and the only therapeutic approach holding any promise is psychotherapy. If the disorder is related to a specific partner, and is therefore not generalized, changing the partner may be the only viable solution.

DISORDERS OF SEXUAL AROUSAL

Two disorders are subsumed under this category: (a) male erectile disorder; (b) female sexual arousal disorder. In both instances the necessary physiological prerequisites to successful intercourse either do not occur, or, if they do occur initially, they are not sustained. In addition to the lack or inadequacy of physiological response, there is lack of a subjective sense of sexual excitement and pleasure. In men and women the disturbance must cause marked distress and/or significant interpersonal difficulty to qualify as a disorder.

Male Erectile Disorder

Male erectile disorder, also commonly referred to as impotence, is a fairly prevalent sexual dysfunction. It affects 10 million American men and almost all men may experience temporary impotence at some point or points in their life. Recently our understanding of penile physiology and pathology has allowed us to identify the complexity of factors which interact in producing an erection. These are vascular, muscular, cavernosal, hormonal, neurogenic, and psychogenic. In addition, three major pathways of erection have been identified: psychogenic, reflexogenic and nocturnal. Although the end result is the same, the initiation and maintenance of each pathway differs. It is beyond the scope of this chapter to provide details about the physiology and pathophysiology of penile erection. The reader is referred to the article by Carrier et al. (1993) for an overview.

The causes of erectile dysfunction are numerous. They can be roughly classified as organic and psychogenic. It behoves the physician to explore thoroughly all possible organic causes before zeroing in on psychogenic causes. Even when a psychogenic factor appears to be obvious, at least the most common endocrinologic causes of impotence should be carefully assessed. These include pituitary problems, adrenal problems, thyroid dysfunction, gonadal dysfunction and diabetes mellitus. Diabetes mellitus is the most common endocrino-pathy associated with impotence due to the complications it produces, rather than the insulin deficiency *per se*.

The role of androgens in erectile function still remains somewhat unclear. The local erectile response may not be androgen-dependent. On the other hand, androgens are essential for sexual maturation. Androgen receptors have been localized in the limbic system and the hypothalamus (Sar and Stump, 1977; Rees and Michael, 1982) indicating a probable central control of erection. The production of androgens in the testes may be under the influence of corticotropin-releasing factor (CRF) which is also secreted by the testes and stimulated by luteinizing hormone (LH) via $5HT_2$ receptors (Dufau et al., 1993). The possible role of serotonin receptors opens up new ways of conceptualizing the central mediation of sexual desire and sexual arousal. The $5HT_2$ receptor in particular has been more closely linked to depression. Also blockade of the same serotonin receptor appears to be important in mediating an antipsychotic effect. Sexual dysfunction is fairly common in depressive illness and with use of antidepressant and antipsychotic medications.

It was stated above that hyperprolactinaemia is associated with hypoactive sexual desire. It is also associated with erectile dysfunc-tion possibly secondary to hypogonadism induced by high levels of prolactin. The cause of high prolactin levels must be identified and corrected since testosterone replacement in the presence of hyper-prolactinaemia will not reverse the dysfunction (Leonard et al., 1989).

The mechanisms of central and peripheral transmission mediating erection have not yet been clearly elucidated. Until this occurs, our understanding of erectile dysfunction will remain incomplete and hence the development of definitive pharmacological strategies to correct such dysfunctions will be delayed. Indirect ways of under-standing erectile function will continue to rely on drug-induced dysfunction because we can draw inferences from the known mech-anism of action of drugs that induce dysfunction as one of their side-effects. It must again be underscored that erectile function is a complex phenomenon with central and peripheral components. The recent discovery of high concentrations of nitric oxide synthetase, the enzyme that catalyses the synthesis of nitric oxide from L-argi-nine in penile neurones (Nozaki et al., 1993), indicates that nitric oxide may be the most likely main neurotransmitter mediating penile erection. If this proves to be the case, it will pave the way for the development of specific therapeutic agents to correct, at least in some cases, erectile dysfunction.

Presently, the available pharmacological approaches to correct erectile dysfunction are unsatisfactory. Yohimbine, an α_2 receptor antagonist, was mentioned above as a possible agent to correct hypoactive sexual desire. It may also be used to enhance penile erections by inhibiting penile venous outflow (Mazo and Sonda, 1984; Margolis et al., 1971; Morales et al., 1987). The dose is the same (6 mg orally three times per day). Another approach to diagnose and to treat certain types of erectile dysfunction is the injection of papaverine and phentolamine, separately or in combination, into the corpora cavernosa of the penis (Orvis and Lue, 1987). Impotence due to neurogenic and vasculogenic causes and, in some instances, psychogenic impotence unresponsive to psychological interventions, may respond to self-injections of these agents. Aside from the inconvenience, the pain associated with the injection and local complications make this approach cumbersome, at least. However, it may be of help to some men.

An interesting study by Segraves et al. (1991) implicates a central dopaminergic effect in inducing penile erections. In a double-blind design using physiological recording of penile tumescence, subcutaneous injections of apomorphine hydrochloride into the arm elicited penile erections in men with psychogenic impotence. The dose of apomorphine ranged from 0.25 to 0.75 mg and maximal erection ranged from 0.3 to 3 cm. Side-effects included nausea, drowsiness and yawning. The authors concluded that their finding is compatible with the assumption that agents which modify central dopaminergic activity lower response thresholds for erectile and ejaculatory reflexes (Foreman and Hall, 1987). Although they do not suggest a widespread use of apomorphine for the treatment of idiopathic erectile disorder, they do suggest that other dopaminergic drugs may be useful for the treatment of erectile dysfunction.

Female Sexual Arousal Disorder

The normal female arousal response consists of vaginal lubrication and expansion, pelvic vasocongestion, clitoral engorgement and swelling of the external genitalia. Failure to attain or sustain these changes until completion of the sexual activity is the main diagnostic criterion of this disorder. Organic causes of female sexual arousal disorder have not been studied as extensively. However, it is safe to assume that many of the factors that are responsible for erectile dysfunction can also contribute to female arousal disorder. Such factors include pituitary, thyroid and adrenal disorders, cardiovascular disease, neurologic disorders and, of course, psychiatric disorders and psychological factors. Pelvic disease, tumors of the female genital tract and trauma are important factors to consider in evaluating female sexual arousal disorder.

Psychological factors contributing to sexual arousal disorder have not been studied in women as extensively as in men. However, most clinicians believe that the findings in men very likely apply to women as well. The most common psychological factor that inhibits sexual arousal in men and women is depression. By inhibiting arousal through a presumed central mechanism as yet not well understood, depression interferes with erections in men and with lubrication in women. Similarly, anxiety either as generalized anxiety disorder or 'performance anxiety' can inhibit sexual response in both sexes. A host of factors can stimulate anxiety specifically related to the partner or the sexual act itself. A common pathway then leads to inhibition of sexual arousal and orgasmic release. If a clinical depressive or anxiety disorder is diagnosed, then the treatment of choice should be antidepressant or antianxiety medication. However, it should be borne in mind that the very agents which can bring about relief of these conditions may of themselves induce inhibition of sexual desire and arousal. Making the distinction here is not easy, as was indicated above. Many pharmacologic agents are known to inhibit sexual arousal in men and women. They will be reviewed in a later section of this chapter.

ORGASMIC DISORDERS

This category includes three disorders: male and female orgasmic disorder (formerly inhibited male and female orgasm) and premature ejaculation. As defined in DSM-IV, the hallmark of the first two disorders is a persistent or recurrent delay in, or absence of, orgasm following a normal sexual excitement phase. In both sexes the disorder must cause marked distress. We will first deal with orgasmic disorder.

Male and Female Orgasmic Disorder

Both male and female orgasmic disorder could be associated with a general medical condition, such as spinal cord lesion, sensory neuropathies or hyperprolactinaemia. Substance-induced orgasmic disorder is fairly common in both sexes. Here the offending agent must be identified. Depending on the nature of the condition that is being treated, the offending agent may be discontinued and replaced with another similarly acting agent. However, this is not always possible and the physician may have to make the difficult decision of allowing the orgasmic disorder to continue if a more serious problem, e.g. suicidal depression or a crippling panic disorder, must be brought under control with the agent that caused the orgasmic disorder. Outside of these two situations, there are no common organic causes of primary *orgasmic* inhibition in either sex. Psychological factors must therefore be considered in all other instances and the appropriate psychological/psychotherapeutic interventions must be expertly administered.

As will be elaborated on below, certain psychotropic compounds induce an orgasmic disorder in men and women. In an effort to reverse this type of antidepressant-induced anorgasmia, four different agents have been reported to have some success. These are bethanechol (for tricyclic-induced anorgasmia), cyproheptadine, yohimbine and amantadine. I am not aware of any studies in which these agents, with the exception of yohimbine, have been given to men or women suffering from primary anorgasmia. The usefulness of yohimbine remains to be established in more extensive well controlled studies. Until then, any reports of their efficacy will remain anecdotal.

Premature Ejaculation

This disorder is defined in DSM-IV as 'the persistent or recurrent onset of orgasm and ejaculation with minimal stimulation before, on, or shortly after penetration and before the person wishes it', and the 'disturbance must cause marked distress or interpersonal difficulty'. It is the most prevalent male sexual dysfunction affecting nearly one in three males and it may be a lifelong and generalized dysfunction. A situational subtype also exists and its prevalence is hard to estimate. It is safe to assume that almost all men will experience isolated incidents of premature ejaculation due to anxiety, stress, interpersonal conflict, partner novelty and a host of related factors. Isolated occurrences do not qualify to be labelled as a disorder and they rarely come to the attention of the physician or mental health specialist.

The causes of premature ejaculation are diverse and multi-faceted. Unquestionably psychological factors play a prominent role. Physiological, neurological and urological causes do play a role too, but their contribution to the overall incidence of the disorder appears to be less than 10%. A host of theories – psychoanalytic, transactional, personality, gestalt, and learning theory – have been proposed to explain the disorder. It is safe to say that, although they sound plausible and they do at times explain some cases of premature ejaculation, none of them has offered a universally applicable understanding of the disorder or, for that matter, a universally applicable treatment approach. It is now understood that ejaculation results from an interplay between the sympathetic and the parasympathetic nervous system. The sympathetic system regulates the delivery of semen into the posterior urethra while the parasympathetic system mediates the emission of the ejaculate. This 'dual mediation theory' (Shiloh et al., 1984) is supported by the finding that administration of phenoxybenzamine, a potent adrenergic blocking agent, will interrupt the emission of semen into the urethra without abolishing the ejaculatory experience by the subject. For a more detailed review of this topic the reader is referred to the excellent article by St. Lawrence and Madakasira (1992).

We will now focus on pharmacological approaches to the problem of premature ejaculation. It should be stated at the outset that there is no known cure for this disorder. All available pharmacological approaches are palliative in nature, they are inconsistent in their action, and may cause undesirable side-effects that preclude their use. Phenoxybenzamine was mentioned above as an alpha-adrenergic blocking agent that delays ejaculation (and erection) with tolerable side-effects (Shiloh et al., 1984). In daily doses of 20–30 mg it can be used temporarily. Prolonged use may impair fertility by abolishing the peristalsis of the vas deferens, the seminal vesicles, and the ejaculatory ducts (Murphy and Lipshultz, 1987). Tricyclic antidepressants had been noted to cause ejaculatory delay (and at times inhibition) presumably due to their anticholinergic activity, and have therefore been tried, in lower doses, to delay ejaculation (Goodman, 1981; Hawton, 1988). Amitriptyline is usually given 3–5 hours before coitus initially at a dose of 25 mg and gradually increasing until the desired effect is obtained or until limiting side-effects ensue. The antipsychotic drug, thioridazine, has been used for many years to delay ejaculation. It combines anticholinergic and alpha-adrenergic blocking activity, and both of these mechanisms are assumed to work synergistically. Doses start at 10–25 mg and are increased as necessary or until side-effects emerge. Prolonged use of this agent is not recommended since it is an antipsychotic with a complex side-effect profile.

The other tricyclic that has been used successfully for the treatment of premature ejaculation is clomipramine (Eaton, 1973; Goodman,

1980; Klug, 1984). In a double-blind crossover study with 50 subjects, clomipramine was found superior to placebo without significant side-effects (Girgis et al., 1982). More recently, Segraves et al. (1993) reevaluated clomipramine as a possible treatment for premature ejaculation, if administered six hours prior to coitus. They found that 25 mg increased the average estimated time to ejaculation after vaginal penetration to 6.1 minutes and a dose of 50 mg increased the interval to 8.4 minutes. These times were significantly different compared to placebo (51 seconds). Ratings of libido, erections, ejaculatory timing, ejaculatory quality, and overall sexual satisfaction all significantly improved in the clomipramine group. It is not clear exactly how clomipramine produces this effect. It appears that anticholinergic activity may not be the only mechanism responsible for ejaculatory delay. A serotonergic component should also be considered based on the widespread observation that serotonin re-uptake inhibitors (SSRIs) also produce a similar effect which may be dose dependent. Varying degrees of ejaculatory delay or inhibition have been reported with SSRIs, and this side-effect at times may necessitate discontinuation of treatment for depressive illness with these agents. This side-effect of SSRIs, if given in lower doses, may be used advantageously for the treatment of premature ejaculation. In a randomized, double-blind placebo-controlled trial of 52 heterosexual males with self-reported premature ejaculation, Mendels et al. (1995) studied the possible beneficial effect of sertraline. Treatment was initiated at 50 mg per day and was titrated to a maximum of 200 mg per day, as needed, over a period of eight weeks. On a mean final daily dose of 131 mg per day, sertraline-treated patients experienced significant increases in estimated latency to ejaculation and successful attempts at intercourse. This study, although interesting, is by no means definitive. Dosing and timing parameters must be determined before sertraline, or any of the other SSRIs, can be formally approved as an added indication for premature ejaculation. What is intriguing to ascertain is whether an SSRI can be used in the lowest possible dose at a specified interval prior to anticipated coitus to achieve a sufficient delay in ejaculatory response to provide a satisfactory sexual experience for the couple. Chronic administration of any agent should be avoided unless ejaculatory dysfunction is associated with depressive illness, in which case the chronic use of an SSRI is justified.

Finally, monoamine oxidase inhibitors and benzodiazepines may have potential beneficial effects. A case report by Segraves (1987) is worthy of note in a subject who successfully used lorazepam at a dose of 1 mg approximately 30 minutes before sexual activity to achieve a 4–5 minute delay in ejaculation. Clearly, systematic and well designed studies are needed to determine proper procedures with those agents that hold promise to correct this highly prevalent disorder.

DRUG-INDUCED SEXUAL DYSFUNCTION

Dyfunction in this category must be clinically significant and it should result in marked distress to the patient and/or interpersonal difficulty. The offending agent must be clearly identified and a causal relationship should be established. This may not be possible until the suspected agent has been removed; symptoms may persist for a period of time, which may be lengthy, but eventually they must subside. If they do not, then the dysfunction must be reclassified as a primary sexual dysfunction. Chemicals interfere with one or, usually, more phases of the sexual response cycle, or they may cause pain associated with intercourse as the predominant feature. Thus, drug-induced sexual dysfunction can manifest itself predominantly as a disorder of sexual desire, or sexual arousal (e.g. erectile dysfunction or impaired lubrication), or as anorgasmia. At times pain may be associated with intercourse which secondarily may inhibit desire, arousal or orgasm.

A large number of chemicals, including abused substances, therapeutic agents and hormones can cause sexual dysfunction. Space does not permit the listing of and elaboration on, all agents that are known to induce sexual dysfunction. For detailed description the reader is referred to some excellent review articles in the literature (Segraves, 1989; 1993; Halvorsen and Metz, 1992; Brock and Lue, 1993). One should distinguish between sexual dysfunction occurring in association with acute intoxication or chronic use/abuse of substances of abuse and sexual dysfunction occurring in association with therapeutic agents or hormones. The following classes of abused substances are known to decrease sexual desire and to cause arousal problems in both sexes: alcohol, stimulants (amphetamines, cocaine and related substances), opioids, sedative-hypnotics and benzodiazepines. Alcohol may ultimately inhibit desire after an initial stimulatory and disinhibitory phase; it definitely inhibits the arousal and orgasmic phases. However, there is enormous individual variability, and the amount of consumed alcohol and adaptive responses all play a role in the degree of resulting dysfunction. Stimulants do not generally interfere with the desire phase but they do inhibit arousal and orgasmic responses. Opioids exert an inhibitory effect on all phases. Sedative-hypnotics resemble alcohol in their inhibitory effects on all phases. Benzo-diazepines dampen sexual desire (with the possible exception of alpra-zolam); they do not inhibit the arousal phase but they do delay or inhibit the orgasmic responses. The latter effect may be utilized ther-apeutically to assist with premature ejaculation, as noted earlier.

A host of therapeutically used agents can cause sexual dysfunction of one kind or another. The major categories and representative agents will be reviewed briefly.

Antihypertensives

Diuretics

Inhibition of desire is variable but inhibition of arousal is signifi-cant. This is attributed to a direct smooth muscle effect, particularly with thiazides. The latter may also inhibit ejaculation. Spironolactone has an antiandrogenic effect and is known to cause low sexual desire, erectile failure and gynecomastia.

Adrenergic blockers (alpha type)

They do not generally affect libido, but they do interfere with the arousal phase and delay/inhibit orgasmic response. The latter effect can be used therapeutically for premature ejaculation. Prazosin rarely causes ejaculatory problems but has been reported to cause erectile dysfunction.

Adrenergic blockers (beta type)

Animal experiments have strongly indicated that beta-blockers inter-fere with sexual behaviour in the rat, possibly through a seroton-ergic mechanism involving the $5HT_{1A}$ receptor (Smith et al., 1990). Abramowicz (1987) has confirmed loss of libido and impairment of sexual function with these agents. Rosen et al. (1988) have shown that beta-blockers reduce serum testosterone and this may be the mechanism by which these drugs cause sexual dysfunction; propra-nolol is probably the worst offender in this regard. Sexual dysfunction caused by propranolol has been estimated to affect about 15% of patients. However, the newer agents (pindolol, atenolol and nadolol) have much lower rates of sexual impairment.

Sympatholytics

This category includes centrally (alpha-methyldopa, clonidine, guanfacine, reserpine), and peripherally acting (guanethidine, reserpine) drugs. All are known to interfere with sexual desire and sexual arousal. The incidence of impotence and ejaculatory failure averages 20–30% but can be as high as 80%. The centrally acting drugs interfere with the tumescence mechanism, whereas the peripherally acting drugs cause erectile failure and ejaculatory disturbance.

Angiotensin converting enzyme inhibitors

This class of antihypertensives includes drugs such as captopril, enalapril, lisinopril and quinapril. They are not known to affect the sexual desire phase but they may interfere with sexual arousal, although to a much lesser degree than most other antihypertensive agents. Orgasmic response is not affected by these drugs.

Psychotropic Drugs

Antipsychotics

Sexual dysfunction associated with this class of agents is highly prevalent, averaging 25% of all patients receiving these drugs, but it may be as high as 80% (Segraves, 1988). All phases of the sexual response cycle can be affected, although to varying degrees depending on the agent. The reason is that this class of drugs displays different degrees of anticholinergic, alpha-adrenergic blocking activity and a fairly uniform antidopaminergic activity. The latter induces elevations in circulating prolactin which exerts an inhibitory effect on sexual response, as noted earlier. The worst offenders among these agents are chlorpromazine, thioridazine, haloperidol and pimozide. However, there is individual variability and perhaps a dose relationship. The newer agents, e.g. clozapine, risperidone, olanzapine and sertindole, may be somewhat less troublesome in this regard.

Antidepressants

Most of commonly used antidepressants cause treatment-emergent sexual dysfunction across all phases of the sexual response cycle. Sexual desire may be less affected by the monoamine oxidase inhibitors, but arousal and orgasmic response is affected just as much as with the other drugs. Bupropion and trazodone may be less offensive and switching to one of these agents is an option. However, trazodone has been linked to priapism and its use, especially in younger males, is problematic. The picture becomes more complicated since sexual dysfunction very often accompanies affective illness. Distinguishing between dysfunction related to the underlying illness versus a drug-induced side-effect is not always easy and requires taking a careful sexual history. The physician is often faced with the dilemma to choose between continuing to prescribe an agent that may be life-saving versus discontinuing such a drug due to a bothersome side-effect. Segraves (1993) has outlined some strategies to deal with antidepressant-induced sexual dysfunction. They include the following approaches: waiting for tolerance to develop, dose reduction, switching to a secondary tricyclic, switching to bupropion, addition of bethanechol, cyproheptadine or yohimbine.

CONCLUSION

The above list is far from exhaustive; it was not meant to be. Rather, a sample of some of the most commonly used drugs and their potential to cause sexual dysfunction was presented to the reader. Again, there are comprehensive reviews in the literature that the reader is referred to. It should be underscored, however, that sexual dysfunction, whether spontaneous or drug-induced, is highly prevalent in the population. In spite of the high prevalence of these disorders, research is relatively sparse. In particular, research with women is notably lacking and the reasons are probably complex and varied.

References

Abramowicz, M. (1987) Drugs that cause sexual dysfunction. *Medical Letters on Drugs and Therapeutics* **29**: 65–70.

Alexander, B. (1993) Disorders of sexual desire: diagnosis and treatment of decreased libido. *American Family Physician* **47**: 832–838.

American Psychiatric Association Press (1994) *Diagnostic and Statistical Manual of Mental Disorders*, 4th edn. Washington, DC: American Psychiatric Association Press.

Brock, G.B., Lue, T.F. (1993) Drug-induced male sexual dysfunction. *Drug Safety* **8**: 414–426.

Carrier, S., Brock, G., Kour, N.W., Lue, T.E. (1993) Pathophysiology of erectile dysfunction. *Urology* **42**: 468–481.

Dufau, M.L., Tinajero, J.C., Fabbri, A. (1993) Corticotropin-releasing factor: an antireproductive hormone of the testis. *FASEB Journal*, **7**, 299–307.

Eaton, H. (1973) Clomipramine in the treatment of premature ejaculation. *Journal of Internal Medicine*, **1**: 432–434.

Foreman, M.M., Hall, J.L. (1987) Effects of D2-dopaminergic receptor stimulation on male rat sexual behaviour. *Journal of Neural Transmission* **68**: 153.

Frank, E., Anderson, C., Rubenstein, D. (1978) Frequency of sexual dysfunction in 'normal' couples. *New England Journal of Medicine*, **299**: 111–115.

Girgis, S.M., El-Haggen, S., El-Hermouzy (1982) A double blind trial of clomipramine in premature ejaculation. *Andrologia*, **14**: 364–368.

Goodman, R.E. (1980) An assessment of clomipramine (Anafranil) in the treatment of premature ejaculation. *Journal of International Medical Research*, **8** (Suppl. 3) 53–59.

Goodman, R.E. (1981) Premature ejaculation. *British Medical Journal* **282**: 1796–1797.

Greene, B.L. (1970) *A Clinical Approach to Marital Problems: Evaluation and Management*. Springfield, IL: Charles C. Thomas.

Halvorsen, J.G., Metz, M.E. (1992a) Sexual dysfunction. Part I: Classification, etiology, and pathogenesis. *Journal of the American Board of Family Practitioners*, **5**: 51–61.

Halvorsen, J.G., Metz, M.E. (1992b) Sexual dysfunction, Part II: Diagnosis, management and prognosis. *Journal of the American Board of Family Practitioners*, **5**: 177–192.

Harrison, W.M., Rabkin, J.G., Ehrhardt, A.A. (1986) Effects of antidepressant medication on sexual function: a controlled study. *Journal of Clinical Psychopharmacology* **6**: 144–149.

Hawton, K. (1988) Erectile dysfunction and premature ejaculation. *British Journal of Hospital Medicine*, **40**: 428–436.

Jacobsen, F.M. (1992) Fluoxetine-induced sexual dysfunction and an open trial of yohimbine. *Journal of Clinical Psychiatry*, **53**: 119–122.

Klug, B. (1984). Clomipramine in premature ejaculation. *Medical Journal of Australia*, **141**: 71.

Leonard, M.P., Nickel, C.J., Morales, A. (1989) Hyperprolactinemia and impotence: why, when and how to investigate. *Journal of Urology*, **142**: 992–994.

LoPiccalo, J., Friedman, J.M. (1988) Broad-spectrum treatment of low sexual desire: integration of cognitive, behavioral, and systematic therapy. In Leiblum S.R., Rosen R.C. (eds), *Sexual Desire Disorders*, pp. 107–144. New York: Guilford.

Margolis R., Prieto, P., Stein, L., Chinn, S. (1971) Statistical summary of 10,000 male cases using Afrodex in treatment of impotence. *Current Therapeutic Research*, **13**: 616–622.

Masters, W.H., Johnson, V.E. (1970) *Human Sexual Inadequacy*. Boston: Little, Brown.

Mazo, R., Sonda, L.P. (1984) A prospective double-blind trial of yohimbine for erectile impotence. *Journal of Urology* **131** (Suppl.): 234A.

Mendels, J., Camera, A. and Sikes, C. (1995) Sertraline treatment for premature ejaculation. *Journal of Clinical Psychopharmacology* **15**: 341–346.

Morales, A., Condra, M., Owen, J.A. et al. (1987) Is yohimbine effective in the treatment of organic impotence? Results of a controlled trial. *Journal Urology* **137**: 1168–1172.

Murphy, J.B., Lipshultz, L.I. (1987) Abnormalities of ejaculation. *Urological Clinics of North America* **14**: 583–596.

Nozaki, K., Moskowitz, M.A., Maynard, K.I. et al. (1993) Possible origins and distribution of immunoreactive nitric oxide synthetase-containing nerve fibers in cerebral arteries. *Journal of Cerebral Blood Flow and Metabolism* **13**: 70–79.

Orvis, B.R., Lue, T.F. (1987) New therapy for impotence. *Urology Clinics of North America* **14**: 569–581.

Rees, H.D., Michael, R.P. (1982) Brain cells of the male rhesus monkey accumulate 3H-testosterone or its metabolites. *Journal of Comparative Neurology* **206**: 273–277.

Rosen, R.C., Kostis, J.B., Jekelis, A.W. (1988) Beta-blocker effects on sexual function in normal males. *Archives of Sexual Behaviour* **17**: 241–255.

Sager, C.J. (1974) Sexual dysfunctions and marital discord. In Kaplan, H.S. (ed.) *The New Sex Therapy: Active Treatment of Sexual Dysfunctions*, pp. 501–516. New York: Time Books.

Sar, M., Stumpf, W.E. (1977) Distribution of androgen target cells in rat forebrain and pituitary after (3H)-dihydrotestosterone administration. *J. Steroid Biochemistry* **8**: 1111–1135.

Schubert, D.S.P. (1992) Reversal of doxepine-induced hypoactive sexual desire by substitution of nortriptyline. *Journal of Sex Education and Therapy* **18**: 42–44.

Segraves, R.T. (1987) Treatment of premature ejaculation with lorazepam. *American Journal of Psychiatry* **144**: 1240.

Segraves, R.T. (1988) Sexual side effects of psychiatric drugs. *International Journal of Psychiatry in Medicine* **18**: 243–252.

Segraves, R.T. (1989) Effects of psychotropic drugs on human erection and ejaculation. *Archives of General Psychiatry* **46**: 275–284.

Segraves, R.T. (1993) Treatment-emergent sexual dysfunction in affective disorder: a review and management strategies. *Journal of Clinical Psychiatry Monograph* **11**: 57–60.

Segraves, K.B., Segraves, R.T. (1991) Hypoactive sexual desire disorder: prevalence and comorbidity in 906 subjects. *Journal of Sex and Marital Therapy* **17**: 55–58.

Segraves, R.T., Bari, M., Segraves, K., Spirnak, P. (1991) Effect of apomorphine on penile tumescence in men with psychogenic impotence. *The Journal of Urology* **145**: 1174–1175.

Segraves, R.T., Saran, A., Segraves, K., Maguire, E. (1993) Clomipramine versus placebo in the treatment of premature ejaculation: a pilot study. *Journal of Sex and Marital Therapy* **19**: 198–200.

Shiloh, M., Paz, C.F., Homanni, Z.T. (1984) The use of phenoxybenzamine treatment in premature ejaculation. *Fertility and Sterility* **42**: 659–661.

Smith, E.R., Maurice, J., Richardson, R., Walter, T., Davidson, J.M. (1990) Effects of four beta-adrenergic receptor antagonists on male sexual behaviour. *Pharmacology, Biochemistry and Behavior* **36**: 1713–1717.

St. Lawrence, J.S., Madakasira, S. (1992) Evaluation and treatment of premature ejaculation: a critical review. *International Journal of Psychiatry in Medicine* **22**: 77–97.

11

Antioxidants in Psychiatric Practice

Sukdeb Mukherjee and Sahebarao P. Mahadik

INTRODUCTION

Antioxidants are chemical compounds that counter the effects of oxygen free radicals (oxyradicals). Free radicals are chemical species that have an unpaired electron in one of their orbits. Production of oxyradicals is ubiquitous during cellular aerobic metabolism. If produced in excess, or not removed effectively, oxyradicals result in cellular damage, such as peroxidation of membrane lipids, oxidation of proteins, and damage to DNA. Under physiological conditions, damage to cellular elements from oxyradicals is prevented by a complex antioxidant defence comprising antioxidant enzymes as well as non-enzymatic elements. During recent years there has been an increasing interest in the role of oxidative injury and adjunctive antioxidant treatment in various medical disorders. The chemistry and physiology of oxyradical metabolism have been comprehensively reviewed, and only a few salient features will be mentioned below.

First, the meaning of certain terms needs to be clear. Oxidative tone refers to the actual rate of oxyradical production. In humans, this cannot be measured directly *in vivo*. Oxidative stress refers to a situation where oxidative tone exceeds the capacity of the antioxidant defence, either because of excessive production of oxyradicals or because the antioxidant defence is impaired. Finally, oxidative injury refers to the actual damage to cellular elements caused by oxidative stress. It is this that will be reflected in clinical manifestations and complications. Thus, what is of main interest to the clinician is the prevention and treatment of oxidative injury.

DEFENCE AGAINST OXIDATIVE INJURY

There are primarily three sources of defence against oxidative injury: (1) an enzymatic antioxidant defence system; (2) a non-enzymatic antioxidant defence system; and (3) conditions that decrease the production of excess oxyradicals.

The major antioxidant enzymes comprise superoxide dismutase (SOD), glutathione peroxidase (GPx), and catalase (CAT), which work in a sequential and concerted manner. All of these are metalloenzymes. SOD exists in two forms: Cu-Zn SOD which is a cellular enzyme and Mn-SOD which is located in mitochondria. GPx requires selenium as a co-factor, while CAT requires the presence of iron. SOD dismutates superoxide ($\cdot O_2^-$) to form hydrogen peroxide (H_2O_2) and oxygen ($2\cdot O_2^- + 2H^+ = H_2O_2 + O_2$). H_2O_2 is also formed during the oxidation of amino acids by amino acid oxidase, monoamine oxidase, and xanthine oxidase. H_2O_2 is not *per se* an oxyradical because it does not have an unpaired electron, but it must be promptly removed by either GPx or CAT. Otherwise, in the presence of transition metals, such as iron, it is converted to hydroxyl ion ($\cdot OH$) ($Fe^{2+} + H_2O_2 = Fe^{3+} + \cdot OH + OH^-$), the most toxic radical known. In the presence of transition metals, $\cdot O_2^-$ can be directly converted to $\cdot OH^-$. $\cdot O_2^-$ also reacts with nitric oxide to form the oxyradical peroxynitrite ($\cdot ONOO$) which on further metabolism yields $\cdot OH$. Thus, high SOD activity, which results in increased H_2O_2 production, must be accompanied by increased GPx and/or CAT activity to limit injury to cellular elements by $\cdot OH$ radicals. On the other hand, low SOD activity will result in inefficient removal of $\cdot O_2^-$ and increased oxidative injury to cellular elements by $\cdot OH$ and $\cdot ONOO$.

The non-enzymatic antioxidant defence is comprised mainly of urate and glutathione (G-SH), which can be synthesized by the body, and dietary antioxidants such as ascorbic acid (vitamin C), α-tocopherol (vitamin E), β-carotene, and quinones. Their antioxidant roles operate in a hierarchical progression. Vitamin C and urate are the first lines of defence. Next comes G-SH, and only when SH radicals are reduced to 50% or less is vitamin E, which is primarily effective against membrane lipid peroxidation, called upon. Vitamin C plays an additional role in recycling vitamin E from its peroxidized state to make it further available as an antioxidant. There are also other non-enzymatic antioxidants, especially from dietary sources, whose roles have not yet been elucidated.

Finally, there is the issue of oxyradical production. This is dependent mainly on caloric intake because it is energy metabolism along the electron transport chain that determines oxidative tone or the amount of oxyradical production. There is now compelling evidence from animal studies that caloric restriction markedly decreases injury from oxyradicals. The relationship between caloric intake and disease processes in humans is currently an important subject of research and remains to be clarified. The issue of caloric intake is a subject that has received no attention where psychiatric disorders are concerned. Other factors commonly encountered in psychiatric patients, especially those with psychosis or severe depression, are very low dietary intake (starvation), and heavy cigarette smoking and excessive consumption of alcohol, both of which increase oxidative tone.

CONSEQUENCES OF OXIDATIVE INJURY

The fundamental issue is the consequence of oxidative injury on cellular structure and function. The cellular elements most vulnerable to injury are the cell membrane lipids that are peroxidized by oxyradicals, especially ˙OH. The degree of vulnerability is determined by the nature of the fatty acids in membrane phospholipids – the more unsaturated the fatty acids the greater likelihood of peroxidative damage. Because of its very high content of long-chain polyunsaturated essential fatty acid derivatives (PUFAs), the brain is particularly prone to oxidative injury. The situation is complicated further by high energy consumption, high turnover of fatty acids, and relatively low levels of antioxidant enzymes in the brain. The net outcome will be determined by the ability of he brain to remove peroxidized PUFAs and replace them efficiently with normal PUFAs.

If compensatory mechanisms are not adequate and oxidative injury leads to the loss of PUFAs, this can have important adverse consequences for brain function. The most abundant PUFAs in the brain are arachidonic acid (AA) and docosahexaenoic acid (DHA). In addition to its known role as a precursor of prostaglandins, AA is now known to play an important role as a second messenger in a number of neurotransmitter systems as well as for trophic factors that are critical for normal brain development and protection against neurodegeneration. Thus, excessive loss of AA from oxidative injury would impair many aspects of normal neuronal function. The role of DHA is less well understood. However, studies in animals indicate that DHA deprivation in early life affects brain development and, subsequently, results in behavioural and learning abnormalities.

OXIDATIVE INJURY IN PSYCHIATRIC DISORDERS

There has been little systematic research on oxidative injury in psychiatric disorders. One study found increased levels of membrane lipid peroxidation products in the cerebrospinal fluid (CSF) of neuroleptic-treated patients, especially those with parkinsonism. Subsequently, increased membrane lipid peroxidation products were reported in the CSF as well as plasma of patients with tardive dyskinesia. Because tardive dykinesia is commonly assumed to be an adverse effect of neuroleptic treatment, the focus came to rest on oxidative injury as a consequence of neuroleptic treatment. These findings appear to be consonant with a number of studies that found the activities of one or more of the antioxidant enzymes to be abnormal in neurolepic-treated schizophrenic patients as well as animals.

The assumption that neuroleptic treatment may be associated with oxidative injury, particularly in those who develop tardive dyskinesia, led to a number of therapeutic trials of vitamin E, a potent membrane-protecting antioxidant, in patients with tardive dyskinesia. With few exceptions, these studies reported amelioration of dyskinesia severity after such treatment. This has led to the recent initiation of a multicentre placebo-controlled study at nine Department of Veterans Administration Medical Centers to examine more systematically the therapeutic potential of vitamin E in patients with tardive dyskinesia.

However, more recent evidence from a study of never-medicated first-episode psychosis patients indicate that the enzymatic antioxidant defence is impaired and plasma levels of membrane lipid peroxidation products are elevated at the onset of psychosis before initiation of neuroleptic treatment. Thus, regardless of neuroleptic effects, oxidative injury appears to be present at the onset of non-affective psychosis.

Unfortunately, there has been no methodologically acceptable investigation of oxidative stress and oxidative injury in other psychiatric disorders, and no investigation of oxidative injury to cellular proteins or DNA in any psychiatric disorder.

ANTIOXIDANTS IN PSYCHIATRIC PRACTICE

Based on the preliminary evidence available, what can one conclude about the use of antioxidants in psychiatric practice? Related questions are – if antioxidants are indicated, what antioxidant should be used, in whom, and when?

Clearly the adverse effects of oxidative stress are not specific to psychiatric disorders and have been implicated in a host of medical disorders, such as Parkinson's disease, Alzheimer's disease, non-insulin-dependent diabetes mellitus, and amyotrophic lateral sclerosis. This 'non-specificity' should not be an issue if one considers the possibility that oxidative stress or oxidative injury does not play a causal role in these disorders but, rather, modifies in an adverse manner their course and outcome. If this position is assumed, better control of oxidative stress might contribute to avoiding a deteriorating course or a refractory clinical state.

Insofar as schizophrenia is concerned, there is compelling evidence of an impaired endogenous enzymatic antioxidant defence system and increased peroxidative damage to cell plasma membrane lipids. Whether or not neuroleptic treatment aggravates or ameliorates the problem has not be systematically investigated. Regardless, the problem of oxidative injury appears to be present both in untreated and in neuroleptic-treated schizophrenic patients.

It is well documented that the typical American diet is seriously deficient in antioxidants. To add to this, a high caloric diet and intake of red meats will increase oxidative tone, exacerbating the oxidative stress. On the other hand, the reduced appetite and poor caloric intake of a depressed patient might also increase oxidative stress. Also, there is the heavy cigarette smoking and excessive use of alcohol that are associated with both schizophrenic and mood disorders. While it might be ideal to advocate a major dietary overhaul with cessation of smoking, avoidance of excess alcohol, etc., this approach is likely to fail in most cases where patients with serious mental disorders are concerned, at least during the initial stages of treatment.

Admittedly the suggestions proposed below rest on preliminary evidence. However, the dictum 'above all, do no harm' is not violated. The use of pharmacological doses of antioxidants should not be associated with adverse effects. On the other hand, they may provide benefits by protecting cells against oxidative injury. Also, it must be noted that prevention is better than cure. It is on these bases that the following therapeutic approaches are proposed.

For all patients with major psychiatric disorders, a careful dietary evaluation should be made to determine caloric intake and dietary intake of antioxidants and pro-oxidants. Every patient should be considered as a unique individual and a Procrustean bed should not be the goal. Where schizophrenic psychosis is concerned, the available evidence indicates the use of adjunctive antioxidant treatment from the very beginning of treatment. This should be complemented by advice regarding dietary improvement, smoking cessation, and avoidance of alcohol. A similar approach may be taken with other disorders.

Adjunctive antioxidant treatments should comprise at least vitamin E at daily doses of 1000–1200 IU along with vitamin C 1000 mg daily. It might be easier to prescribe one capsule of 25 000 IU of β-carotene daily than to convince the patient to eat half a cup of carrots daily. To decrease oxidative tone, the patient should be advised to limit the intake of red meats. This may be difficult. There are as yet no clear guidelines as to how much red meat is safe and acceptable for those with an impaired antioxidant defence. In our experience, the most difficult task is to get patients to reduce their caloric intake to a reasonable level. Caloric restriction which has been shown to decrease oxidative stress is a daily intake of about 1600 calories for those living a sedentary life. A dietary survey at our centre revealed that most schizophrenic patients have a daily caloric intake of around 2400–2800 per day. Smoking cessation is probably the most difficult step of all. Regrettably, there has been very little done to reduce the heavy smoking of psychotic patients.

The two final questions are probably the most easy to answer. To limit oxidative stress should be a goal for all psychiatric patients, and this should be implemented as early as possible during the course of their illness. One can argue that there is insufficient empirical evidence to support such a therapeutic approach. We would agree with that. However, there is one body of evidence that has gone ignored that supports this approach. Cross-national studies co-ordinated by the World Health Organization – the International Pilot Study of Schizophrenia and Determinants of Outcomes of Severe

Mental Disorders – found the outcome to be far better for patients in India than for patients in industrialized urbanized countries, such as the USA, UK, and Denmark. This was so even though very few of the patients in India followed through with maintenance treatment. Using data from the Food and Agricultural Organization and an ecological approach, Danish investigators found that more than 80% of the cross-national variance in outcome could be accounted for by the ratio of dietary intake of fats from animal and bird sources to dietary intake of fats from fish and vegatable sources. Little attention has been paid to this finding. High intake of fats from animal sources is associated with increased oxidative tone. Higher intake of fats from fish and vegetable sources is associated with lower oxidative tone and greater intake of omega-3 essential fatty acids. Thus, it remains a viable possibility that dietary factors that reduce oxidative tone and provide a more balanced essential fatty acid composition might influence the outcome of severe mental disorders.

We do not wish to detract from the importance of developing safer and more efficient neuroleptic and antidepressent drugs. However, conventional pharmacotherapy alone might not be sufficient to contain the course of severe mental disorders, if indeed, as the emerging data are indicating, there is ongoing insult from oxidative stress and impaired essential fatty acid metabolism. These must be addressed, or we can ignore them to the peril of our patients.

Suggested Further Reading

Adler, L.A., Peselow, E., Rotrosen, J. et al. (1993) Vitamin E treatment of tardive dyskinesia. *American Journal of Psychiatry* **150**: 1405–1407.

Allen, R.G. (1991) Oxygen-reactive species and antioxidant responses during development: the metabolic paradox of cellular differentiation. *Proceedings of the Society for Experimental Biology and Medicine* **196**: 117–129.

Bourre, J.-M., Francois, M., Youyou, A. et al. (1989) The effects of dietary α-linolenic acid on the composition of nerve membranes, enzymatic activity, amplitude of electropysiological parameters, resistance to poisons and performance of learning tasks in rats. *Journal of Nutrition* **119**: 1880–1892.

Cadet, J.L., Lohr, J.B. (1987) Free radicals and the developmental pathology of schizophrenic burnout. *Integrative Psychiatry* **5**: 40–48.

Crawford, M.A. (1993) The role of essential fatty acids in neural development: implications for perinatal nutrition. *American Journal of Clinical Nutrition* **57** (Suppl): 703S-710S.

Halliwell, B., Gutteridge, J.M.C. (1989) *Free Radicals in Biology and Medicine*, 2nd edn. Oxford: Clarendon Press.

Miguel, A., Quintanilha, A.T., Weber, H. (eds) (1989) *CRC Handbook of Free*

Radicals and Antioxidants in Biomedicine, Vols I–III. Boca Raton, FL: CRC Press.

Neuringer, M., Connor, W.E., Lin, D.S. et al. (1986) Biochemical and functional effect of prenatal and postnatal ω-3 fatty acid deficiency on retina and brain in rhesus monkeys. *Proceedings of the National Academy of Sciences, USA* **83**: 4021–4025.

Reddy, R., Mahadik, S.P., Mukherjee, S. et al. (1991) Enzymes of the antioxidant defense system in chronic schizophrenic patients. *Biological Psychiatry* **30**: 409–412.

Wainwright, P.E. (1992) Do essential fatty acids play a role in brain and behavioral development? *Neuroscience and Biobehavioral Reviews* **16**: 193–205.

12

Transcultural Psychiatry

Eric Johnson-Sabine

INTRODUCTION

Transcultural psychiatry is a difficult term to define. It has come to embrace the understanding of mental illness from different cultural perspectives. It also includes how the presentation of mental illness may result from the interaction of different cultures. A further factor complicating the relationship between culture and mental illness is the effect of racism.

Culture has been defined as 'that complex whole which includes knowledge, belief, art, morals, law, custom, and any other capabilities and habits acquired by man as a member of society' (Tyler, 1874) and, more simply, as 'a blueprint for living' (Kluckholm, 1944).

Fernando explains the complex interrelationship of culture, race and ethnicity:

> [Culture] is often compared with race both in common parlance and in professional thinking, mainly because people who are seen as racially different are conceptualized as having different cultures, and the term culture is used to conceal racism. The concept of ethnicity in social science literature and in popular thinking has replaced, to some degree, both race or culture as a basis for defining, meaningfully, groups of people who feel themselves to be separate in multiracial and multicultural societies. Ethnicity has both racial and cultural connotations but its main characteristic is that it implies a sense of belonging.
>
> (Fernando, 1988)

MIGRATION AND MENTAL ILLNESS

For an individual the experience of confronting and adjusting to a different culture is met after migration. The migration from one distinct environment to another (e.g. rural to urban) and, in particular, across significant geographical distances, is likely to be accompanied by psychological sequelae. However, how such psychological reactions are manifested is dependent on factors associated with the migrant, the circumstances of migration and the society to which he migrates.

Migration may be associated with *culture shock*. This is the initial destabilizing stage of adjustment to living in another culture without customary cues governing social behaviour. The adjustment reaction has also been called *uprooting disorder* (Zwingmann and Gunn, 1983). The disorder develops if social relationships continue to be unpredictable; there are feelings of nostalgia and a sense of loss of familiar supports. Ideally there should be gradual resolution of these difficulties in due course when a greater sense of integration and security develops that is allied to a sense of belonging. Where there is no resolution of feelings the migrant may go on to develop psychiatric illness.

Rack (1982) categorizes migrants into three groups that sometimes overlap: the settler, the exile and the gastarbeiter or migrant worker. These have different combinations of push and pull factors accounting for their desire to migrate. Of these groups, the exiles, or political refugees, have often been separated from their families and exposed to severe psychological trauma and even torture. They may develop psychiatric symptoms after migration including post-traumatic stress disorder (Turner and Gorst-Unsworth, 1990) and affective psychosis (King et al., 1994).

Acculturation is the process of settling and adaption by the migrant to the host community and the reaction of the host community to the migrant. If the migrant values and adopts the new culture and discards his old cultural values then assimilation takes place. If old cultural values are retained and the host community respects alternative cultural values then integration can occur. If neither the migrant nor the host community value each other's culture then there will be pressures to marginalize, separate from or reject the migrant by the host community (Rack, 1982; Mavreas and Bebbington, 1990).

Two main theories have been advanced to explain increased rates of mental illness in some migrant groups. The first is based on the hypothesis that the stress of migration combined with the hostility of the host community leads to a psychological reaction which may develop into a major psychiatric illness (the stress hypothesis). The second is based on the hypothesis that people who are liable to develop a mental illness and are unsettled in their native environment are more likely than others to migrate (the selection hypothesis).

Murphy (1977) has postulated a third hypothesis that the observed differences in rates of mental illness, rather than resulting from migration itself, may represent a different pattern of disorder in the migrant's culture of origin. The selection hypothesis appeared to be supported by early work showing higher rates of mental disorder in Norwegian immigrants to America compared with non-migrant Norwegians and other Americans (Ødegaard, 1932). However, rates of mental illness appeared to reduce towards the population norms for descendants of immigrants, which supported the stress hypothesis (Sanua, 1969).

Later studies have shown that the psychological reaction to migration is more complicated and varies between different ethnic groups who have different reasons for migration and are differentially accepted into their new environment. It has been strongly argued that racist attitudes of the host community are of paramount importance in provoking mental illness in migrants (Fernando, 1988; Burke, 1986). Burke (1986) identifies racism as the means by which social deprivation in its victims is generated and maintained. He argues that institutional racism then prevents those who have impaired mental health from receiving proper care and finally the host society uses methods of social control including false diagnosis and inappropriate use of psychiatric treatments to enforce subordination.

Other factors have been identified which affect the likelihood of migration being accompanied by psychiatric illness. The circumstances of migration, including its legality and whether it was voluntary or imposed, affect the subsequent adjustment of the migrant (Littlewood and Lipsedge, 1982). Isolation, separation from family, communication difficulties and social hardship all contribute to psychological impairment (Cox, 1977; Herz, 1988).

PSYCHIATRIC ILLNESS AMONG MINORITY GROUPS IN THE UK

There have been many studies of migrants from various parts of the world to the UK. These studies often group together migrants who come from very different cultural backgrounds, e.g. West Indies and Africa. Some of the studies have poor control groups which have failed to correct for the younger age structure and excess of males in migrant groups and studies have often ignored the confounding effects of racism.

Hospital admissions in the UK for psychotic disorders in people from the Indian sub-continent have been reported as being both higher and lower than those in the base population (Teague, 1993; Thomas et al 1993). Dean et al. (1981b) showed that Asians of Indian origin had three times the expected rate of schizophrenia. The Asians of Pakistani origin had rates of schizophrenia similar to the native population. In contrast, Cochrane (1977) showed an over-representation of Pakistanis admitted with a diagnosis of schizophrenia. Cochrane and Bal (1987) showed high rates of first admissions for schizophrenia for Pakistani men and Indian women, but Pakistani women appeared to have significantly lower rates. These conflicting findings are difficult to interpret, but it appears that major differences may exist within the Asian community. Brewin (1980) has suggested that living in an extended family in a close community may be an important protective factor against severe mental illness in the British Asian community. However, sound evidence for this cultural stereotype is lacking (Sashidharan, 1993) and Fernando (1988) warns that the stereotype of the supportive, closeknit Asian family may result in their being denied services.

Studies of depression in Asian patients show rates similar to the general population (Dean et al., 1981b), although some studies have reported lower rates (Cochrane, 1977).

Investigations of neurosis in British Asians also fail to show consistent results. Ndetei and Vadher (1984) showed high scores for somatic symptoms in Asian immigrants along with African and Caribbean patients but Brewin (1980) showed that Asian patients consulted general practitioners at the same rates as an English sample for all types of complaints. Johnson (1986) found that Asians consulted their general practitioners more often than did other groups, but did not find evidence to support excess somatization. Dean et al. (1981b) showed that, on their in-patient sample, Pakistanis had significantly lower rates than the base population for alcoholism and personality disorders for men and lower rates of neurosis for men and women.

Attempted suicide was formerly reported as being below the rate of the general population for Asian patients (Burke 1976a). Subsequently, there has been an increase in overdoses in young Asian women. One study showed the rate for patients treated in Casualty Departments was double that for young white women (Merrill and Owens, 1988). Young British Asian females have also been shown to have higher rates of symptoms of bulimia nervosa compared with white females (Whitehouse and Mumford, 1988).

Community studies undertaken by Cochrane and Stopes-Roe (1977, 1981) and Stopes-Roe and Cochrane (1980) showed inconsistent rates for minor neurotic symptoms in Asians compared with white groups. Overall, Cochrane (1983) considered that Asians suffered less psychiatric morbidity than the general population.

Psychiatric illness among Africans in the UK has been examined in a number of studies. One study identified African patients, of all minority groups, as having proportionately the greatest contact with specialist psychiatric services (Bagley, 1971). An apparent high incidence of schizophrenia has been identified among African immigrants (Rwegellera, 1977; Littlewood and Lipsedge, 1981). Studies appeared to show an earlier onset of symptoms compared with other immigrant groups and an over-representation of male admissions. Rwegellera (1980) showed high rates of compulsory admissions in this patient group. These studies are flawed by the heterogeneous composition of the patient groups and by having small numbers.

The rates for depression and neurosis among African immigrants are inconsistent.

For Irish-born patients in the UK, Dean et al. (1981a) showed that, for first admissions, the rate of schizophrenia was 2.4 times the expected number. They also showed 5.3 times the expected rate of admission for alcoholism in males and four times the expected rate for females. Murphy (1986) has suggested that social insecurity may account for the high rates of alcoholism.

For neurosis, one study showed Irish patients to have more symptoms than English patients (Kelleher, 1972) but the reverse was found by another study (Cochrane and Stopes-Roe, 1979). Relatively high rates of suicide and attempted suicide among Irish-born patients have been reported compared with English patients (Burke, 1976b; Cochrane, 1977).

Afro-Caribbeans in the UK have consistently been shown to have higher rates of admission to hospital and more often receive a diagnosis of schizophrenia than do members of other ethnic groups.

Two studies have adopted a prospective methodology: Harrison et al. (1988) found an increased rate of schizophrenia in Afro-Caribbean migrants which was larger again for British born, second generation Afro-Caribbean patients; King et al. (1994) also showed high rates for Afro-Caribbean patients who were all British born but also showed high rates for all other ethnic minority groups.

Wessely et al. (1991) used a case control methodology to avoid problems with inaccurate denominators (i.e. the numbers of British Afro-Caribbean people in the general population). They calculated the odds ratio for schizophrenia in Afro-Caribbean and white patients over a 20-year period up to 1984. They showed that Afro-Caribbeans were at an elevated risk of schizophrenia and that this risk had increased over the study period.

Criticisms have been levelled against the validity of the repeated findings of high rates of schizophrenia in Afro-Caribbean patients. Numbers of patients in these studies are small so that slight increases have major effects on rates. Even the well-designed studies have had difficulties with calculating the numbers of Afro-Caribbean people in the general population which has been complicated by a low registration of young black males in the National Census.

Littlewood and Lipsedge (1981) have drawn attention to the over-diagnosis of schizophrenia in black patients. They have reported that patients with religious delusions and possibly suffering from an 'acute psychotic reaction' are likely to be diagnosed as having schizophrenia, especially if they are of Caribbean origin. Other studies that have paid particular attention to diagnosis have failed to identify an 'atypical psychosis' among patients of Afro-Caribbean origin (Harvey et al., 1990; King et al., 1994) and the criticism that UK psychiatrists would overdiagnose schizophrenia in Afro-Caribbeans is disputed (Lewis et al., 1990).

There remains the possibility of a category fallacy as described by Kleinman (1987), namely that European diagnostic concepts are inappropriately applied to patients with different cultural backgrounds. Outcome studies could help answer this criticism. Littlewood and Lipsedge (1982) have pointed out that twice as many black patients compared with whites had their diagnosis changed during the course of their psychiatric career, which may indicate a different pattern or course of the disorder among apparently psychotic black patients.

Littlewood and Lipsedge (1988) have also observed that black patients present with schizophrenia at a younger age. This was confirmed in the prospective study of King et al. (1994). The *lifetime* incidence of Afro-Caribbean patients may therefore be closer to the incidence of the base population. Glover et al. (1994), using data from admissions to three London health districts, suggests that the high incidence of schizophrenia in British, Afro-Caribbeans could be explained by a cohort effect. Those with high risk of schizophrenia appear mainly to have been born before 1966 and after 1950 suggesting that they are in a tightly delineated birth cohort.

Hickling (1991a) has studied the prevalence of schizophrenia in Jamaica where he found an admission rate for schizophrenia five to six times lower than the rate reported for Afro-Caribbeans in the UK. In another study, he compared the psychopathology of a group of Afro-Caribbean migrants who returned to Jamaica after an average of 12 years abroad with a matched control sample of Jamaicans who had never migrated (Hickling, 1991b). These were selected samples and not representative of their respective populations but nevertheless showed a higher frequency of mental hospital admissions for the ex-migrants. Ninety-four percent of the admissions had been for schizophrenia. The ex-migrants continued to show significant psychopathology and experienced significant social stress both abroad and after returning home. In Hickling's view, his findings taken together 'suggest that high admission rates of schizophrenia for Caribbean migrants to the UK and elsewhere is peculiar to that group'.

Sashidharan (1993) points out that if apparent rates of schizophrenia are not declining with successive generations of Afro-Caribbeans in the UK (McGovern and Cope, 1987; Harrison et al., 1988; King et al., 1994) it suggests that the direct psychological effects of migration are not applicable. He argues that the most important determinant of mental health in black patients in the UK is the condition under which they live and that social and demographic factors prevalent in the black community could account for the higher rates. He expresses concern that scientific interest in high rates of mental disorder in one ethnic group which is then attributed to cultural factors is an abandonment of cultural relativism and perhaps is driven by the ideas of 'race science'. Historically, race science sought to identify biological weakness in non-European races. Sashidharan suggests that the concept of 'ethnic vulnerability' to schizophrenia is close to a belief in a biological vulnerability.

With these observations borne in mind, Eagles (1991) has explored the biological hypothesis that might explain the apparent increased rates of schizophrenia among Afro-Caribbean immigrants. He raises the possibility that aetiological factors may include viral and other infective agents, obstetric complications and, least convincingly, genetic mutations.

Rates of affective disorders among Afro-Caribbean patients appear to be similar to the base population. Rates of less severe psychiatric disorder are inconsistent and are affected by service provision and utilization.

Littlewood and Lipsedge (1989) argue that attention is directed mainly towards mental health problems in black patients rather than towards what might be learned from areas where they have better mental health. There is a continual focus on the negative aspects of mental health problems of Afro-Caribbeans. In this respect there is a link between black patients having a problem and being a problem.

Both rates of alcoholism and attempted suicide appear to be low in the British Afro-Caribbean population but these disorders have not been extensively studied in the black British population.

Halpern (1993) suggested that, for most ethnic minority groups, their psychiatric morbidity is related to the ethnic density of the area in which they live. Members of ethnic minorities living in areas of low density suffer more prejudice and less support which may contribute to their developing psychiatric illness.

USE OF MENTAL HEALTH SERVICES BY ETHNIC MINORITY GROUPS

Ethnic minorities in Britain do not appear to make full use of available mental health services. There may be a reluctance to use existing services and those services may be unsuited to meet the mental health needs of patients from ethnic minority groups. Additionally help for mental health problems may be available from religious or traditional healers.

Littlewood and Lipsedge quote a dissertation by Bal (1984) who examined Asian patients attending their general practitioner. They report that Bal found that physical complaints formed part of the presentation of psychological and social difficulties. He suggested that Asian patients used a communication that they perceived as acceptable to the doctor and one which did not involve or implicate the family. Leff (1986) has suggested that some languages use somatic images more readily to indicate psychological distress. Fernando (1988) views 'somatization' as part of the presentation of emotional distress which can only be understood in the context of the patient's beliefs and expectations.

Studies have consistently shown an over-representation of black patients admitted to hospital on an involuntary basis (McGovern and Cope, 1987; Thomas et al., 1993). This may be related to the higher rates of schizophrenia diagnosed in this population. However, King et al. (1994) failed to show a significantly greater police involvement or use of compulsory admission for black patients during a *first* admission to hospital although there was a trend in this direction. Burke (1986) considers that the enforcement of treatment on black patients is part of institutional racism aimed at subjugating disadvantaged patients whose mental health needs have never been properly addressed. Perkins and Moodley (1993) argue that the poor relationship between black patients and psychiatric services may account for their finding that one third of black patients admitted to a London psychiatric unit denied that they had anything wrong with them, in contrast to the white patients, all of whom perceived themselves to have some sort of problem accounting for their admission.

There has been relatively little examination of compulsory admission of Asian patients. One study (Thomas et al., 1993) showed similar or lower rates for Asian patients compared with whites.

INTERNATIONAL EPIDEMIOLOGY OF MENTAL ILLNESS

It is unclear how mental illness is manifested around the world and whether diagnoses made in different countries and in different cultures are compatible with each other.

An attempt to explore whether schizophrenia could be meaningfully identified in different parts of the world was undertaken by the World Health Organization (WHO). The International Pilot Study of Schizophrenia (IPSS) (WHO, 1973) was set up to examine diagnostic practice in nine centres across the world using a standardized diagnostic method (the Present State Examination (PSE)). Results showed that patterns of symptoms in all the countries involved were similar. Diagnostic practice was very similar in seven of the nine centres: Aarhus (Denmark), Agra (India), Cali (Colombia), Ibaden (Nigeria), London (UK), Prague (Czechoslovakia), Taipeh (Taiwan). In the remaining two centres (Moscow and Washington) there appeared to be a broader definition of schizophrenia.

Following the IPSS it was considered feasible to set up cross-cultural epidemiological studies of schizophrenia. The patients seen in the original IPSS study were followed up after two years (Sartorius et al., 1977). There were marked variations between different countries in the course and outcome of schizophrenia but a better course and prognosis were observed in the developing countries. These findings have been replicated, but have also been challenged on method-ological grounds including selection factors, and attention has been drawn to the hazard of attributing unexplained variance to culture (Edgerton and Cohen, 1994).

The WHO incidence study of schizophrenia was carried out in Aarhus, Chandigarh (urban and rural regions), Dublin, Honolulu, Moscow, Nagasaki and Nottingham (Sartorius et al., 1986). Incidence rates for broad definitions of schizophrenia varied between 1.5 (Aarhus) and 4.2 (Chandigarh) per 100 000 population aged 15–54. Rates for a narrowly defined diagnosis of schizophrenia ranged between 0.7 (Aarhus) and 1.4 (Nottingham) per 100 000 population. This last finding of a similar incidence of narrowly defined schizo-phrenia in a variety of cultures, according to Leff, suggests that aetiological factors are common to all the cultures studied (Leff, 1988), implying that this may indicate a biological aetiology.

Torry (1987) argues that no disorder, either of biological or social aetiology, occurs at the same rates across the globe. It is likely, there-fore, that the centres are selective and known areas with unusual rates of schizophrenia, e.g. Northern Scandinavia or Western Ireland were not recruited into the study.

Kleinman (1987) has criticized the IPSS for demonstrating a 'cate-gory fallacy', that is the inappropriate application to one culture of a culturally based construct from another. A Western diagnostic tool, the PSE, was applied without validation in other cultures. Symptoms of psychosis may have been reliably identified but the validity of the diagnoses made has not been established. In Kleinman's view, the IPSS methodology cannot be employed to examine the impact of cultural factors on schizophrenia because its rigid diagnostic template has excluded any cultural diversity.

The IPSS study has been the most carefully designed cross-cultural study to date. If its findings are partially invalidated by category fallacy then other studies examining psychiatric illness in different cultures according to Western diagnostic concepts are likely to be less helpful. Kleinman suggests that an anthropological approach attempting to elicit local explanatory models of mental illness might be more useful. In anthropologically based cross-cultural studies there would be an attempt to compare symptom terms and illness labels without the requirement of a unified framework.

CROSS-CULTURAL STUDIES USING COMMUNITY SAMPLES

Cross-cultural studies of depression are confounded by the fact that symptoms associated with mood states are themselves culturally determined. Depression is a personal experience in a social context. Not only may its presentation vary but depression as a concept may not be transferable across cultures (Marsella, 1978). Murphy et al. (1964) explored symptom patterns associated with depression in 30 different countries. Suicidal ideas and somatic manifestations were inversely linked in North America but not in Latin America. Among Christians guilt and intensity of religious beliefs were linked but not among Muslims. Murphy (1973a) suggests that guilt is culturally pathoplastic and a sense of failure in different cultures may lead to either guilt or shame. The contribution of somatic symptoms to the presentation of depression also appears to vary between different cultural groups (Teja et al., 1971; Tseng, 1975; Racy, 1970). There is probably little value in trying to redefine local belief systems and patterns of symptoms according to Western nosological models unless there is the intention of imposing Western psychiatric treatment.

Two notable studies have attempted to elicit symptoms while recognizing that there were likely to be local patterns of presentation.

Carstairs and Kapur (1976) studied three South Indian rural communities using locally devised measures (The Indian Psychiatric Survey Schedule). They showed a high prevalence of psychiatric symptoms, especially in women, and variations of symptomatology related to age and class.

Leighton et al. (1963) used measures employed in a rural population survey of Stirling County, North America to explore a rural and urban Yoruba population in Nigeria. An attempt was made to standardize the means on which caseness was judged by providing clinical templates. There were more symptoms but fewer cases (23%) in the Yoruba population compared with the Stirling County population (where 31% were identified as cases).

CULTURE BOUND SYNDROMES

These disorders are defined as being confined to one culture and particular to the beliefs of that culture. They had been regarded from the ethnocentric viewpoint as 'exotic' disorders in remote places, although the concept can be applied to disorders of Western or 'dominant' cultures. Littlewood and Lipsedge (1986) have suggested that many culture bound syndromes follow a triphasic pattern – initially dislocation of the individual as a representative of a particular group, then emergence of symptoms as an exaggerated form of this extrusion, finally restitution into normal relationships. Typically, culture bound syndromes occur among young men or women who are powerless and socially neglected. Culture bound syndromes are also usually dramatic, the individual is unaware or not responsible for the disorder, the disorder has symbolic cultural significance and there may be 'mystical pressure' associated with the behaviour.

The following are the most often described culture bound syndromes.

- *Koro* (head of turtle) or *suk-yeong* (shrinking penis). This is a syndrome characterized by the belief that the penis is shrinking and will disappear into the abdomen, resulting in death. It is accompanied by a panic state and behaviour aimed at preventing the penis retracting any further. It was thought to be confined to the Chinese population in South East Asia. The syndrome has been seen in individuals and groups, where rules governing sexual behaviour have been violated. Isolated cases have been described in Europeans and in Afro-Caribbeans (Berrios and Morley, 1984; Ang and Weller; 1984). Two of these cases had a psychotic illness and Ang and Weller suggest the symptom is not specific to a particular category of mental illness.
- *Wihtigo* (Witiko, Windigo). This has been described in North American Indians who suffer harsh winters and shortages of food. The sufferer develops nausea and a loss of appetite. He fears that he may turn into a Wihtigo, a giant cannibalistic spirit. A sufferer may sometimes act out a craving for human flesh and may ask to be killed to prevent the transformation. Littlewood and Lipsedge (1982) describe this condition as occurring in a society where young men are expected to become adult hunters after initiation tests which include fasting in order to obtain supernatural powers.
- *Amok*. This has been reported as occurring in Malaysia. A male leaves his community after an insult and returns in a frenzied state attempting to kill anyone he sees. It seems that this behaviour may have represented an extreme way of dealing with tension and in earlier times the sufferer was admired and thought

to be acting in a quite understandable way in reaction to an unacceptable injury (Murphy, 1973b).

- *Latah*. This disorder has been observed in South East Asia, Siberia, Lapland and Japan. Female sufferers develop echolalia and echopraxia and sometimes coprolalia, often precipitated by some sudden shock. The syndrome may have an equivalence to hysteria in Western cultures but is not regarded as an illness among some of the communities in which it occurs (Leff, 1988).
- *Sar*. This is a possession state seen in Somali women. The Sar spirits are said to hate men. The condition may legitimize outrageous behaviour in women who have felt neglected by their husbands (Littlewood and Lipsedge, 1986).
- *Piblokto*. This is a brief disorder affecting Eskimo females who tear off their clothes and rush into the snow. The behaviour is followed by amnesia and withdrawal (Kiev, 1972).
- *Anorexia nervosa*. This condition is mainly diagnosed in Western societies, although sporadic cases have been described elsewhere. Young females with anorexia nervosa have symptoms of starvation, which exempt the sufferer from adulthood and separation from the family. They also parody cultural demands to diet and to be slim.

Littlewood and Lipsedge (1986) also suggest that overdosing and shoplifting fit the criteria for culture bound syndromes.

CLINICAL APPLICATIONS

Many authors have argued that racism may interfere in individual therapy between a black patient and a white therapist. Marcella and Pedersen (1981) recommend experiential teaching of cultural issues and personal insight into the therapist's cultural background. Therapists who participate in Race Awareness Training groups can gain a better recognition of their own prejudices.

Research into ethnic matching of patients and therapist in America (Marcella and Pedersen, 1981) suggests that this is preferred by patients from ethnic minorities regardless of the therapist's style. Bavington and Majid (1986) have described a 'culturally consonant' psychotherapeutic approach for patients of Asian origin in Britain and they also report on the successful running of a multicultural psychodynamic group.

Lau (1986) has provided an account of family therapy in different cultures in Britain. She shows the importance of being aware of the family belief system, 'respecting the pre-eminence of the family in extended families and avoiding an ethnocentric view of family systems'. However, Fernando (1988) suggests that formal family therapy may be impossible when the therapist and family do not share common cultural beliefs, although family meetings to explore the context in which symptoms have emerged may be helpful.

Fernando (1991) recommends that Western psychiatry should develop by trying to incorporate techniques to maintain mental health used by other cultures. These techniques should be learned through an equal exchange of information between cultures.

Rack has identified particular needs when providing a mental health service for ethnic minorities (Rack, 1982). These include the provision of interpreters (or, better still, bilingual clinicians), understanding naming systems and food prohibitions and recognizing that hospital routines may be unfamiliar. In addition, a knowledge of different explanatory models of mental illness is important for a proper understanding of the individual patient. Advocates who can communicate on behalf of patients may also help remedy the sense of powerlessness experienced by many patients from ethnic minorities, and providers of psychiatric services to minorities should also consult their local communities about the nature of those services.

CONCLUSION

Historically, transcultural psychiatry was concerned with how European models of mental illness compared with other manifestations of mental illness across the world. There had been an attempt to look for 'universals' in mental illness, but according to a predetermined model. One culture had been placed above the others and its values had been the norm against which others were judged. The danger of this ethnocentric approach is the tendency to discard differences or regard them as anomalous.

In contrast, 'cultural psychiatry' developed from an anthropological standpoint where apparent differences were important and not discounted. Underlying the anthropological approach is a belief that cultures should not be judged in relation to each other but are capable of being understood and explained in their own terms. This approach aims to avoid the category fallacy of inappropriately applying diagnostic concepts derived from one culture to another (Kleinman, 1977).

Sashidharan (1986) has warned that there is also a built-in ethnocentrism to the study of transcultural psychiatry itself. Complex social phenomena, which constitute a culture, may be condensed into manageable problems that can be contained within the expertise of culturally informed practitioners. Such practitioners produce solutions to these 'problems' divorced from the lives and needs of the people concerned.

Nevertheless, most critics of the concept of transcultural psychiatry agree that, within its field of activity, there are important issues which have been raised. These are to do with understanding the origin, manifestation and treatment of psychiatric disorder in different cultures. In addition, an exploration of the processes which are involved in the relationship between dominant and subordinated cultures throws up questions about psychiatry in general, including its nosology and conceptual framework.

References

Ang, P.C., Weller, M.P.I. (1984) Koro and psychosis. *British Journal of Psychiatry* **145**: 335.

Bagley, C. (1971) Mental illness in immigrant minorities in London. *Journal of Biosocial Science* **3**: 449–459.

Bal, S. (1984) The symptomatology of mental illness among Asians in the West Midlands. BA Dissertation, Department of Economics and Social Sciences, Wolverhampton Polytechnic. In Littlewood, R., Lipsedge, M. (eds) (1989) *Aliens and Alienists*, 2nd edn. London: Routledge.

Bavington, J., Majid, A. (1986) Psychiatric services for ethnic minority groups. In Cox, J.L. (ed.) *Transcultural Psychiatry*, pp. 87–106. London: Croom Helm.

Berrios, G.E., Morely, S.J. (1984) Koro-like symptoms in a non-Chinese subject. *British Journal of Psychiatry* **145**: 331–334.

Brewin, C. (1980) Explaining the lower rates of psychiatric treatment among Asian immigrants in the United Kingdom: a preliminary study. *Social Psychiatry* **15**: 17–19.

Burke, A.W. (1976a) Attempted suicide among Asian immigrants in Birmingham. *British Journal of Psychiatry* **128**: 528–533.

Burke, A.W. (1976b) Attempted suicide among the Irish-born population in Birmingham. *British Journal of Psychiatry* **128**: 534–537.

Burke, A.W. (1986) Racism, prejudice and mental illness. In Cox, J.L. (ed.) *Transcultural Psychiatry*, pp. 139–157. London: Croom Helm.

Carstairs, G.M., Kapur, R.C. (1976) *The Great Universe of Kota: Stress Change and Mental Disorder in an Indian Village*. London: Hogarth Press.

Cochrane, R. (1977) Mental illness in immigrants to England and Wales: an analysis of mental hospital admissions, 1971. *Social Psychiatry* **12**: 23–35.

Cochrane, R. (1983) *The Social Creation of Mental Illness*. London: Longman.

Cochrane, R., Bal, S.S. (1987) Migration and schizophrenia: an examination of five hypotheses. *Social Psychiatry* **22**: 181–191.

Cochrane, R., Stopes-Roe, M. (1977) Psychological and social adjustment of Asian immigrants to Britain: a community survey. *Social Psychiatry* **12**: 195–206.

Cochrane, R., Stopes-Roe, M. (1979). Psychological disturbance in Ireland, in England and in Irish emigrants to England: a comparative study. *Economic and Social Review* **10**: 301–320.

Cochrane, R., Stopes-Roe, M. (1981) Social class and psychological disorder in natives and immigrants to Britain. *International Journal of Social Psychiatry* **27**: 173–183.

Cox, J.L. (1977) Aspects of transcultural psychiatry. *British Medical Journal* **130**: 211–221.

Dean, G., Downing, H., Shelley, E. (1981a) First admissions to psychiatric hospitals in South-East England in 1976 among immigrants from Ireland. *British Medical Journal* **282**: 1831–1833.

Dean, G., Walsh, D., Downing, H., Shelley, E. (1981b) First admissions of native-born and immigrants to psychiatric hospitals in South East England, 1976. *British Journal of Psychiatry* **139**: 506–512.

Eagles, J.M. (1991) The relationship between schizophrenia and immigration. Are there alternative hypotheses? *British Journal of Psychiatry* **159**: 783–789.

Edgerton, R.B., Cohen, A. (1994) Culture and schizophrenia: the DOSMD challenge. *British Journal of Psychiatry* **164**: 222–231.

Fernando, S. (1988) *Race and Culture in Psychiatry*. London: Croom Helm.

Fernando, S. (1991) *Mental Health, Race and Culture*. London: Macmillan.

Glover, G.R., Flannigan, C.B., Feeney, S.T. et al. (1994) Admission of British Caribbeans to mental hospitals: is it a cohort effect? *Social Psychiatry and Psychiatric Epidemiology* **29**: 282–284.

Halpern, D. (1993) Minorities and mental health. *Social Science Medicine* **36**: 597–607.

Harrison, G., Owen, D., Holton, A., Neilson, D., Boot, D. (1988) A prospective study of severe mental disorder in Afro-Caribbean patients. *Psychological Medicine* **18**: 643–657.

Harvey, I., Williams, M., McGuffin, P., Toone, B.K. (1990) The functional psychoses in Afro-Caribbeans. *British Journal of Psychiatry* **157**: 515–522.

Herz, D.G. (1988) Identity – lost and found: patterns of migration and psychological and psychosocial adjustment of migrants. *Acta Psychiatrica Scandanavica* **78** (Suppl.): 159–165.

Hickling, F.W. (1991a) Psychiatric hospital admission rates in Jamaica, 1971 and 1988. *British Journal of Psychiatry* **159**: 817–821.

Hickling, F.W. (1991b) Double jeopardy: psychopathology of black mentally ill returned migrants to Jamaica. *International Journal of Social Psychiatry* **37**: 80–89.

Johnson, M.R.D. (1986) Inner-city residents: ethnic minorities and primary care. In Rothwell, T. Phillips, D. (eds) *Health, Race and Ethnicity*. London: Croom Helm.

Kelleher, M.J. (1972) Cross-national (Anglo-Irish) differences is obsessional symptoms and traits of personality. *Psychological Medicine* **2**: 33–41.

Kiev, A. (1972) *Transcultural Psychiatry*. Harmondsworth: Penguin.

King, M., Coker, E., Leavey, G., Hoare, A., Johnson-Sabine, E. (1994) Incidence of psychotic illness in London: comparison of ethnic groups. *British Medical Journal* **309**: 1115–1119.

Kleinman, A. (1977) Depression, somatization and the 'new cross-cultural psychiatry', *Social Science and Medicine* **11**: 3–10.

Kleinman, A. (1987) Anthropology and psychiatry. The role of culture in cross-cultural research on illness. *British Journal of Psychiatry* **151**: 447–454.

Kluckholm, C. (1944) *Mirror for Man*. McGraw Hill: New York.

Lau, A. (1986) Family therapy across cultures. In Cox, J.L. (ed.) *Transcultural Psychiatry* pp. 234–252. London: Croom Helm.

Leff, J.P. (1986) The epidemiology of mental illness across cultures. In Cox J.L. (ed.) *Transcultural Psychiatry*, pp. 23–36. London: Croom Helm.

Leff, J.P. (1988) *Psychiatry Around the Globe: A Transcultural View*. London: Gaskell.

Leighton, A.H., Lambo, T.A., Hughes, C.C. et al. (1963) *Psychiatric Disorder among the Yoruba*. New York: Cornell University Press.

Lewis, G., Croft-Jeffreys, C., David, A. (1990) Are British psychiatrists racist? *British Journal of Psychiatry* **157**: 410–415.

Littlewood, R., Lipsedge, M. (1981) Some social and phenomenological characteristics of psychotic immigrants. *Psychological Medicine* **11**: 289–302.

Littlewood, R., Lipsedge, M. (1982) *Aliens and Alienists*. Harmondsworth: Penguin.

Littlewood, R., Lipsedge, M. (1986) The 'culture-bound syndromes' of the dominant culture: culture, psychopathology and biomedicine. In Cox, J.L. (ed.) *Transcultural Psychiatry*, pp. 253–273. London: Croom Helm.

Littlewood, R., Lipsedge, M., (1988) Psychiatric illness among British Afro-Caribbeans. *British Medical Journal* **296**: 950–951.

Littlewood, R., Lipsedge, M. (1989) *Aliens and Alienists*, 2nd edn. London: Routledge.

Marsella, A.J. (1978) Thoughts on cross-cultural studies on the epidemiology of depression. *Culture, Medicine and Psychiatry*, **2**: 343–357.

Marsella, A.J., Pedersen, P.B. (ed.) (1981) *Cross-cultural Counselling and Psychotherapy*. New York: Pergamon Press.

Mavreas, V., Bebbington, P. (1990) Acculturation and psychiatric disorder: a study of Greek Cypriot immigrants. *Psychological Medicine* **10**: 941–951.

McGovern, D., Cope, R.V. (1987) First admission rates for first and second generation Afro-Caribbeans. *Social Psychiatry* **22**: 139–149.

Merrill, J., Owens, J. (1988) Self-poisoning among four immigrant groups. *Acta Psychiatrica Scandinavica* **77**: 77–80.

Murphy, H.B.M. (1973a) Current trends in transcultural psychiatry. *Proceedings of the Royal Society of Medicine* **66**: 711–716.

Murphy, H.B.M. (1973b) History and evolution of syndromes: the striking case of Latah and Amok. In Hamner, M. (ed.) *Psychopathology.* New York: Wiley.

Murphy, H.B.M. (1977) Migration, culture and mental health. *Psychological Medicine* **7**: 677–684.

Murphy, H.B.M. (1986) The mental health impact of British cultural traditions. In Cox, J.L. (ed.) *Transcultural Psychiatry*, pp. 179–195. London: Croom Helm.

Murphy, H.B.M., Wittkower, E.D., Chance, N.E. (1964) A cross-cultural enquiry into symptomatology of depression. *Transcultural Psychiatric Research Review* **1**: 5–18.

Ndetei, D.M., Vadher, A. (1984) Patterns of anxiety in a cross-cultural hospital population. *Acta Psychiatrica Scandanavica* **70**: 69–72.

Ødegaard, O. (1932) Emigration and insanity. *Acta Psychiatrica Scandanavica* (Copenhagen Suppl.), No. 4.

Perkins, R.E., Moodley, P. (1993) Perceptions of problems in psychiatric inpatients: denial, race and service usage. *Social Psychiatry and Psychiatric Epidemiology* **28**: 189–193.

Rack, P. (1982) *Race, Culture and Mental Disorder.* London: Tavistock.

Racy, J. (1970) Psychiatry in the Arab East. *Acta Psychiatrica Scandanavica* (Suppl.) **211**: 1–171.

Rwegellera, G.G.C. (1977) Psychiatric morbidity among West Africans and West Indians living in London. *Psychological Medicine* **7**: 317–329.

Rwegellera, G.G.C. (1980) Differential use of psychiatric services by West Indians, West Africans and English in London. *British Journal of Psychiatry* **137**: 428–432.

Sanua, V.D. (1969) Immigration, migration and mental illness: a review of the literature. In Brody, E.B. (ed.) *Behaviour in New Environments.* California: Sage.

Sartorius, N., Jablensky, A., Shapiro, R. (1977) Two year follow-up of the patients included in the WHO international pilot study of schizophrenia. *Psychological Medicine* **7**: 529–541.

Sartorius, N., Jablensky, A., Korten, A. et al. (1986) Early manifestations and first-contact incidence of schizophrenia in different cultures: a preliminary report on the initial evaluation phase of the WHO collaborative study on determinants of outcome of severe mental disorders. *Psychological Medicine* **16**: 909–928.

Sashidharan, S.P. (1986) Ideology and politics in transcultural psychiatry. In Cox, J.L. (ed.) *Transcultural Psychiatry*, pp. 158–178. London: Croom Helm.

Sashidharan, S.P. (1993) Afro-Caribbeans and schizophrenia: the ethnic vulnerability hypothesis re-examined. *International Review of Psychiatry* **5**: 129–144.

Stopes-Roe, M., Cochrane, R. (1980) Mental health and immigration: a comparison of Indian, Pakistani and Irish immigration to England. *Ethnic and Racial Studies* **3**: 316–341.

Teague, A. (1993) Ethnic group: first results from the 1991 census. *Population Trends* **72**: 12–17.

Teja, J.S., Narang, R.L., Aggarwal, A.K., (1971) Depression across cultures. *British Journal of Psychiatry* **119**: 253–260.

Thomas, C.S., Stone, K., Osborn, M., Thomas, P.F., Fisher, M. (1993) Psychiatric morbidity and compulsory admission among UK-born Europeans, Afro-Caribbeans and Asians in central Manchester. *British Journal of Psychiatry* **163**: 91–99.

Torry, E.F. (1987) Similar incidence worldwide of schizophrenia: case not proven. *British Journal of Psychiatry* **151**: 132–133.

Tseng, W. (1975) The nature of somatic complaints among psychiatric patients: the Chinese case. *Comprehensive Psychiatry* **116**: 237–245.

Turner, S., Gorst-Unsworth, C. (1990) Psychological sequelae of torture: a descriptive model. *British Journal of Psychiatry* **157**: 475–480.

Tyler, E.B. (1874) *Primitive Culture: Researches into the Development of Mythology, Philosophy, Religion, Language, Art and Custom.* (Reprinted 1958 as *The Origins of Culture.*) New York: Harper and Row.

Wessely, S., Castle, D., Der, G., Murray, R. (1991) Schizophrenia and Afro-Caribbeans. A case control study. *British Journal of Psychiatry* **159**: 795–801.

Whitehouse, A.M., Mumford, D.B. (1988) Increased prevalence of bulimia nervosa amongst Asian schoolgirls. *British Medical Journal* **297**: 718.

WHO (1973) *Report of the International Pilot Study of Schizophrenia* Vol. 1. Geneva: World Health Organization.

Zwingmann, C.A.A., Gunn, A.D.G. (1983) *Uprooting and Health; Psychosocial Problems of Students from Abroad.* Geneva: World Health Organization.

Index